VASCULAR ULTRASOUND

To Wendy, Tony and June

Commissioning Editor: Claire Wilson
Development Editor: Catherine Jackson
Project Manager: Srikumar Narayanan and Anne Dickie
Designer: Kirsteen Wright
Illustration Manager: Merlyn Harvey
Illustrator: Cactus Design

VASCULAR ULTRASOUND

THIRD EDITION

How, Why and When

Abigail Thrush Msc
Medical Physicist, Department of Clinical Physics, St Bartholomew's Hospital, Bart's and the London NHS Trust, London, UK

Tim Hartshorne AVS
Vascular Technologist, Department of Surgery, Leicester Royal Infirmary, University Hospitals of Leicester NHS Trust, Leicester, UK

With contributions from
Colin Deane PhD **and David Goss** PhD
Clinical Scientists, Vascular Laboratory, Department of Medical Engineering and Physics, King's College Hospital, London, UK

CHURCHILL LIVINGSTONE

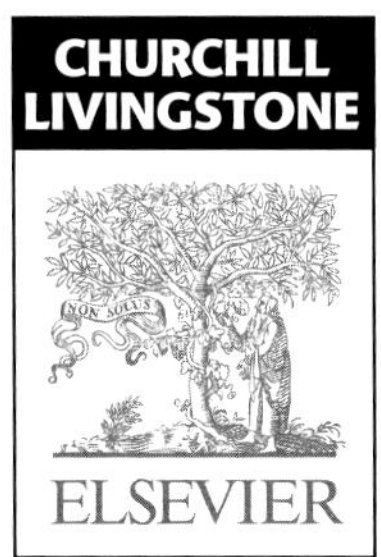

Edinburgh • London • New York • Oxford • Philadelphia • St Louis • Sydney • Toronto 2010

CHURCHILL
LIVINGSTONE
ELSEVIER

First edition 1999
Second edition 2005
Third edition 2010
Reprinted 2010 (twice), 2011

ISBN 978 0 443 06918 5

British Library Cataloguing in Publication Data
A catalogue record for this book is available from the British Library

Library of Congress Cataloging in Publication Data
A catalog record for this book is available from the Library of Congress

Notice
Knowledge and best practice in this field are constantly changing. As new research and experience broaden our knowledge, changes in practice, treatment and drug therapy may become necessary or appropriate. Readers are advised to check the most current information provided (i) on procedures featured or (ii) by the manufacturer of each product to be administered, to verify the recommended dose or formula, the method and duration of administration, and contraindications. It is the responsibility of the practitioner, relying on their own experience and knowledge of the patient, to make diagnoses, to determine dosages and the best treatment for each individual patient, and to take all appropriate safety precautions. To the fullest extent of the law, neither the Publisher nor the Authors assumes any liability for any injury and/or damage to persons or property arising out of or related to any use of the material contained in this book.

The Publisher

Printed in China

Contents

Preface

Vascular ultrasound is a speciality in its own right and vascular surgeons are highly dependent on the skills of vascular sonographers for the investigation of patients suffering from peripheral vascular disease. This book aims to provide an understanding of the principles and practice of vascular ultrasound.

An introduction to some of the basic theory behind the science and technology of ultrasound is included. This will help sonographers to understand the function of scanner controls and enable them to obtain optimal images and Doppler recordings. B-mode imaging, color flow images and spectral Doppler recordings are all prone to artefacts and it is essential that their presence is recognized. The potential sources of errors in any measurements made by ultrasound should be understood. Specific disorders of the arterial and venous system are covered, and the techniques for diagnosing these problems are described. Examples of normal and abnormal images and Doppler recordings are included and interpretation of these discussed. We are extremely grateful to Dr Colin Deane and Dr David Goss who have contributed additional chapters and material for this edition, extending the scope of this text.

We hope this book will serve as a useful resource to sonographers and clinician new to the field and as a reference for more experienced staff.

Abigail Thrush
Tim Hartshorne

Acknowledgments

We would like to thank Yasin Akil, Mustapha Azzam, Helen Dawson, David Evans, Pouran Khodabakhsh, Nick London, May Naylor, Ross Naylor, Ria Sharpe and Jo Walker for their help and support in the preparation of this book.

1 Introduction

Since the first edition of this book there have been significant developments in ultrasound technology, magnetic resonance angiography (MRA), and computed tomographic angiography (CTA) scanning. The latest generation of duplex systems produces higher-resolution images, with the availability of techniques such as harmonic imaging and compound imaging. The images produced by MRA can be visually stunning, and it has been suggested that MRA and spiral CT may replace duplex investigations in the future. However, duplex scanning still has many advantages. Apart from improvements in image resolution, it is the ability to visualize flow in real time, make quantitative measurements of blood velocity, and detect flow direction that will insure duplex scanning will remain an important imaging technique for the foreseeable future. Ultrasound imaging remains a relatively inexpensive imaging modality. For instance, it is not cost-effective to screen patients for aortic aneurysm or carotid artery disease with MRA. The low risk associated with ultrasound makes it suitable for regular posttreatment follow-up. However, MRA or CT scanning is essential for planning endovascular repair of an aortic aneurysm.

Therefore, each modality has its part to play in the management of patients with vascular disorders. In many centers, diagnostic angiography and venography have been largely replaced by the use of duplex ultrasound investigations. This has the advantage of allowing surgeons and physicians to select patients for surgical treatment or conservative management without the need for invasive investigations. In addition, vascular radiologists can spend more time performing therapeutic procedures, such as angioplasty, rather than diagnostic angiograms.

Treatment of vascular disease is also changing with the development of minimally invasive endovascular surgical procedures such as endovascular aortic aneurysm repair (EVAR) and endovenous laser treatment (EVLT) for varicose veins. Some surgeons and radiologists use ultrasound to help guide catheter placement during such treatments. Portable scanners are relatively inexpensive and can be used in the community setting for screening and simple assessments, avoiding the need for patents to travel to large hospitals.

Vascular ultrasound examinations rely on the use of ultrasound to produce a black and white anatomical image that can demonstrate the presence of disease along an arterial wall or the presence of thrombus in a vein. Doppler ultrasound can provide a functional map in the form of a color flow image, which displays the blood flow in arteries and veins. Spectral Doppler analysis enables Doppler waveforms to be recorded from vessels. It is then possible to visualize changes in flow patterns in vessels and calculate velocity measurements, enabling the sonographer to grade the severity of the vascular disease (Fig. 1.1).

Arterial disease is one of the major causes of morbidity and mortality in the developed world. There are many risk factors associated with the development of arterial disease, but it is widely accepted that tobacco smoking is one of the primary causes. Atherosclerotic plaques develop over time, leading to arterial obstruction or embolization. Radiologists and surgeons are able to perform a variety of procedures to treat arterial disorders. An example is angioplasty, which involves the use of a balloon mounted on the end of a catheter that is guided, using angiography, to the area of stenosis (narrowing) or occlusion (blockage). The balloon is then positioned across the stenosis or occlusion and inflated for a short period of time, to dilate the lesion, increasing the diameter of the lumen (Fig. 1.2). Surgical

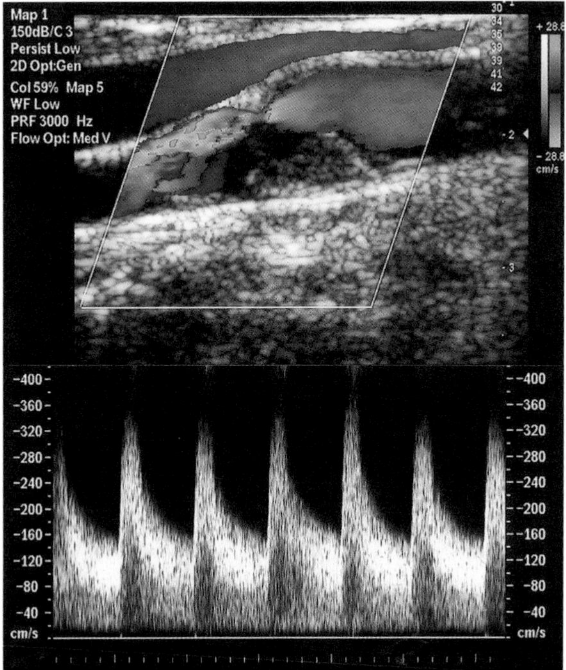

Figure 1.1 • An example of a carotid ultrasound scan showing how B-mode imaging, color flow imaging, and spectral Doppler are used to investigate a stenosis.

bypass or endarterectomy can be performed when angioplasty is not possible or is not suitable to treat specific problems. Endovascular or minimally invasive procedures can now be used to treat a range of vascular disorders, including the repair of aortic aneurysms, and are less traumatic for the patient. Duplex scanning has a role to play in the follow-up of patients who have undergone these techniques.

Ultrasound has also had a significant impact on the investigation of venous disorders. Ultrasound allows the detection of deep-vein thrombosis, which can lead to fatal pulmonary embolism. The investigation of venous insufficiency in the superficial and deep veins has proved extremely useful for assessing patients with varicose veins and venous ulcers. This enables surgeons to select patients for venous surgery, minimally invasive techniques, or nonsurgical treatments, such as compression dressings.

It is recommended that the reader obtain an overview of other imaging modalities in order to have an understanding of the role of vascular ultrasound in relation to these other techniques for investigating vascular disorders. In addition, it is

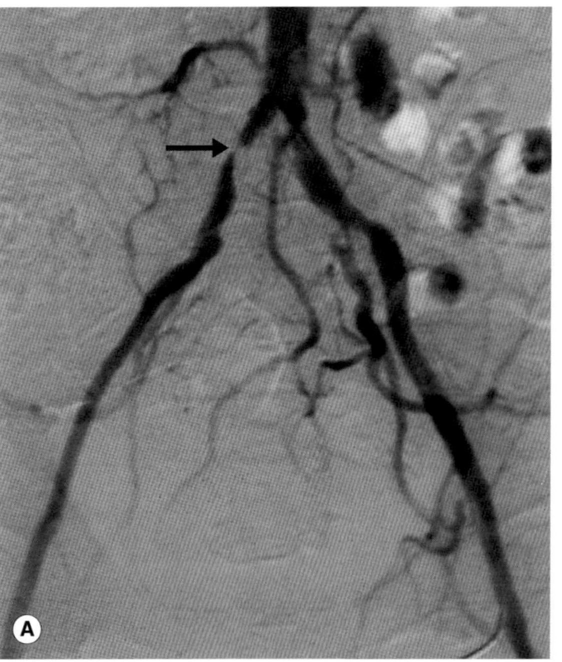

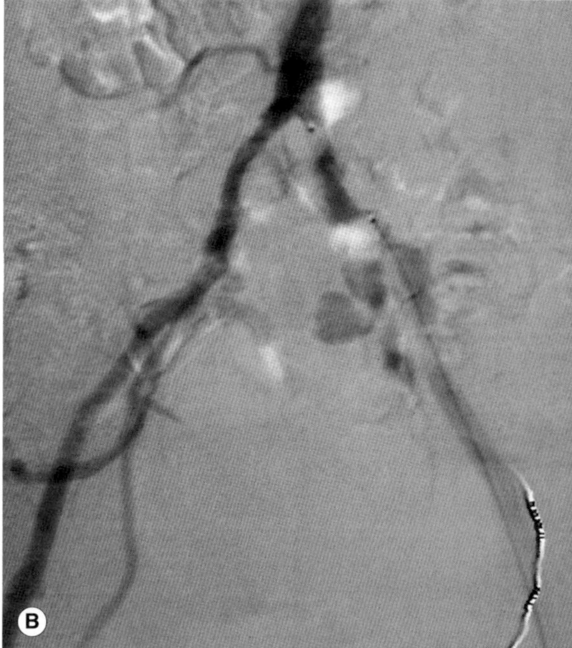

Figure 1.2 • (A) An angiogram demonstrating a significant stenosis in the right common iliac artery (arrow). (B) The stenosis has been dilated by percutaneous balloon angioplasty.

important to know about the different radiological and surgical techniques used to treat peripheral vascular disease. Over the years the role of ultrasound has developed to include screening, diagnosis, guidance of treatment procedures, and follow-up after surgical or minimally invasive treatment. Future developments may see an increasing role for three-dimensional technology to provide more comprehensive information about plaques and aneurysms.

2 Ultrasound and imaging

CONTENTS

INTRODUCTION

It is important to understand how ultrasound interacts with tissue to be able to interpret ultrasound images and to identify artifacts. Knowledge of how an image is produced allows optimal use of the scanner controls. The aim of this and the next two chapters is to give a simple explanation of the process involved in producing images and blood flow measurements.

NATURE OF ULTRASOUND

Ultrasound, as the name implies, is high-frequency sound. Sound waves travel through a medium by causing local displacement of particles within the medium; however, there is no overall movement of the medium. Unlike light, sound cannot travel through a vacuum as sound waves need a supporting medium. Consider a piece of string held at both ends: with one end briefly shaken, the vibration caused will travel along the string and in so doing transmit energy from one end of the string to the other. This is known as a transverse wave, as the movement of the string is at right angles to the direction in which the wave has moved. Ultrasound is a longitudinal wave, as the displacement of the particles within the medium is in the same direction as that in which the wave is travelling. Figure 2.1 shows a medium with particles distributed evenly within it. The position of the particles within the medium will change as a sound wave passes through it, causing local periodic displacement of these particles (Fig. 2.1B). The size, or amplitude, of these displacements is shown in Figure 2.1C. As the particles move within the medium, local increases and decreases in pressure are generated (Fig. 2.1D).

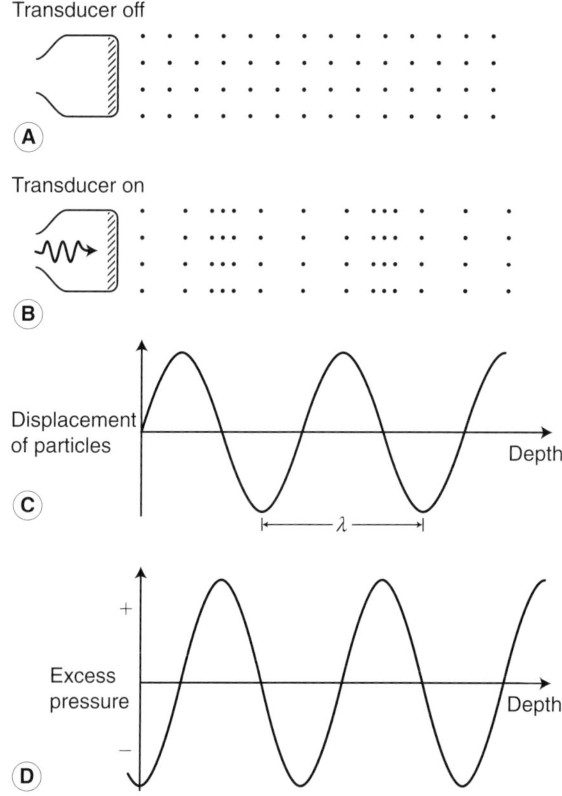

Figure 2.1 • (A) A medium consisting of evenly distributed particles. (B) The positions of the particles change (shown here at a given point in time) as the ultrasound wave passes through the medium. (C) The amplitude of the particle displacement. (D) Excess pressure.

Wavelength and frequency

Ultrasound is usually described by its frequency, which is related to the length of the wave produced. The wavelength of a sound wave is the distance between consecutive points where the size and direction of the displacement are identical and the direction in which the particles are travelling is the same. The wavelength is represented by the symbol λ and is shown in Figure 2.1C. The time taken for the wave to move forwards through the medium by one wavelength is known as the period (τ). The frequency, *f*, is the number of cycles of displacements passing through a point in the medium during 1 second (s) and is given by:

$$f = 1/\tau \quad (2.1)$$

MEDIUM	SPEED OF SOUND (m/s)
Air	330
Water (20°C)	1480
Fat	1450
Blood	1570
Muscle	1580
Bone	3500
Soft tissue (average)	1540

Table 2.1 Speed of sound in different tissues

The unit of frequency is the hertz (Hz), with 1 Hz being one complete cycle per second. Audible sound waves are in the range of 20 Hz to 20 kHz, whereas medical ultrasound scanners typically use high frequencies of between 2 and 15 MHz (i.e., between 2 000 000 and 15 000 000 Hz).

Speed of ultrasound

Sound travels through different media at different speeds (e.g., sound travels faster through water than it does through air). The speed of a sound wave, *c*, is given by the distance traveled by the disturbance during a given time and is constant in any specific material. The speed can be found by multiplying the frequency by the wavelength and is usually measured in meters per second (m/s):

$$c = \lambda f \quad (2.2)$$

The speed of sound through a material depends both on the density and the compressibility of the material. The more dense and the more compressible the material, the slower the wave will travel through it. The speed of sound is different for the various tissues in the body (Table 2.1). Knowledge of the speed of sound is needed to determine how far an ultrasound wave has traveled. This is required in both imaging and pulsed Doppler (as will be seen later), but ultrasound systems usually make an estimate by assuming that the speed of sound is the same in all tissues: 1540 m/s. This can lead to small errors in the estimated distance traveled because of the variations in the speed of sound in different tissues.

GENERATION OF ULTRASOUND WAVES

The term 'transducer' simply means a device that converts one form of energy into another. In the case of an ultrasound transducer, this conversion is from electrical energy to mechanical vibration. The piezoelectric effect is the method by which most medical ultrasound is generated. Piezoelectric materials will vibrate mechanically when a varying voltage is applied across them. The frequency of the voltage applied will affect the frequency with which the material vibrates. The thickness of the piezoelectric element will determine the frequency at which the element will vibrate most efficiently; this is known as the resonant frequency of the transducer. The speed of sound within the element will depend on the material from which it is made. A resonant frequency occurs when the thickness of the element is half the wavelength of the sound wave generated within it. At this frequency, the reflected waves from the front and back faces of the element act to reinforce each other, so increasing the size of the vibration produced. When an appropriate coupling medium is used (e.g., ultrasound gel), this vibration will be transmitted into a surrounding medium, such as the body. The named frequency of a transducer is its resonant frequency. This is not to say that the transducer will not function at a different frequency, but it will be much less efficient at those frequencies. Most modern imaging transducers are designed as broad-band transducers, meaning that they will function efficiently over a wide range of frequencies, and these are usually labeled with the frequency range over which they operate (e.g., 3–9 MHz). Figure 2.2 shows how the transducer output of narrow-band and broad-band transducers varies with the frequency of the excitation voltage. A broad-band transducer is more efficient over a wider range of frequencies than a narrow-band transducer. Ultrasound transducers also use the piezoelectric effect to convert the returning ultrasound vibrations back into electrical signals. These signals can then be amplified, analyzed, and displayed to provide anatomical images together with flow information.

Pulsed ultrasound

Simple Doppler systems operate with a continuous single-frequency excitation voltage, but all imaging systems and pulsed Doppler systems use pulsed excitation signals. If ultrasound is continuously transmitted along a particular path, the energy will also be continuously reflected back from any boundary in the path of the beam, and it will not be possible to predict where the returning echoes have come from. However, when a pulse of ultrasound is transmitted it is possible to predict the distance (d) of a reflecting surface from the transducer if the time (t) between transmission and reception of the pulse is measured and the velocity (c) of the ultrasound along the path is known, as follows:

$$d = \frac{tc}{2} \qquad (2.3)$$

The factor 2 arises from the fact that the pulse travels along the path twice, once on transmission and once on its return. This can be used to predict where returning echoes have originated from within the body.

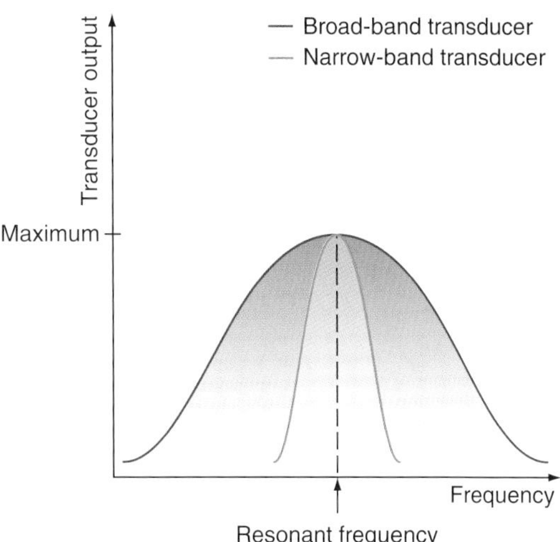

Figure 2.2 • Plot of transducer output versus frequency for a broad-band and a narrow-band transducer. A broad-band transducer will be more efficient over a wider range of frequencies than a narrow-band transducer.

Frequency content of pulses

Typically, the pulses used in imaging ultrasound are very short and will only contain 1–3 cycles in order that reflections from boundaries that are close together can be easily separated. Pulsed

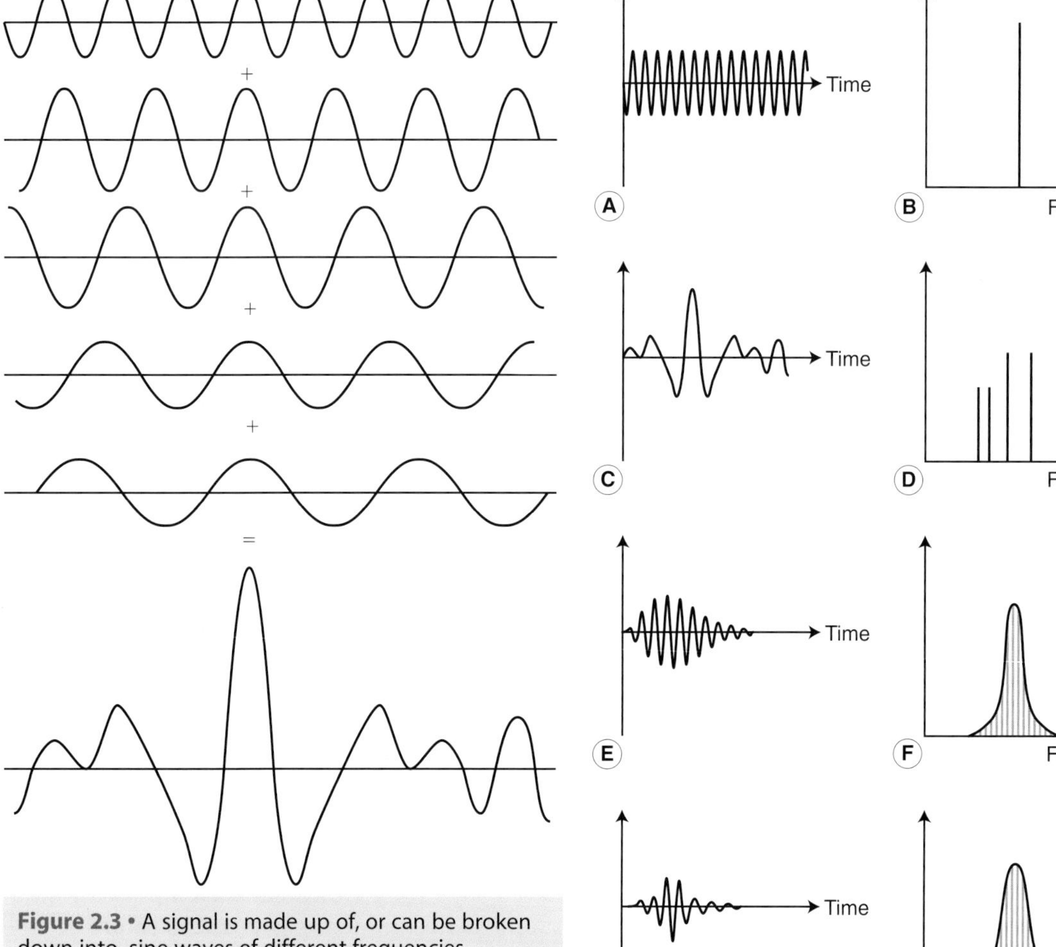

Figure 2.3 • A signal is made up of, or can be broken down into, sine waves of different frequencies, different amplitudes and phases. (From Fish 1990, with permission.)

Figure 2.4 • Four different signals (amplitude plotted against time) and their corresponding frequency spectra (power plotted against frequency). (A, B) For a continuous single frequency. (C, D) Signal shown in Figure 2.3. (E, F) A long pulse. (G, H) A short pulse. The shorter the pulse, the greater the range of frequencies within the pulse. (After Fish 1990, with permission.)

Doppler signals are longer and contain several cycles. In fact, a pulse is made up not of a single frequency but of a range of frequencies of different amplitudes. Different-shaped pulses will have different frequency contents. Figure 2.3 illustrates how a signal can be made up of the sum of several different frequencies. The frequency content of a signal can be displayed on a graph, such as those shown in Figure 2.4 (right panels). This is known as a frequency spectrum and displays the frequencies present within the signal against the relative amplitudes of these frequencies. Figure 2.4A provides an example of a continuous signal consisting of a single frequency. As only one frequency is present in the signal, the frequency spectrum displays a single line at that frequency (Fig. 2.4B). Figure 2.4C, E, and G give examples of three differently shaped signals along with their frequency spectra (Fig. 2.4D, F, and H), showing the range of frequencies present in each of the different signals. As ultrasound imaging uses pulsed ultrasound, the transducer is not transmitting a single frequency but a range of frequencies.

Beam shape

The shape of the ultrasound beam produced by a transducer will depend on the shape of the element(s), on the transmitted frequency, and on whether the beam is focused. The shape of the beam will affect the region of tissue that will be insonated and from which returning echoes will be received. Multi-element array transducers use several elements to produce the beam, as discussed later in this chapter.

INTERACTION OF ULTRASOUND WITH SURFACES

The creation of an ultrasound image depends on the way in which ultrasound energy interacts with the tissue as it passes through the body. When an ultrasound wave meets a large smooth interface between two different media, some of the energy will be reflected back, and this is known as specular reflection. The relative proportions of the energy reflected and transmitted depend on the change in the acoustic impedance between the two materials (Fig. 2.5). The acoustic impedance of a medium is the impedance (similar to resistance) the material offers against the passage of the sound wave through it and depends on the density and compressibility of the medium. The greater the change in the acoustic impedance across a boundary, the greater the proportion of the ultrasound that is reflected. There is, for example, a large difference in acoustic impedance between soft tissue and bone, or between soft tissue and air, and such interfaces will produce large reflections. This is the reason why ultrasound cannot be used to image beyond lung or bone, except in limited situations, as only a small proportion of the ultrasound is transmitted. It is also the reason for the loss of both imaging and Doppler information beyond calcified arterial walls, bone (Fig. 10.13), and bowel gas, leading to an acoustic shadow beyond. Table 2.2 shows the ratio of the reflected to incident wave amplitude for a range of reflecting interfaces.

The path along which the reflected ultrasound travels will also affect the amplitude of the signal detected by the transducer. If the beam is perpendicular to the interface, the reflected ultrasound will travel back along the same path to the transducer. If, however, the beam intercepts the interface at an angle of less than 90°, then the beam will be reflected along a different path. Figure 2.6 shows that the angle of incidence (θ_i) is the same as the angle of reflection (θ_r) measured from a line perpendicular to the interface. This means that

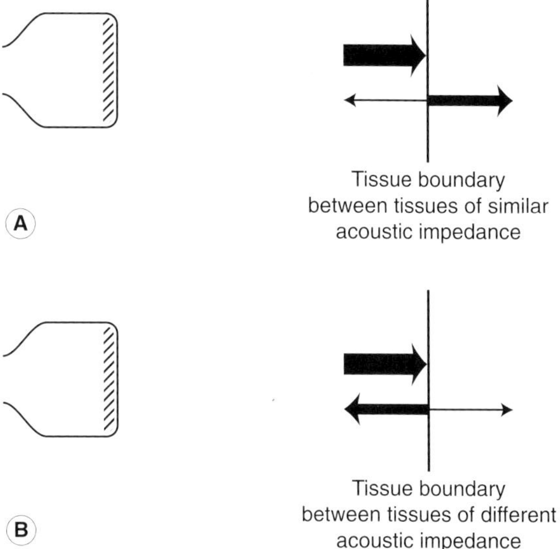

Figure 2.5 • When the ultrasound beam meets a boundary between two media, some of the ultrasound will be transmitted and some will be reflected. (A) When the two media have similar acoustic impedances, the majority of the ultrasound will be transmitted across the boundary. (B) When the two media have different acoustic impedances, most of the ultrasound will be reflected.

REFLECTING INTERFACE	RATIO OF REFLECTED TO INCIDENT WAVE AMPLITUDE
Muscle/blood	0.03
Soft tissue/water	0.05
Fat/muscle	0.10
Bone/muscle	0.64
Soft tissue/air	0.9995

Table 2.2 The ratio of reflected to incident wave amplitude for an ultrasound beam perpendicular to different reflecting interfaces (after McDicken 1981, with permission)

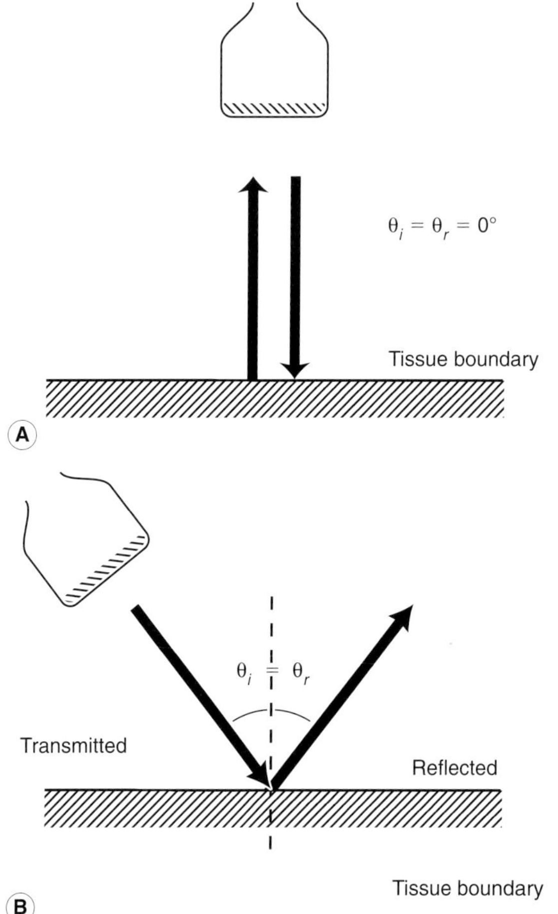

Figure 2.6 • (A) When an ultrasound beam is perpendicular to an interface, the reflected ultrasound will return by the same path. (B) If the interface is not perpendicular to the beam then the reflected ultrasound will travel along a different path. The angle of incidence of the beam (θ_i) is equal to the angle of reflection (θ_r).

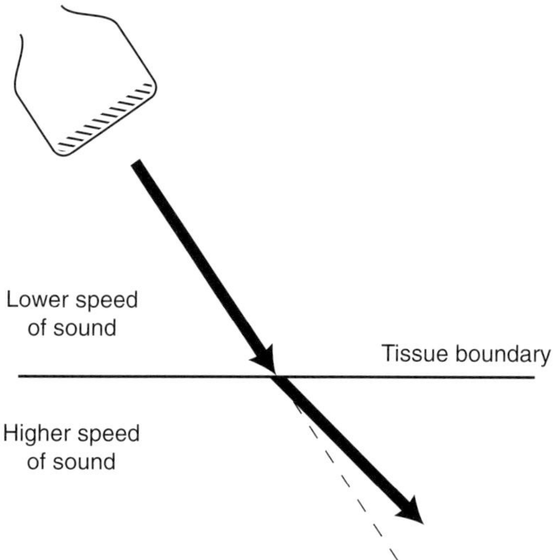

Figure 2.7 • Refraction. When a beam is transmitted through an interface between two media in which the sound travels at different speeds and the beam is not perpendicular to the interface, the path of the beam will be bent.

when the beam is at 90° to the interface, all the reflected ultrasound will travel back towards the transducer, but as the angle of incidence becomes smaller, the beam will be reflected away from the transducer and therefore the transducer will receive less of the reflected ultrasound. The best image of an interface will be obtained when the interface is at right angles to the beam, and likewise the poorest image will be obtained when the interface is parallel to the beam. Thus, when an artery is imaged in transverse section, the anterior and posterior walls can be seen more clearly than the side, or lateral, walls which are parallel to the beam (Fig. 8.5).

If the ultrasound beam is not perpendicular to the interface and there is a change in the speed of sound in the media on either side of the interface, the path of the beam will be bent. This is known as refraction and is illustrated in Figure 2.7. Refraction causes the beam to change its direction of travel and can lead to artifacts whereby the signal detected by the transducer has originated from a different point in the tissue than that displayed on the image. This is most important where there are large changes in the velocity of sound between media, such as the interface between the uterus and amniotic fluid. It is not usually a major problem in vascular ultrasound, with the exception of the presence of the skull bone in the path of a transcranial Doppler beam.

Although specular reflection occurs at large, smooth boundaries, the majority of signals returning from tissue are made up of ultrasound energy that has been back-scattered from rough surfaces or small structures within the tissue. When the ultrasound beam interacts with a rough surface or small structure it will be scattered in all directions rather than reflected back along one path.

Figure 2.8 shows the difference between specular reflection and scattering from rough surfaces and small structures. Scattering occurs when the small structures are of a similar size to or smaller than the wavelength of the ultrasound and will result in less of the ultrasound returning to the transducer along the original beam path. The amount of energy lost from the beam by scattering is highly dependent on the frequency [proportional to the fourth power of the frequency (i.e., f^4) for structures that are much smaller than the wavelength of the ultrasound]. In the case of peripheral vascular ultrasound, specular reflection will occur at the vessel walls, which are often perpendicular to the beam, leading to large reflected signals. However, ultrasound will be scattered by groups of red blood cells within the lumen, leading to much smaller returning signals, which will not normally be visible on an image.

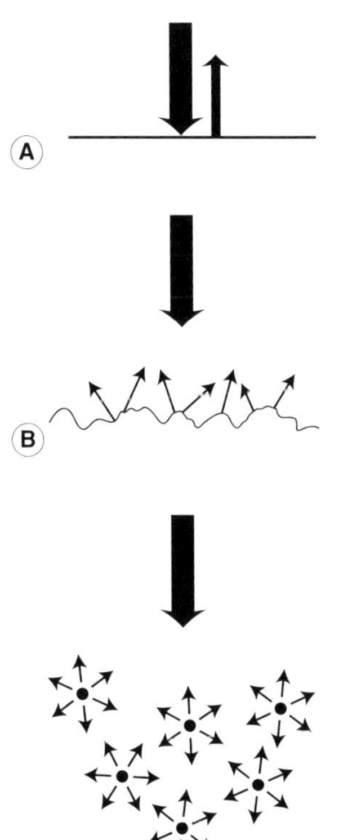

Figure 2.8 • Specular reflections occur at large smooth interfaces (A), whereas ultrasound is scattered by rough surfaces (B) and small structures (C).

LOSS OF ULTRASOUND ENERGY IN TISSUE

Attenuation is the loss of energy from the ultrasound beam as it passes through tissue. The more the ultrasound energy is attenuated by the tissue, the less energy will be available to return to the transducer or to penetrate deeper into the tissue. Attenuation is caused by several different processes. These include absorption, scattering, reflection, and beam divergence. Absorption causes ultrasound energy to be converted into heat as the beam passes through the tissue. The rate of absorption varies in different types of tissue. Ultrasound energy can also be lost by scattering from small structures within the tissue or reflection from large boundaries that are not perpendicular to the beam, preventing the ultrasound from returning to the transducer. The attenuation coefficients of various tissues are presented in Table 2.3, from which it can be seen that muscle attenuates the ultrasound more quickly than fat. The units of the coefficient of attenuation are in dB $MHz^{-1}cm^{-1}$, showing that the rate of attenuation depends on frequency of ultrasound, with higher frequencies being attenuated more quickly than lower frequencies. This is why higher ultrasound frequencies penetrate tissue less effectively than lower ultrasound frequencies and can only be used for imaging superficial structures. This is similar to the situation in which you can hear your neighbor's hi-fi bass through the partition wall better than the treble.

MEDIUM	ATTENUATION COEFFICIENT AT 1 MHz (dB cm^{-1})
Water (20°C)	0.2
Fat	60
Blood	20
Muscle	150
Bone	1000
Soft tissue (average)	70

Table 2.3 Attenuation coefficients of different tissues

PRODUCING AN ULTRASOUND IMAGE

Ultrasound imaging uses information contained in reflected and scattered signals received by the transducer. If it is assumed that the speed of the ultrasound through the tissue is constant, it is possible to predict the distance from a reflective boundary or scattering particle to the transducer. When an ultrasound pulse returns to the transducer, it will cause the transducer to vibrate, and this will generate a voltage across the piezoelectric element. The amplitude of the returning pulse will depend on the proportion of the ultrasound reflected or back-scattered to the transducer and the amount by which the signal has been attenuated along its path. The amplitude of the pulse received back at the transducer can be displayed against time. This display can be calibrated such that the time delay of the returning pulse represents the distance of the boundary from the transducer, thus showing the depth of the boundary in the tissue. The varying amplitude of the signal can be displayed as a spot of varying brightness that travels down the display with time. This type of display is known as a B-mode or brightness scan. If the group of transducer elements used to form the beam is moved slightly so that the beam now passes through the tissue along a path that is adjacent to the first, and the returning signal is displayed next to that from the first pulse, a B-mode image can be produced, as shown diagrammatically in Figure 2.9A. In this display the distance traveled by the pulse is shown along the vertical axis and the distance between adjacent pulses is shown along the horizontal axis, with the amplitude of the received signal represented by the brightness on the screen. An example of a B-mode image showing a bifurcating artery is presented in Figure 2.9B.

Ultrasound scanners use electronic multi-element array transducers that typically comprise 128 or more piezoelectric elements, capable of producing many adjacent beams or scan lines. The quality of the image depends on the distance between adjacent beam paths, known as the line density. The more closely the scan lines are

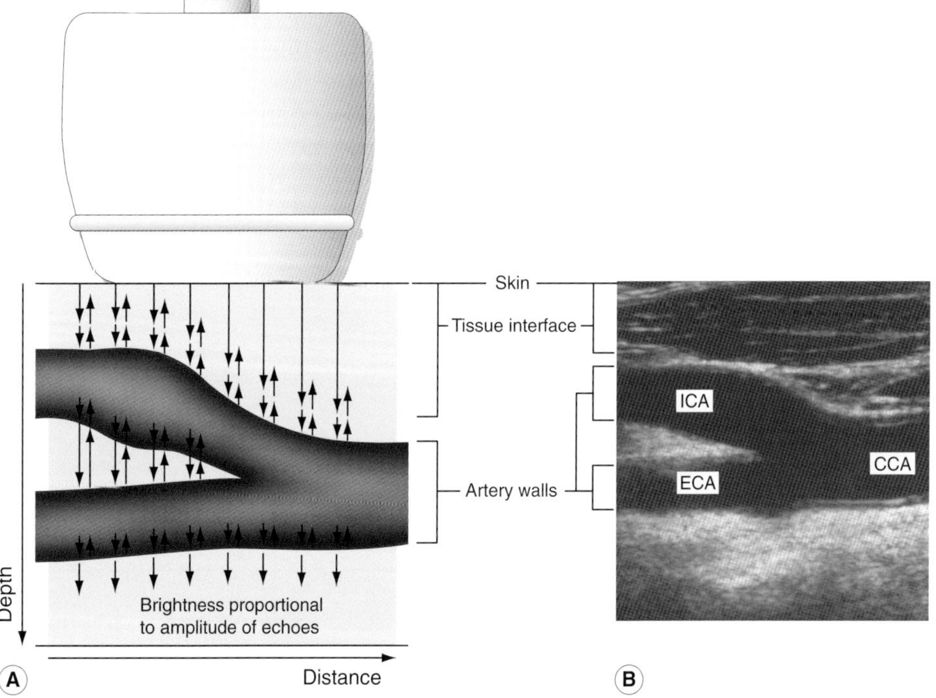

Figure 2.9 • If consecutive ultrasound pulses are transmitted along adjacent paths (A) and displayed in brightness mode in adjacent scan lines, a B-mode image (B) is produced. ICA, internal carotid artery; ECA, external carotid artery; CCA, common carotid artery.

arranged, the more time it will take to produce an image of a given size, which will affect the rate at which the image is updated. This would not be important if a stationary object was being imaged, but most structures in the body are in motion due to cardiac and respiratory movements. The rate at which complete images are produced per second is known as the frame rate and is affected by the number of scan lines and by the width and depth of the region of tissue being imaged. The deeper the tissue being interrogated, the longer it will take for the returning signal to reach the transducer before the next pulse can be transmitted. In B-mode imaging, it is rarely a problem to produce images with a high enough line density and frame rate.

AMPLIFICATION OF RECEIVED ULTRASOUND ECHOES

There are two methods of increasing the amplitude of the returning signal: increasing the output power and increasing the receiver gain. Increasing the voltage of the excitation pulse across the transducer will cause the transducer to transmit a larger-amplitude ultrasound pulse, thus increasing the amplitude of reflections. However, increasing the output power causes the patient to be exposed to more ultrasound energy. The alternative is to amplify the received signal, but there is a limit at which the amplitude of the received signal is no greater than the background noise, and at which no amount of amplification will assist in differentiating the signal from the noise. For a given frequency of transducer, the depth at which the reflected or back-scattered signals are no longer greater than the noise is known as the penetration depth. Increasing the overall gain of the received signal will increase the high-amplitude signals detected near the transducer and the lower-amplitude signals detected from deeper in the tissue, which have been attenuated to a greater extent.

It is useful to be able to image the reflections from similar boundaries that lie at different depths at a similar brightness on the image. Equally, it is useful to image the back-scattered signals from tissues at different depths at a similar level of gray on the B-mode image. Figure 2.10A and B show signals returning from four identical boundaries at different depths in an attenuating medium. It can be seen that the echoes received from the deeper

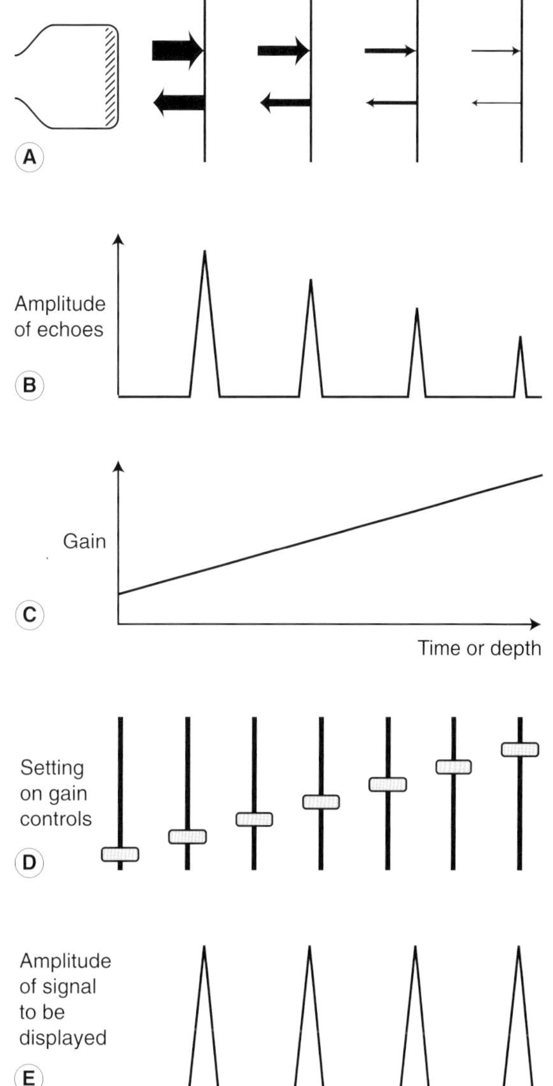

Figure 2.10 • Echoes returning from similar boundaries at different depths (A) will be of different amplitudes (B) due to attenuation. The receiver gain of the scanner can be increased during the time that the echoes are received (C) using the gain controls (D) to produce signals of similar amplitude (E).

boundaries have been attenuated more than those from the shallower boundaries. If the gain of the receiver amplifier is increased over the time during which the pulse is returning to the transducer (Fig. 2.10C), it is possible to use greater amplification for the signal received from the deeper boundaries. By changing the gain over time, the returning echoes from the four boundaries can now be displayed at a similar brightness (Fig. 2.10E). When the next pulse is transmitted, the gain would return to the baseline value and increase with time as before. This method of varying gain over time is known as time gain compensation (TGC) or depth gain compensation (DGC). The TGC control can usually be altered by a set of sliding knobs or paddles to allow different gains to be set for signals returning from different depths, as shown in Figure 2.10D.

DYNAMIC RANGE, COMPRESSION CURVES, AND GRAY-SCALE MAPS

Echoes reflected from tissue–air or tissue–bone interfaces are large compared with the low-amplitude back-scattered signals from small structures within the tissue. The larger signal amplitudes are of an order of 100 000 times greater than the smallest signal detected, just above the noise level of the scanner. This large range of signal amplitudes can best be described using the decibel scale (see Appendix A) as 100 dB. The range of signals that can be displayed by the scanner monitor is much less than 100 dB, typically about 20 dB, and therefore the range of signal amplitudes needs to be reduced in order to be displayed. This can be achieved either by selecting not to display the lowest or the highest signals present or by compressing the signal. The signal can be compressed using a nonlinear amplifier. This applies more gain to lower-amplitude signals than higher-amplitude signals, so reducing the dynamic range of the signal to be displayed. Figure 2.11A gives an example of a compression curve, showing how the amplitude of the signal to be displayed relates to the amplitude of the input signal. The input signal is the received signal, which has already been amplified by the TGC. This compression curve accentuates the differences in lower to mid-range amplitude signals. The choice of compression curve used depends on what aspect of the image is important in a given application, for example, the fine detail of back-scatter from tissue or the presence of large boundaries, such as vessel walls. There are usually a range of compression curves available on modern scanners, and which are often selected automatically by the system, depending on the selected application (e.g., vascular or abdominal). Figure 2.11B and C shows the same carotid plaque imaged using two different compression curves. The dynamic range of signals arriving at the transducer that can be displayed is defined as the ratio of the largest echo amplitude that does not cause saturation, resulting in peak white, to the smallest echo that can be differentiated from noise.

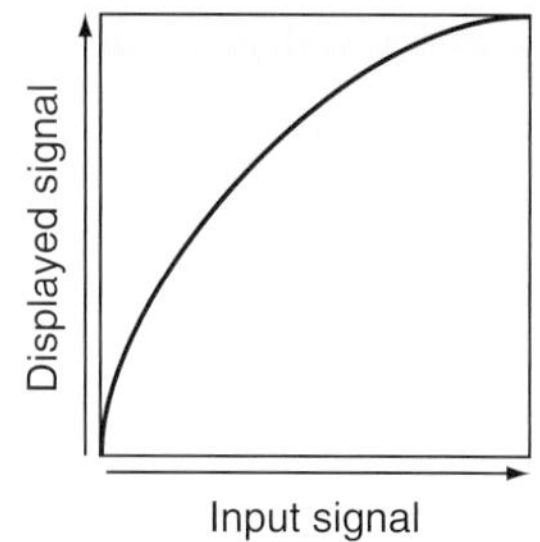

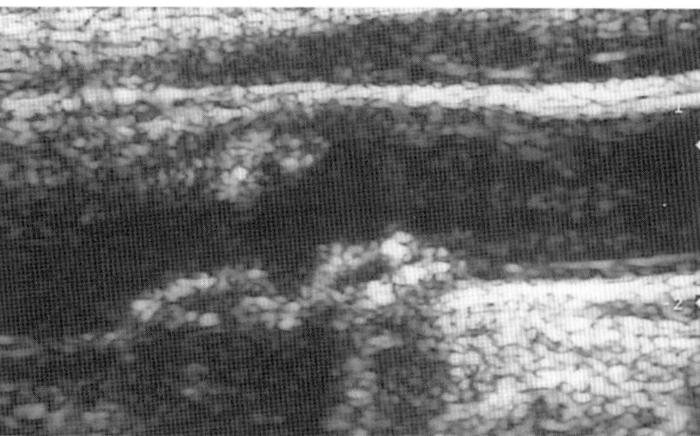

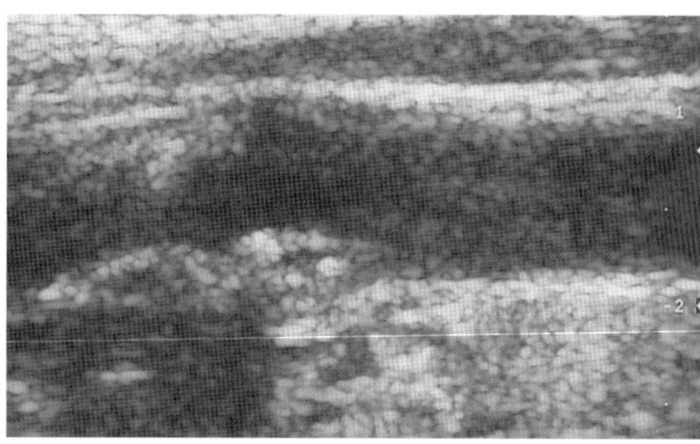

Figure 2.11 • (A) An example of a compression curve, showing how the amplitude of the signal to be displayed relates to the amplitude of the input signal. This compression curve accentuates the differences in the lower to mid-range amplitude signal. (B) and (C) show the same carotid plaque imaged using two different compression curves.

Finally, the scanner uses a gray-scale map to assign a level of gray dependent on the amplitude of the amplified signal, to produce the gray-scale image. Some systems have a choice of gray-scale maps, used in different applications, and these will affect the appearance of the image. It is helpful for the sonographer to refer to the scanner operator manual and to explore the effect of the compression curves and gray-scale maps used on the image obtained.

TRANSDUCER DESIGNS AND BEAM-FORMING

In order to produce a two-dimensional (2D) image, the ultrasound beam has to pass through adjacent areas of the tissue. This can be done by physically moving the transducer, and in early real-time scanners this was performed by rocking or rotating the transducer element. Multi-element electronic imaging transducers are typically made up of 128 or more elements arranged in a row (Fig. 2.12A), often about 4 cm long. These are known as array transducers. If a group of elements are all excited simultaneously (Fig. 2.13A), the wavelets will interfere to produce a beam that is perpendicular to the transducer face. The groups of elements within the array that are excited can be varied to produce ultrasound beams that follow parallel adjacent paths (Fig. 2.13B). For example, elements 1–5 produce the first beam, 2–6 the second, 3–7 the third, and so on. A linear array transducer produces a rectangular image in which the field of view is the same at depth as it is close to the transducer (Fig. 12.12A).

A sector image can be produced by arranging the elements in a curvilinear array (Fig. 2.12B). As the beam paths diverge, the image fans out and therefore the scan lines run more closely in the portion of the image near to the transducer and become more spread out at depth. This leads to some loss of image quality at depth but allows a larger field of view compared with that produced by a linear array transducer. Curvilinear arrays are mainly used for abdominal imaging.

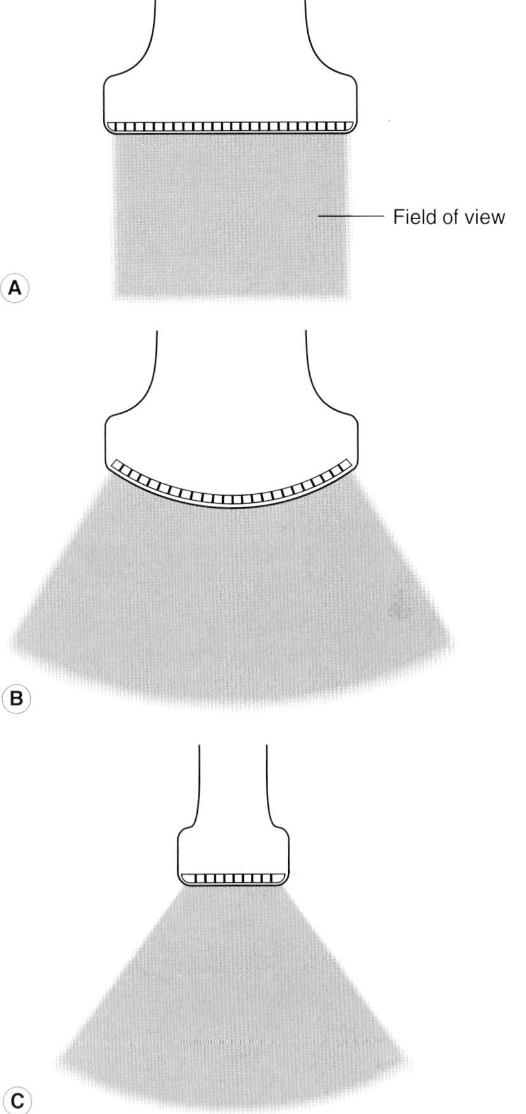

Figure 2.12 • (A) Linear array transducer. This is typically made up of 128 elements in a row and produces a rectangular field of view. (B) Curvilinear array transducer. This produces a sector image, with a field of view that diverges with depth. (C) Phased array transducer. This uses a smaller array of elements and electronically steers the beam to produce a sector image.

Using several elements to form the ultrasound beam enables the beam shape to be manipulated. If the elements used to form the beam are excited at slightly different times, the wavefronts produced by the elements will interfere differently than they would if they were all excited at the same time. For example, if the element on the far right in the array (Fig. 2.14A) is excited first, with the next element excited after a very short delay, and so forth, the wavefronts produced will interfere in such a way

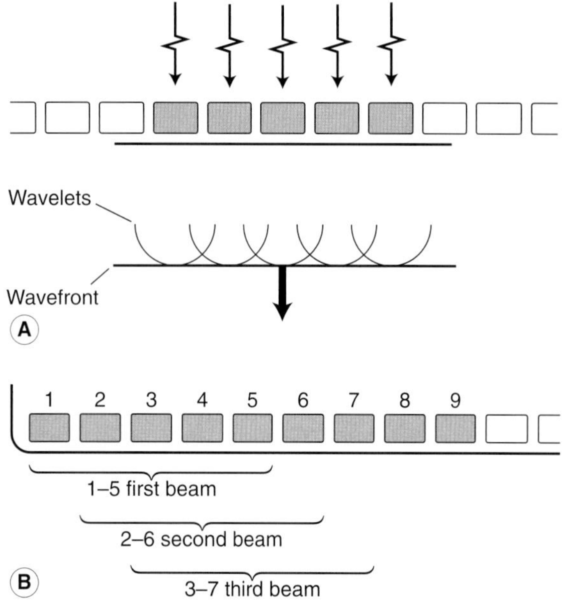

Figure 2.13 • (A) A group of elements within an array can be excited simultaneously, and the resulting wavelets will interfere to produce a wavefront perpendicular to the transducer face. (B) The group of elements excited within an array can be varied to produce beams following parallel adjacent paths.

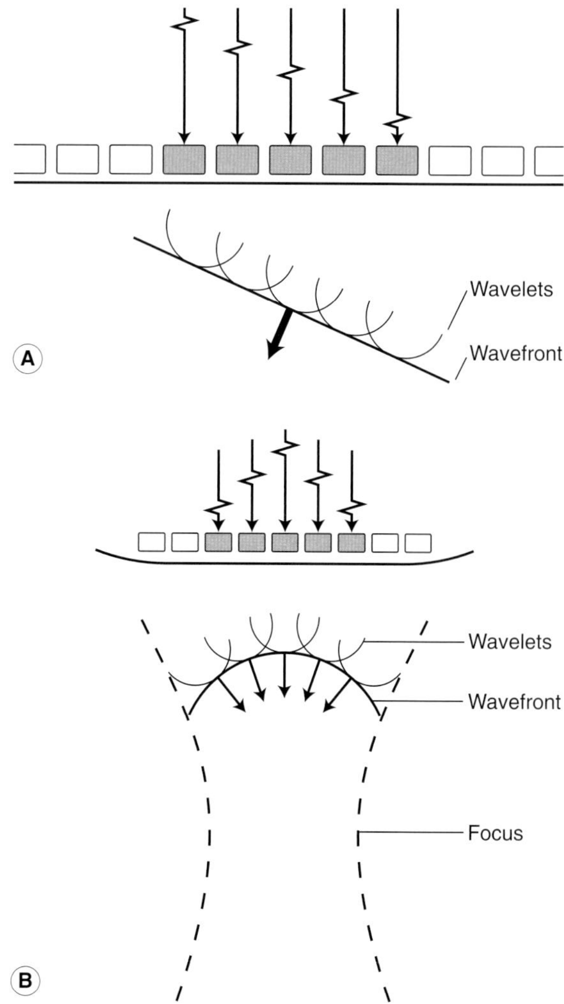

Figure 2.14 • (A) Introducing a time delay between exciting consecutive elements within the array causes the wavelets to interfere in such a way that the beam is steered away from the path perpendicular to the transducer face (e.g., steered left or right). (B) Delays between excitation of the elements in the array can be used to focus the beam.

that the beam is no longer perpendicular to the front of the transducer. The angle at which the beam is produced will depend on the delay between the excitation pulses of the different elements. By changing the delay between each set of excitation pulses, it is possible to steer the beam through a range of angles from left to right.

Phased array transducers use a smaller array of elements and electronically steer the beam in this way to produce a sector image (Fig. 2.12C). This type of transducer produces a large field of view compared with the size of the transducer face, also known as the transducer footprint. Phased array transducers are used, in particular, in cardiac ultrasound, as the heart can only be imaged through small spaces between the ribs, thus requiring a transducer with a small footprint to image a large field of view at depth. Beam steering is also used in linear array transducers when a beam that is not perpendicular to the transducer face is required, such as in Doppler ultrasound (see Chs 3 and 4) and in compound imaging. In compound imaging, the target is insonated several times with the beam steered at several different angles (Fig. 2.15). The returning echoes from these different imaging beams are combined to produce a single image. This gives improved imaging of interfaces that are not parallel to the transducer face, such as the lateral walls of a vessel, and reduces noise and speckle. Figure 2.16 shows the improvement in the image that can be provided when imaging a carotid plaque with compound imaging compared to conventional imaging.

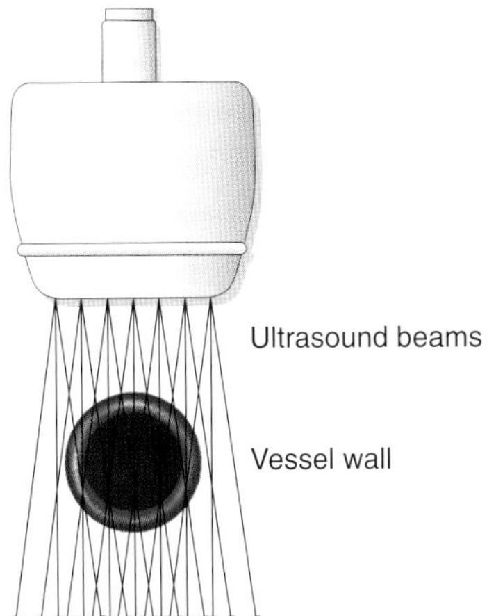

Figure 2.15 • Compound scanning sums several images obtained with the ultrasound beam steered at slightly different angles, to improve imaging of boundaries that are perpendicular to the transducer face and to reduce noise and speckle.

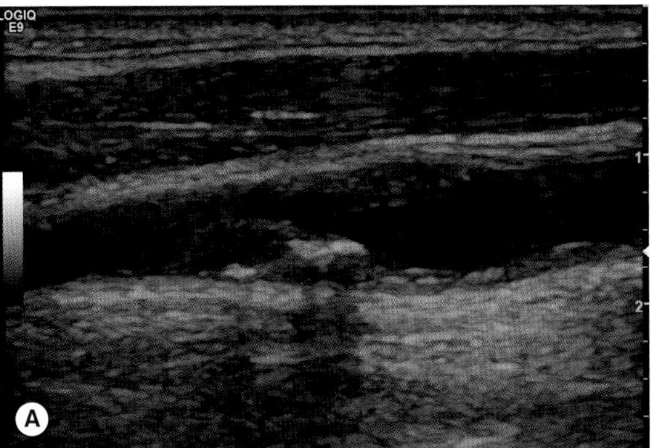

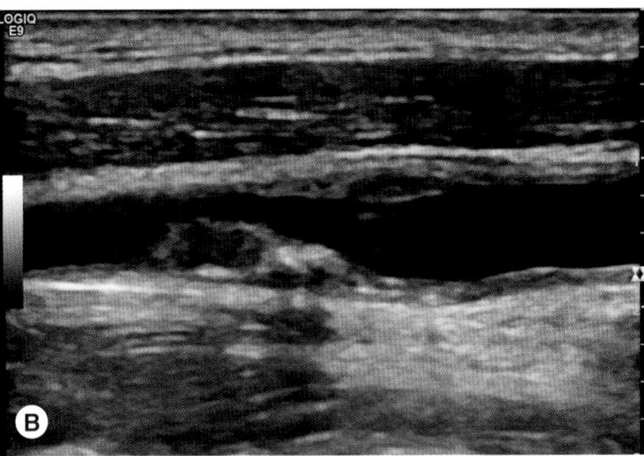

Figure 2.16 • Images showing the improvement that can be provided by compound imaging of a carotid artery plaque (B) compared to conventional imaging (A).

FOCUSING THE BEAM

The ultrasound beam can be focused to improve the image quality within the focal zone. By using several elements, excited with a range of delays, it is possible to focus the beam. Figure 2.14B shows how, if the elements at each end of the group of active elements are excited first, with the next two elements being excited after a short delay, and so forth, the wavelets will interfere to produce a concave wavefront causing the beam to converge at the focal point. The distance of the focal point from the front of the transducer is governed by the length of the delays, with longer delays producing a shorter focal length.

Many modern scanners use multiple zone focusing whereby the image will be created in zones, using different focal lengths for different depths. The upper portion of the image, near to the transducer, will be produced using a short focal length, a second set of scan lines with a longer focal length will be used for the next zone of the image, and so on. The advantage is that image quality is improved throughout the image; however, the disadvantage is that the frame rate is reduced by a factor of 1/(number of focal zones).

The focus of the beam can also be altered during reception. This is known as dynamic focusing. In this case, delays are introduced between consecutive elements on reception, rather than transmission, before the received signals are summed together. With regard to Figure 2.17, dynamic focusing allows the signals that have traveled farther along path B to be added to the signal that has traveled along path A by delaying the signal received by the middle element before summing it with the signals received by the outer elements. The focal point of the received signal again depends on the lengths of the delays introduced. As the delay can be varied while the signal is being received from different depths, the focal length can be optimized through the image without a reduction in frame rate.

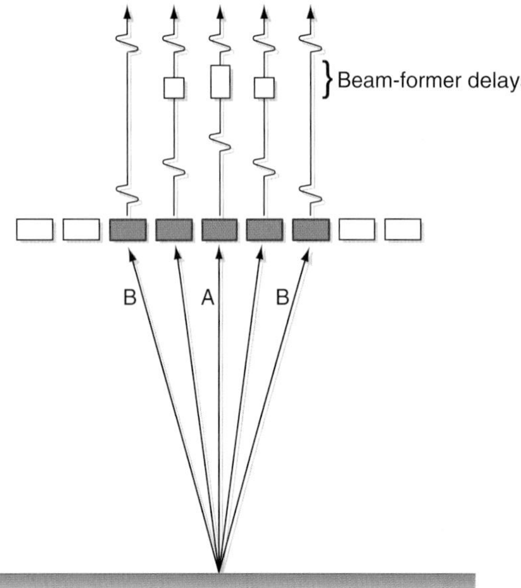

Figure 2.17 • Introducing delays before summing the signals received at different elements allows dynamic focusing of the received beam. In this case, dynamic focusing allows the signals that have traveled farther along path B to be added to the signal that has traveled along path A by delaying the signal received by the middle element before summing it with the signals received by the outer elements.

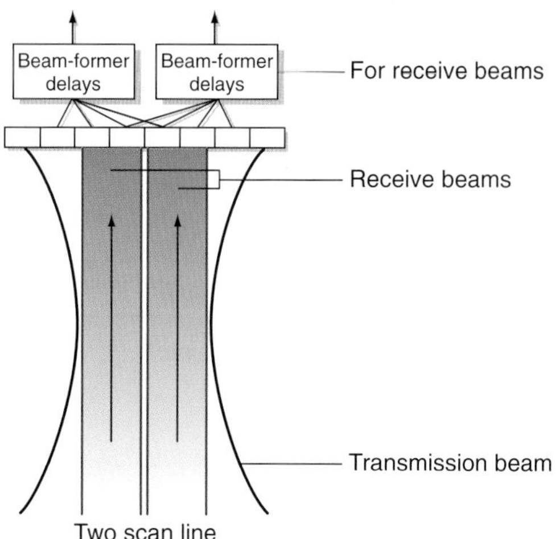

Figure 2.18 • Parallel beam-forming of two or more received beams from a single wide transmitted beam permits improvements in imaging frame rate. (Hoskins, Thrush, Whittingham, Diagnostic Ultrasound 2003. Cambridge University Press)

A technique known as parallel beam-forming may be used to improve the frame rate (i.e., the number of images produced per second). This uses a wide, weakly focused transmitted beam. The received signal produced from this transmitted beam can then be processed using different sets of delays in order to form two or more different received beams, simultaneously, as shown in Figure 2.18 (Whittingham 2003). This allows two or more received signals, producing two or more scan lines, for each transmitted pulse, so enabling higher frame rates.

IMAGE RESOLUTION

The resolution of a system is defined as its ability to distinguish between two adjacent objects. Figure 2.19 demonstrates how the echoes from two reflecting surfaces can be resolved and also how they can no longer be distinguished from each other if the two objects are moved closer together. The resolution of an ultrasound image can be

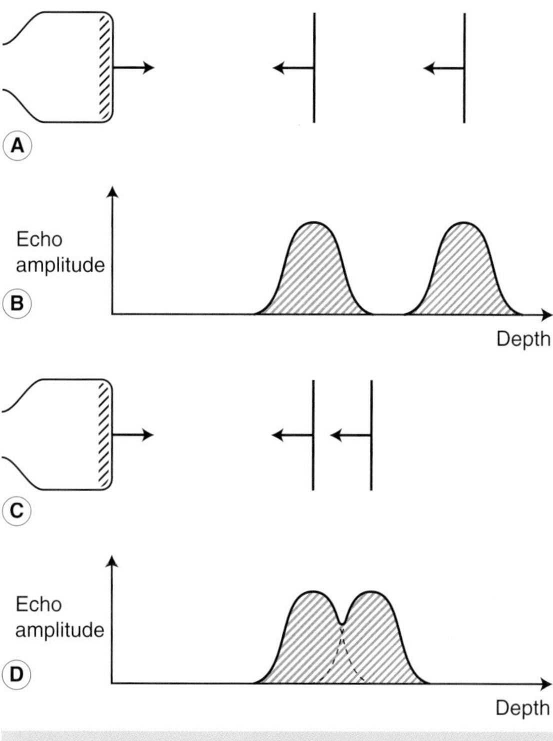

Figure 2.19 • Echoes returning from two boundaries (A) can be resolved (B). However, if the boundaries are close together (C), they can no longer be seen as different echoes (D).

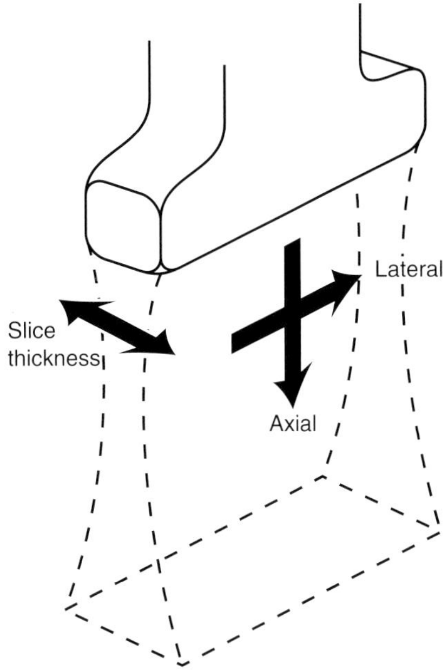

Figure 2.20 • Resolution of a transducer can be described in different planes – axial and lateral. The slice thickness of the beam relates to the width of the beam in the nonimaging plane and governs the thickness of the slice of tissue being imaged.

described in three planes: axial (along the beam), lateral (across the image), and slice thickness – as shown in Figure 2.20. Axial resolution depends on the length of the excitation pulse, which in turn depends on the operating frequency of the transducer. The higher the frequency, the better the resolution. There is, however, a compromise, as the higher the frequency, the greater the attenuation and therefore the poorer the penetration. The lateral resolution depends on factors such as the density of the scan lines and the focusing of the beam. Lateral resolution is poorer than axial resolution.

The out-of-imaging plane beam thickness, or slice thickness, will affect the region perpendicular to the scan plane over which returning echoes will be obtained. Ideally, the slice thickness should be as thin as possible to maintain image quality, so focusing is often used in this plane as well as in the imaging plane. This can be done either by incorporating a fixed lens into the front face of the transducer or by electronic focusing using a 2D array of elements, which allows focusing in both the imaging plane and the plane at right angles to the image. These 2D arrays are often called 1½D arrays as there are relatively few elements along the width of the array compared with the length.

Resolution of an ultrasound system can be assessed using a test object consisting of fine wires embedded in a tissue-mimicking material. The groups of six wires are positioned so the wires are at different distances apart, allowing the user to assess the smallest separation at which the wires can still be resolved. The tissue-mimicking material is designed to have similar attenuation to tissue and to produce a similar back-scattered signal. Figure 2.21A is a schematic diagram of the wires in the test object and in Figure 2.21B and C the images are obtained from the test object with 2.25 MHz phased array and 10 MHz linear array transducers, respectively. It can be seen that the 10 MHz transducer gives better axial resolution, as all six wires are seen, whereas the 2.25 MHz transducer provides better penetration, to 12 cm depth compared with 3 cm for the 10 MHz transducer. Choosing the frequency of transducer to use for a given examination depends on a compromise between the depth of the region to be imaged and the axial resolution that can be obtained. It is preferable to select the highest-frequency transducer that will provide adequate penetration. The ability to visualize objects within an image also depends on the appropriate use of imaging controls, such as gain settings.

TISSUE HARMONIC IMAGING

Tissue harmonic imaging (THI) can improve the image quality in difficult subjects; however, in good subjects poorer images may be obtained than with conventional imaging. THI utilizes the fact that high-amplitude ultrasound pulses undergo nonlinear propagation, whereby the pulse becomes progressively distorted as it passes through tissue (Fig. 2.22; Whittingham 1999). This distortion of the pulse results in the frequency content of the returning pulse being significantly different from that of the transmitted pulse. Figure 2.22D shows how the energy spectrum of the distorted pulse will contain harmonic frequencies ($2f$, $3f$, etc.) that are multiples of the original transmitted frequency, f.

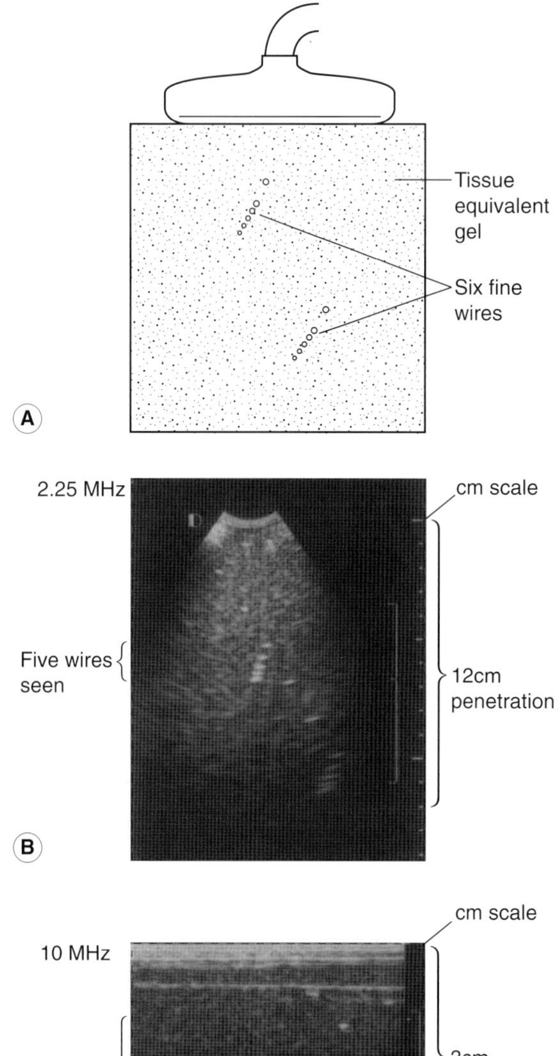

Figure 2.21 • Assessing ultrasound axial resolution. (A) Schematic diagram of a group of six unevenly spaced wires in a test object. (B, C) Images of the test object in (A) obtained with 2.25 and 10 MHz transducers, respectively. The 10 MHz transducer gives better axial resolution and the 2.25 MHz transducer provides better penetration.

For the harmonic frequencies to be used to form the image, the fundamental and harmonic signals need to be separated. This can be done in two ways: either frequency filtering or pulse inversion. Filtering was the method initially used in harmonic imaging, whereby the receiver is tuned to a center frequency that is twice the center frequency of the transmitted pulse, as seen in Figure 2.23. Usually the transmitted pulse used in THI is a lower frequency than that used in conventional imaging. For example, in an abdominal application, a center frequency of 3.5 MHz would typically be used in conventional imaging whereas a center frequency of 1.75 MHz would be used for THI, producing a second harmonic at 3.5 MHz. Improvements in transducer sensitivity over the years have enabled the production of broad-band transducers with large bandwidths, allowing the transducer to transmit ultrasound with a center frequency *f* and selectively receive the returning harmonics with center frequency 2*f*.

The pulse, or phase, inverion approach uses two pulses along each scan line, the second pulse being an inverted version of the first. For linear propagation of these pulses, if the returning pulses are summed they will cancel each other out (Figure 2.24A–C). However if nonlinear propagation has occurred the pulses will not cancel each other out (as nonlinear distortion occurs more for the positive-pressure, compressional part of the cycle than for the negative-pressure, rarefractional part of the cycle), providing the noncanceling harmonic signal (Figure 2.24 D–F). The advantage in pulse inversion harmonics over the filtering method is that shorter pulses can be used, resulting in better axial resolution; however, as two transmitted pulses are required to produce each scan line, the imaging frame rate may be reduced. As nonlinear propagation only occurs in high-amplitude pulses, harmonics are not present in lower-amplitude echoes produced, for example, reverberations by multiply reflected pulses, reverberations, grating lobes, or side lobes. In conventional imaging it is these spurious echoes that cause noisy images. These spurious echoes will contain little or no harmonics and therefore will not be detected when using THI. Figure 2.25 shows the improvement when imaging an aorta using harmonic imaging compared to conventional imaging.

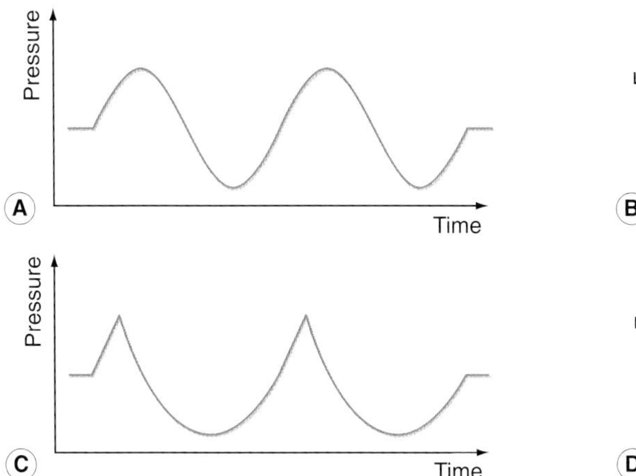

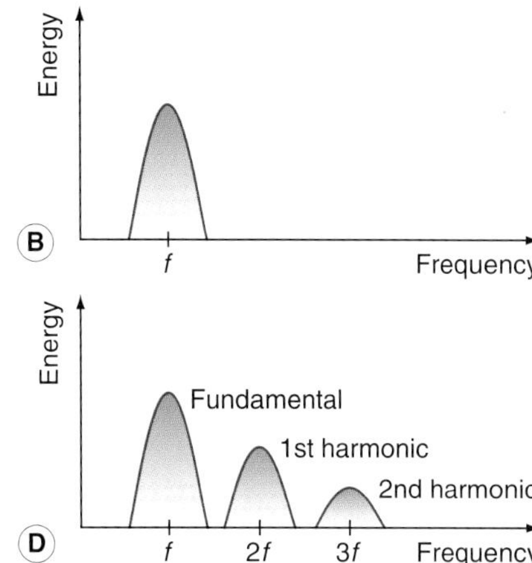

Figure 2.22 • (A) An undistorted pulse with its frequency spectra (B) showing a center frequency *f*. (C) Large-amplitude signals become progressively distorted as they pass through tissue. (D) The distorted pulse contains harmonics (2*f*, 3*f*, etc.) of the fundamental frequency *f*. (With kind permission from Springer Science + Business Media, European Radiology 9 (Suppl 3), Tissue harmonic imaging, 1999, S323–326, T.A. Whittingham.)

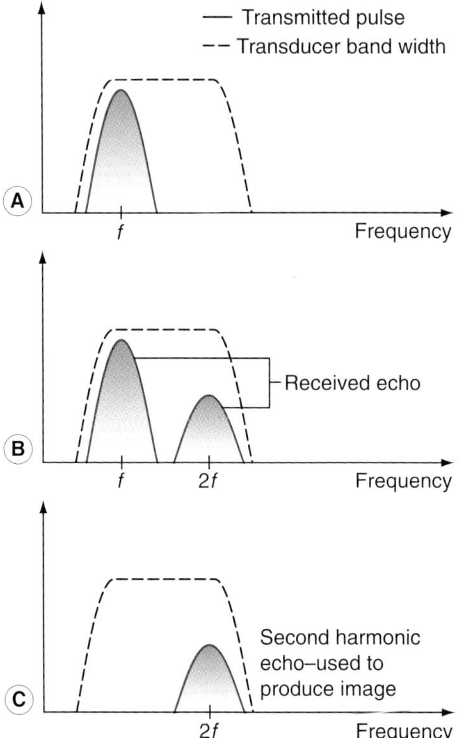

Figure 2.23 • Tissue harmonic imaging. Wide transducer bandwidths enable pulses of center frequency *f* to be transmitted (A) and use only the received harmonic frequencies, center frequency 2*f*, to produce the image (C). (With kind permission from Springer Science + Business Media, European Radiology 9 (Suppl 3), Tissue harmonic imaging, 1999, S323–326, T.A. Whittingham.)

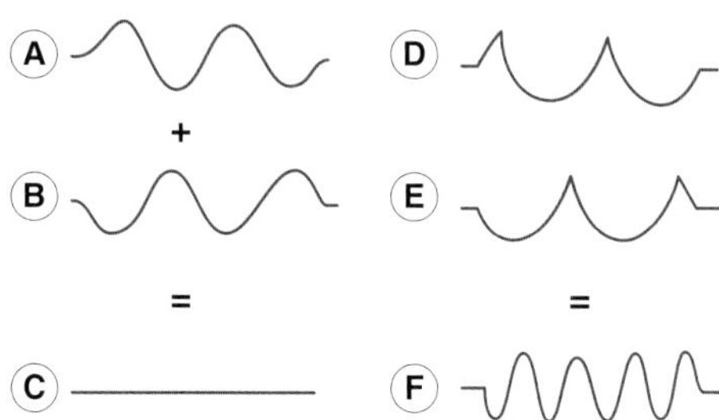

Figure 2.24 • Pulse inversion: if the undistorted echo from a pulse (A) is summed with the undistorted echo from the inverted pulse (B) the two will cancel each other out (C). However, if a distorted echo, due to nonlinear propogation (D), is summed with the distorted echo from the inverted pulse (E), the two signals are not identical so will not cancel out but provide the harmonic component, which is twice the frequency of the fundamental frequency (F).

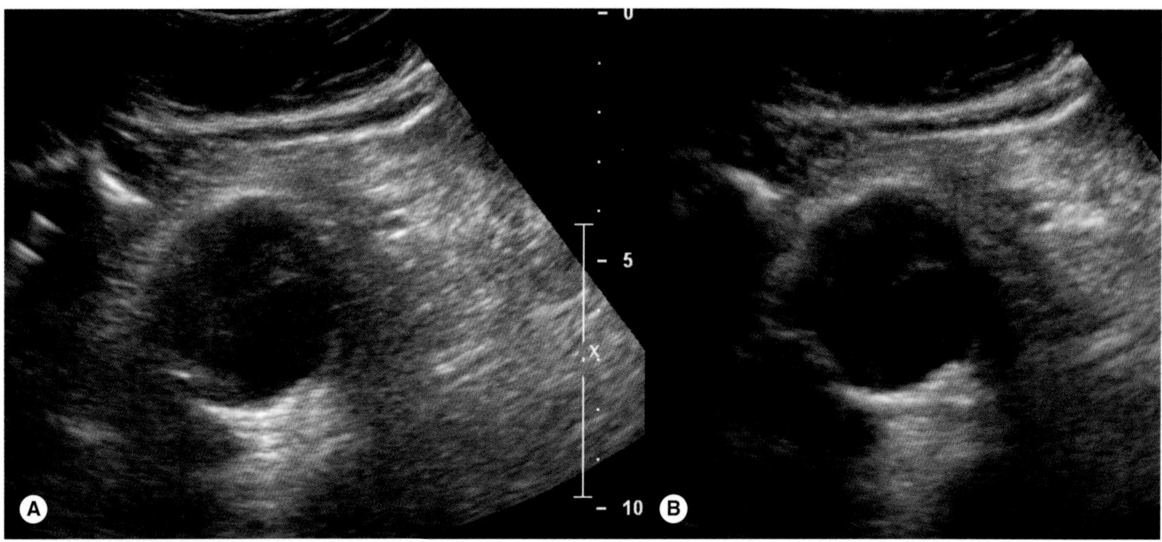

Figure 2.25 • Tissue harmonic imaging can provide improved image quality, as seen by comparing conventional imaging (A) with tissue harmonic imaging (B) of an aorta.

References

Fish P 1990 Physics and instrumentation of diagnostic medical ultrasound. Wiley, Chichester

McDicken W N 1981 Diagnostic ultrasonics: principles and use of instruments, 2nd edn. Wiley, New York

Whittingham T A 1999 Tissue harmonic imaging. European Radiology 9 (Suppl. 3): S323–S326

Whittingham T A 2003 Transducers and beam-forming. In: Hoskins P R, Thrush A, Martin K et al. (eds) Diagnostic ultrasound: physics and equipment. Greenwich Medical Media, London, pp 23–48

Further reading

Hedrick W R, Hykes D L, Starchman D E 2005 Ultrasound: physics and instrumentation, 4th edn. Mosby, St Louis

Kremkau F W 2005 Diagnostic ultrasound – principles and instruments, 5th edn. WB Saunders, Philadelphia

Whittingham T A 1997 New and future developments in ultrasound imaging. British Journal of Radiology 70: S119–S132

Whittingham T A 1999 Section I: New transducers. European Radiology 9 (Suppl. 3): S298–S303

Whittingham T A 1999 Section II: Digital technology. European Radiology 9 (Suppl. 3): S307–S311

Doppler ultrasound

CONTENTS

THE DOPPLER EFFECT

The Doppler effect enables ultrasound to be used to detect blood flow and to quantify vascular disease. The Doppler effect is the change in the observed frequency due to the relative motion of the source and the observer. This effect can be heard when the pitch of a police car's siren changes as the car travels towards you and then away from you. Figure 3.1 helps to explain the effect in more detail. In Figure 3.1A the source of the sound and the observer are both stationary, so the observed sound has the same frequency as the transmitted sound. In Figure 3.1B the source is stationary and the observer is moving toward it, causing the observer to cross the wavefronts of the emitted wave more quickly than when stationary, so that the observer witnesses a higher-frequency wave than that emitted. If, however, the observer is moving away from the source (Fig. 3.1C), the wavefronts will be crossed less often and the frequency witnessed will be lower than that emitted. Figure 3.1D shows the opposite case, in which the source is moving toward a stationary observer. The source will move a short distance toward the observer between the emission of each wave, and in so doing shorten the wavelength, so the observer will therefore witness a higher frequency. Similarly, if the source is moving away from the observer, the wavelength will be increased, leading to observation of a lower frequency (Fig. 3.1E). The resulting change in the observed frequency is known as the Doppler shift, and the magnitude of the Doppler shift frequency is proportional to the relative velocities of the source and the observer.

History behind the discovery of the Doppler effect

This effect was first described by an Austrian physicist named Christian Doppler in 1842. He used the

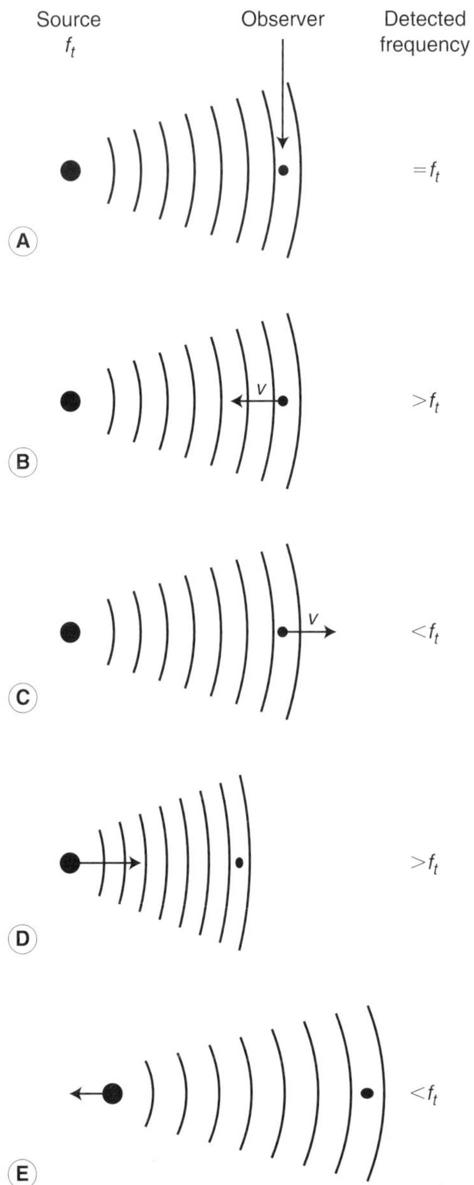

Figure 3.1 • The Doppler effect is the change in the observed frequency due to motion between the source and the observer (A) The source of the sound and the observer are both stationary, so the observed sound has the same frequency as that transmitted (B) The source is stationary and the observer is moving toward the source (with velocity *v*), so that the observer witnesses a higher frequency than that emitted (C) The observer is moving away from the source, so the frequency detected is lower than that emitted (D) The source is moving toward a stationary observer, so the detected frequency is increased. (E) The source is moving away from the observer, thus decreasing the frequency observed.

Doppler effect to explain the "color of double stars." A rival Dutch scientist working at the same time tried to prove Doppler's theory wrong by hiring a train and two trumpeters. One trumpeter stood on the train while the other stood by the track, and an observer compared the pitch of the trumpeter who passed by on the train with that of the stationary trumpeter. This experiment verified Doppler's theory, although Doppler's use of this effect to explain the "color of double stars" was in fact incorrect.

DOPPLER EFFECT APPLIED TO VASCULAR ULTRASOUND

In the case of vascular ultrasound, the Doppler effect is used to study blood flow. The simplest Doppler ultrasound instruments use transducers consisting of two piezoelectric elements, one to transmit ultrasound beams and the other to receive the returning echoes back-scattered from the moving blood cells (Fig. 3.2). In this situation, the Doppler effect occurs twice. First, the transducer is a stationary source while the blood cells are moving receivers of the ultrasound waves (Fig. 3.1B). The ultrasound is then back-scattered from the blood cells, which now act as a moving source, with the transducer acting as a stationary observer (Fig. 3.1D). The Doppler shift observed depends on the frequency of the ultrasound originally transmitted by the transducer and the velocity of the blood

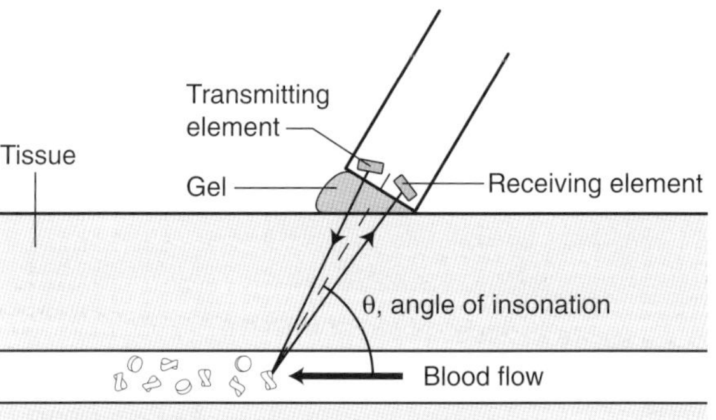

Figure 3.2 • Simple Doppler ultrasound instruments use transducers consisting of two piezoelectric elements, one to transmit ultrasound and the other to receive the returning echoes back-scattered from the moving blood cells.

cells from which the ultrasound is back-scattered. The observed frequency also depends on the angle from which the movement of the blood is observed (i.e., the angle between the ultrasound beam and the direction of the blood flow). The Doppler shift frequency, f_d (i.e., the difference between the transmitted frequency, f_t, and received frequency, f_r) is given by:

$$f_d = f_r - f_t = \frac{2vf_t \cos\theta}{c} \quad (3.1)$$

where v is the velocity of the blood, θ is the angle between the ultrasound beam and the direction of blood flow (also known as the angle of insonation), and c is the speed of sound in tissue. The factor of 2 is present in the Doppler equation as the Doppler effect has occurred twice, as explained above.

Consider, for example, a 5 MHz transducer used to interrogate a blood vessel with a flow velocity of 50 cm/s using an angle of insonation of 60°. Taking the speed of sound in tissue to be 1540 m/s, the Doppler equation can be used to estimate that the Doppler shift frequency produced will be 1.6 kHz. In fact, it is a useful coincidence that the typical values of blood velocity found in the body and the transmitted frequencies used in medical ultrasound result in Doppler shift frequencies that are in the audible range (from 20 Hz to 20 kHz). The simplest Doppler systems can extract the Doppler shift frequency and output it to a loudspeaker, enabling the operator to listen to the Doppler shifts produced from the blood flow.

The Doppler equation shows that the detected Doppler shift depends on the angle of insonation, θ, through the term $\cos\theta$. Table 3.1 shows how the $\cos\theta$ term varies between 0 and 1 as the angle changes from 0° to 90°. When the angle of insonation is 90°, the $\cos\theta$ term is 0, so virtually no Doppler shift is detected. When the angle of insonation is 0° (i.e., the Doppler beam is parallel to the direction of flow), the $\cos\theta$ term is 1, giving the maximum detectable Doppler shift frequency for a given velocity of blood and transmitted frequency. Figure 3.3 shows how the detected Doppler shift frequencies change as the Doppler angle changes. When the transducer is pointing toward the flow, a positive frequency shift is seen, but once the transducer is pointing away from the direction of flow, a negative frequency shift is seen. The smaller the angle of insonation, the larger the frequency shift detected, but as the angle of insonation approaches a right angle, very small frequency shifts are detected.

Θ (°)	cosΘ
0	1
30	0.87
45	0.71
60	0.5
75	0.26
90	0

Table 3.1 Variation of the cosθ term of the Doppler equation with the angle of insonation

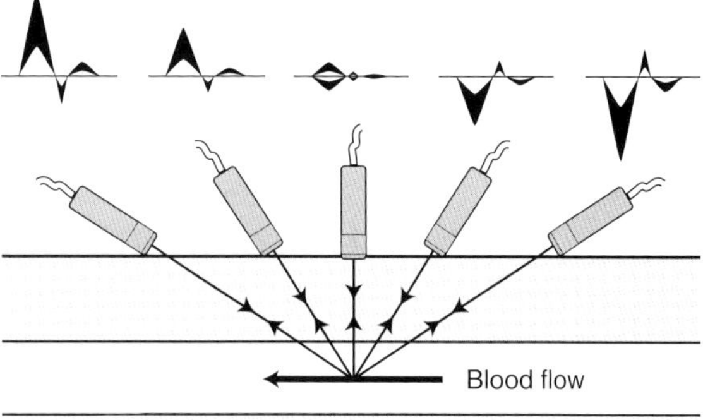

Figure 3.3 • The detected Doppler shift frequency changes as the angle of insonation changes.

Back-scatter from blood

Blood is made up of red blood cells (erythrocytes), white blood cells (leukocytes), and platelets suspended in plasma. Red blood cells occupy between 36% and 54% of the total blood volume. They have a biconcave disc shape and a diameter of 7 µm, which is much smaller than the wavelength of ultrasound used to study blood flow. This means that groups of red blood cells act as scatterers of the ultrasound (see Fig. 2.8).

The back-scattered signal from blood received at the transducer is small, partly due to the back-scattered energy being radiated in all directions, unlike specular reflections, and partly because the effective cross-section of the blood cells is small compared with the width of the beam. The back-scattered power is proportional to the fourth power of the frequency (i.e., f^4), and therefore as the transmitted frequency selected to detect flow is increased, there is an increase in back-scattered power. However, this is offset by the increase in attenuation of the overlying tissue with the increase in frequency. Ultrasound systems will often use a lower transmitted frequency for Doppler than for B-mode imaging, and the imaging and Doppler transmitted frequencies are usually indicated on the image. In situations in which blood velocity is low or blood cells are stationary, such as aneurysms or venous flow, the cells may aggregate into clumps that can sometimes produce sufficiently high-amplitude back-scattered echoes to be displayed on the B-mode image (see Fig. 13.22).

EXTRACTING THE DOPPLER SIGNAL

The simplest Doppler systems consist of a transducer with two piezoelectric elements (Fig. 3.2), one continuously transmitting ultrasound and the other continuously receiving back-scattered signals both from stationary tissue and flowing blood. This received signal therefore consists of the transmitted frequency reflected by stationary objects and the Doppler-shifted frequencies back-scattered from moving blood cells. As the returning echoes are of low amplitude, first they must be amplified. The Doppler shift frequency can then be extracted from the received signal by a process known as demodulation. One method of demodulation used in Doppler systems is shown in Figure 3.4. Here, the received signal is multiplied by the transmitted signal and the product is filtered to remove the high frequencies, thus providing the Doppler shift frequency. The received signal has a different frequency from the transmitted frequency, owing to the Doppler effect, and a lower amplitude, owing to attenuation of the signal by overlying tissue. As mentioned earlier, once the Doppler shift frequency has been extracted (by demodulation) and amplified, it can simply be output to a loudspeaker or investigated using a spectrum analyzer (Fig. 3.5). With experience, it is possible for the operator to recognize the different sounds produced by normal and diseased vessels.

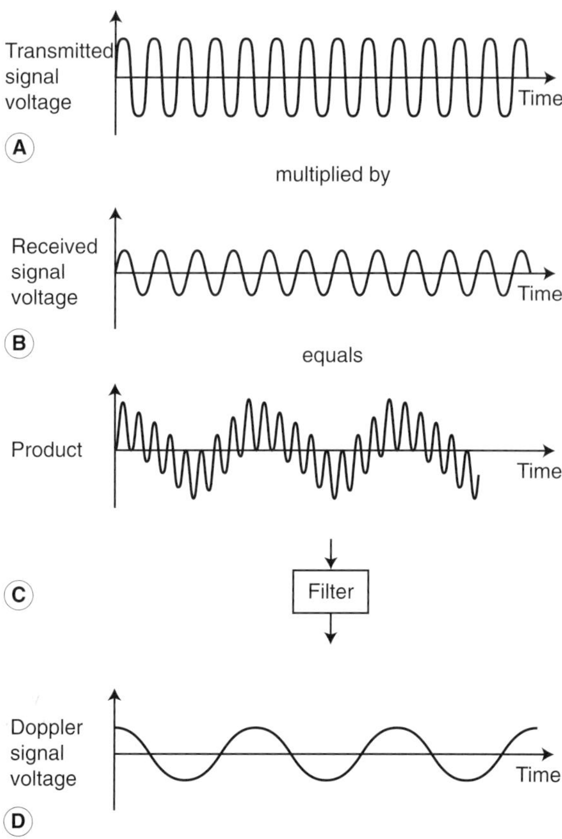

Figure 3.4 • Demodulation. This is used to extract the Doppler frequency, in this case by multiplying the transmitted signal (A) by the received signal (B) and filtering out the high-frequency component (C) to leave the Doppler signal (D). (After Fish 1990, with permission.)

The instruments described so far will not give information about the direction of flow relative to the transducer. This information is available in the returning signal, as objects moving toward the transducer will produce an increase in the detected frequency, while those moving away will produce a decrease in the detected frequency. Extracting directional information from the received Doppler signal requires more sophisticated electronics or software and this will not be explained in this textbook. When the flow directions have been separated, stereo loudspeakers can be used with one channel for forward flow and the other for reverse.

It is preferable to display both the forward and reverse Doppler signals simultaneously on the same spectrum. This is done by displaying the

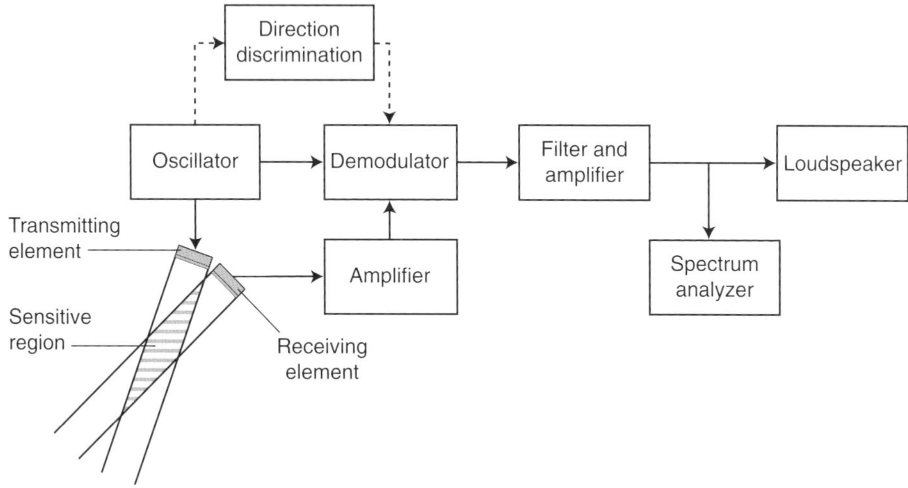

Figure 3.5 • Elements of a simple continuous-wave Doppler system.

signals on either side of a baseline, with flow toward the transducer displayed above the baseline and flow away from the transducer displayed below. Figure 3.6A shows the flow in the vertebral artery and vein displayed in different directions on the spectrum. Most Doppler systems allow the operator to invert this display, if desired, so that the flow away from the transducer can be displayed above the baseline, and it is important that the operator be aware that this has been done in order to interpret any results correctly. The fact that the display is inverted is usually indicated on the screen (Fig. 3.6B). The baseline can also be shifted up and down to make maximum use of the spectral display (Fig. 3.6C).

As well as obtaining Doppler shift frequencies from the flowing blood, the slow moving vessel walls act as large reflective surfaces, producing large-amplitude, low-frequency Doppler shift signals along with the low-amplitude high frequencies obtained from blood. These signals are known as wall thump, due to their sound, and are removed by high-pass filters. The high-pass filter will remove any signals with a frequency below the cut-off frequency of the filter, and this can be controlled by the operator. If this is set too low, the wall thump signal (Fig. 3.7A) will not be removed, whereas if it is set too high, important Doppler information will be removed, possibly altering the waveform shape (Fig. 3.7C) (e.g., by suggesting the absence of diastolic flow). The ideal filter setting (Fig. 3.7B) should remove unwanted signals such as wall thump without removing important blood flow information.

ANALYSIS OF THE DOPPLER SIGNAL

The Doppler signal can be investigated using spectral analysis, allowing waveforms to be displayed (as seen in Fig. 3.6) and blood velocity to be measured. The blood cells flowing through a vessel will be moving at different velocities within the vessel; for example, cells near the vessel wall will be moving more slowly than those in the center (see Ch. 5). The velocity of the blood cells will vary with time, owing to the pulsatile nature of arterial blood flow. This means that the Doppler shift signal obtained from flowing blood will contain a range of frequencies, due to the range of velocities present, and the frequency content will vary with time. It has already been explained in Chapter 2 (Figs 2.3 and 2.4) how a signal is made up of sine waves of different frequencies. Spectral analysis can be used to break down the Doppler signal into its component frequencies and to show how these component frequencies vary with time. Figure 3.8 shows how a spectrum is displayed, with time along the horizontal axis and the Doppler shift frequency along the vertical axis. The third axis, the brightness of the display, relates to the back-scattered power of the signal at each frequency (i.e., the proportion of the blood cells

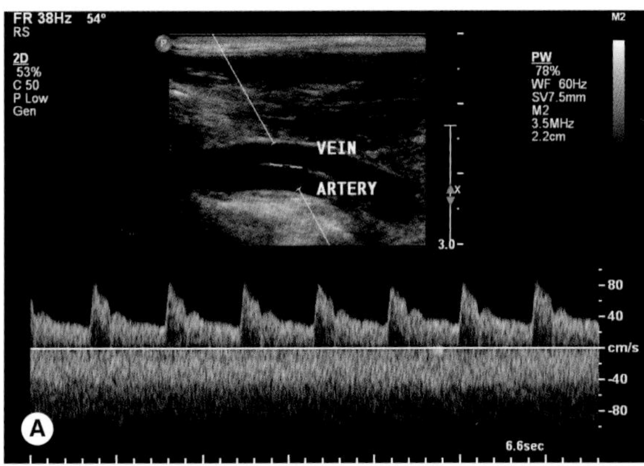

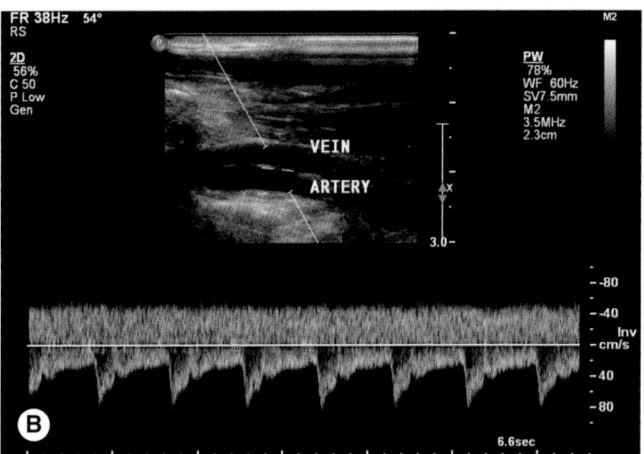

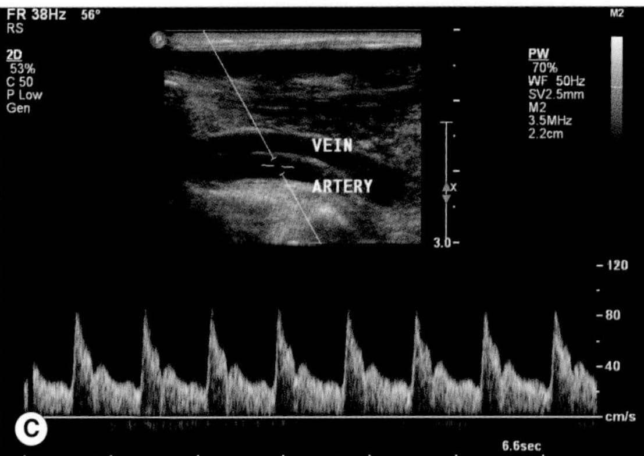

Figure 3.6 • The use of an offset, or baseline, allows both forward and reverse flows to be displayed on the same spectrum (A), which can be inverted if required, shown by negative values of the velocity being displayed above the spectral Doppler baseline (labled 'inv') (B). The baseline can be altered to make maximum use of the spectral display (C). The values of the transmitted imaging and Doppler frequencies are often displayed on the screen.

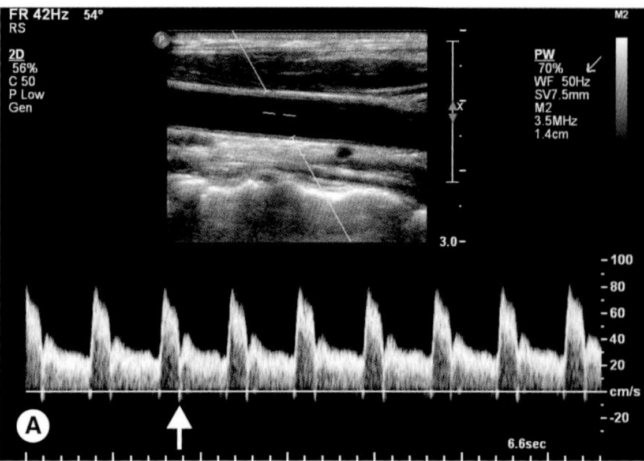

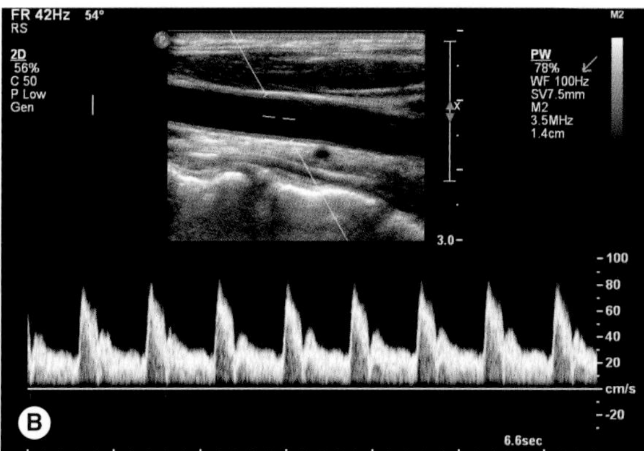

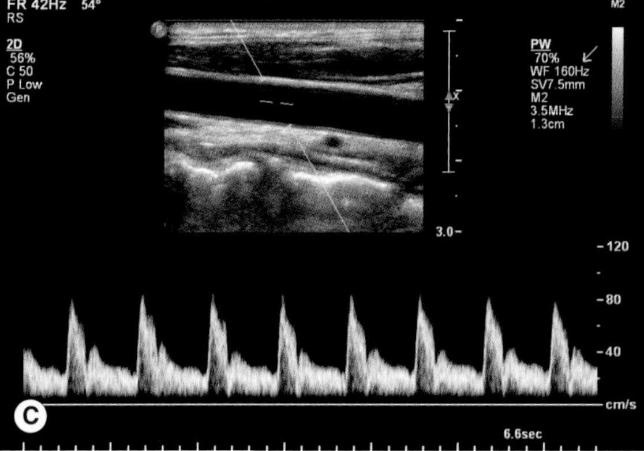

Figure 3.7 • (A) Wall thump gives a low-frequency, high-amplitude signal (large arrows). (B) A filter can be used to remove wall thump from the Doppler signal, but if the filter cut-off frequency is set too high (as in C), this can alter the appearance of the waveform. Small arrow shows wall filter setting in A: 50 Hz, B: 100 Hz and C: 160 Hz.

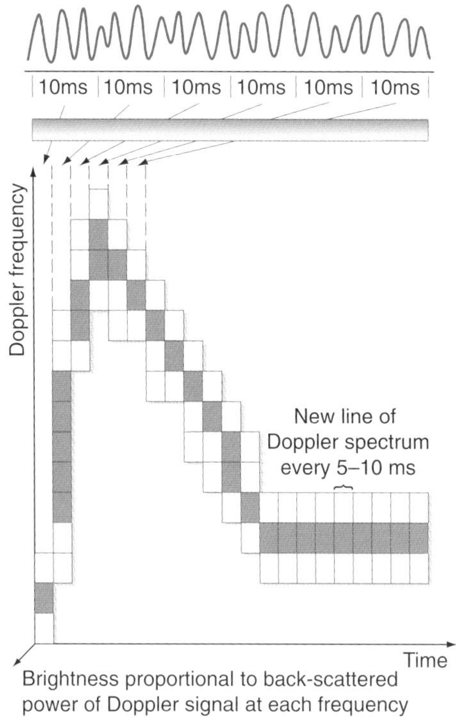

Figure 3.8 • Spectral analysis of the Doppler signal enables the frequencies present within the signal to be displayed as consecutive spectra. This produces a display of the changes in blood velocity over time.

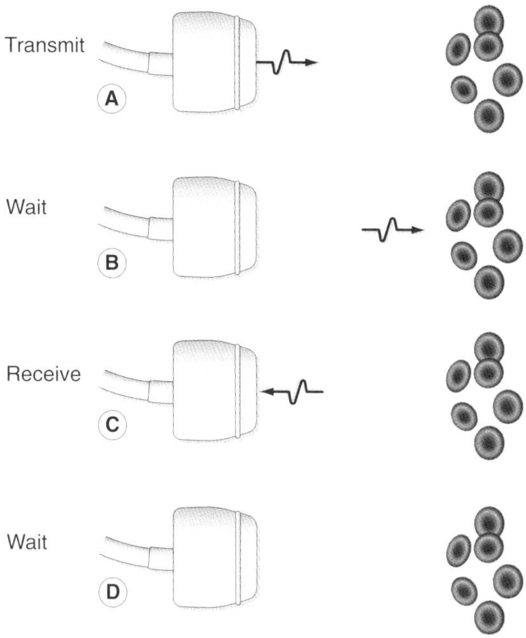

Figure 3.9 • Pulsed Doppler ultrasound. The system transmits a pulse (A), waits for a specified time (B) and then only receives from a given depth (C); it waits again, with the receiver off (D), for all the echoes to return from greater depths before transmitting the next pulse.

moving at a particular velocity). Spectral analysis is carried out using mathematical techniques such as the fast Fourier transform (FFT). Figure 3.6C shows a typical spectral display produced by a Doppler system. In this case, each vertical line of data is produced every 5–10 ms (i.e., 100–200 lines of data per second).

Continuous-wave (CW) Doppler

Continuous-wave (CW) Doppler continuously emits a single frequency while the receiving element continuously detects any echoes from the sensitive region of the beam (i.e., where transmitted and received beams overlap) (shaded region in Fig. 3.5). This region usually covers a depth of a few centimeters, and any flow within this area will be detected. This means that CW Doppler is unable to provide information about the depth from which the Doppler signal is returning. CW Doppler is therefore said to have poor range resolution. Veins often lie adjacent to arteries and so, in many cases, the CW Doppler will simultaneously detect arterial and venous flow.

Pulsed Doppler

The poor range resolution of CW Doppler can be overcome by using a pulse of ultrasound energy and only acquiring the returning signal at a known time after the pulse has been transmitted. Thus, by knowing the speed of sound in tissue, the depth from which the signal has returned can be calculated, in the same way as described for pulsed echo imaging (equation 2.3). As the piezoelectric element is only emitting ultrasound for a short period of time, it is possible to use the same element to receive the returning signal. Figure 3.9 shows how the pulse of ultrasound is transmitted and how the receiver then waits a given time before acquiring the signal over a short period of time. Although the system acquires no further signals, it has to wait for the echoes from greater depths to return before sending the next pulse. The time during which the received signal is acquired is known as the range gate, and this can be altered by the operator in order to determine the sample volume size. The sample volume is the region from which returning signals can be detected. Its size depends not only on the size of the range gate but also on the shape of the transmitted pulse and the shape of the ultrasound beam; it is sometimes described as being teardrop-shaped (Fig. 3.10). The depth of the sample volume is determined by the time the ultrasound system waits before acquiring the signal, which is also controlled by the operator. The size of the sample volume has a significant effect on the Doppler spectrum produced. For example, a large sample volume is required if the operator wishes to record both the fast-moving blood in the center of the vessel and the slower-moving blood near the walls. This is discussed further in Chapter 6.

In order to measure the frequencies present in the blood flow, thousands of pulses are sent along the beam path per second. The frequency at which these pulses are sent is known as the pulse repetition frequency (PRF) and is in the kHz range. The upper limit of the PRF is given by the constraint that the system has to wait for all the returning echoes from the last pulse before transmitting the next one. In fact, the pulsed Doppler method, unlike CW systems, does not actually measure the Doppler shift. However, the shape of the detected signal is similar to the Doppler shift that would be obtained from a CW system, so it can be described by the Doppler equation and is typically referred to as the Doppler signal. The ultrasound pulses enable the changing velocity of the blood to be sampled, and the resulting signal can be analyzed to obtain a frequency spectrum using an FFT. The FFT requires either 64 or 128 consecutive pulses to produce one line of the spectrum, and Doppler systems are able to process these data fast enough to produce real-time Doppler spectra.

The path of the Doppler beam and the size and position of the sample volume are displayed on the pulse echo image. The values of the PRF, sample volume size, and depth are usually displayed at the side of the image, as shown in Figure 3.11. Pulsed Doppler is able to provide good range resolution, but the disadvantage is that pulsed Doppler suffers from an artifact known as aliasing, that puts an upper limit on the maximum frequency that can be detected.

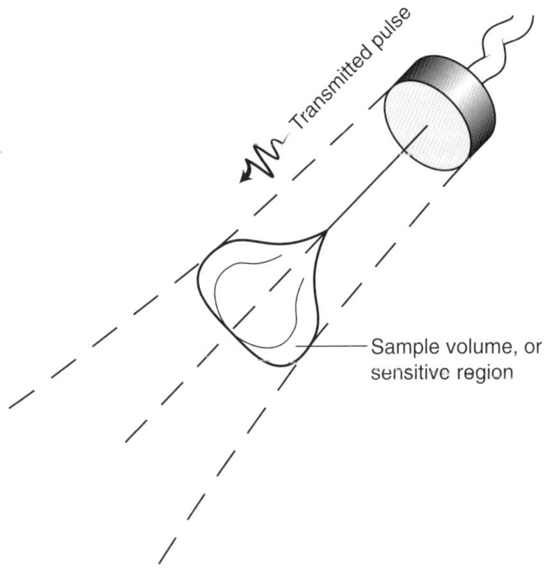

Transmitted pulse

Sample volume, or sensitive region

Figure 3.10 • The sample volume, or sensitive region, of a single-element pulsed Doppler system is shaped like a teardrop.

Aliasing

Aliasing is the incorrect estimation of the frequency of a signal due to insufficient sampling of the

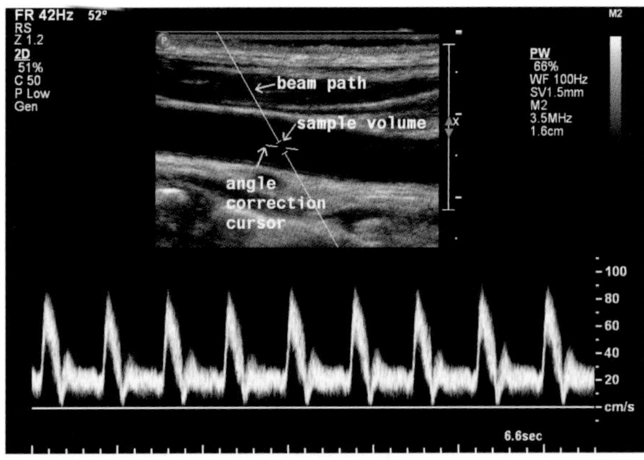

Figure 3.11 • The path of the Doppler ultrasound beam, sample volume size, and position are displayed on the image.

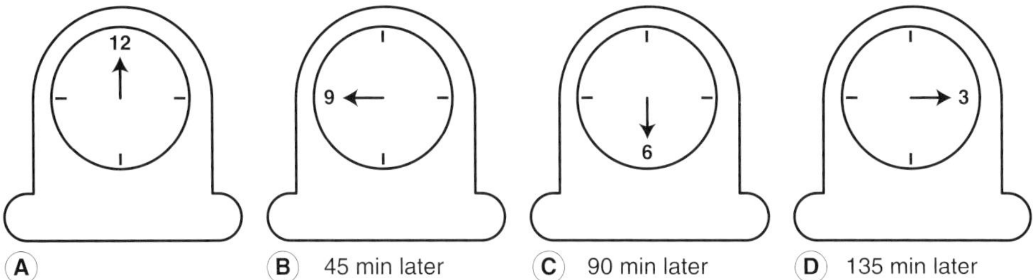

Figure 3.12 • Aliasing. If the speed of a minute hand is observed once every 45 minutes, the hand will appear to be moving slowly anticlockwise.

signal. Imagine that you have a clock with only a minute hand and you wish to estimate the speed at which the hand is moving. If you look at the face every 45 min (Fig. 3.12), starting on the hour, first the hand would point at 12, then, 45 min later, it would point at 9, then at 6, at 3 and at 12 again. This would give the impression that the hand was traveling slowly anticlockwise. The speed of the hand would appear to be one complete revolution every 3 hours rather than, as expected, once an hour. In order to estimate the speed of the hand correctly, the clock would have to be viewed at least twice in a complete cycle (i.e., at least twice an hour).

Figure 3.13 shows how the frequency of a simple sine wave, indicated by the solid line, can be underestimated when the signal is sampled less than twice in a complete cycle. If the dots represent the points at which the signal is sampled, then the lowest-frequency sine wave that would fit the sampled data is that shown by the dashed line. If, instead, the signal is sampled at least twice in a complete cycle, shown by the crosses, it is no longer possible to fit a lower-frequency sine wave to the sampled data and the correct frequency is measured. Aliasing occurs when the sampling frequency is less than twice the frequency to be estimated, a limit known as the Nyquist frequency.

An example of aliasing of a Doppler signal can be seen in Figure 3.14A, where the frequency detected at peak systole is underestimated and displayed below the baseline of the spectrum. Aliasing can be overcome by increasing the sampling rate (i.e., increasing the PRF or scale). There is, however, an upper limit to the PRF that can be used, as the system has to wait for each pulse to return before the next pulse can be transmitted, in order to prevent confusion as to where a returning signal has originated. Therefore, there is also a limit to the maximum Doppler shift frequency that can be detected. This limits the maximum detectable Doppler frequency ($f_{d\max}$) and velocity ($V_{\max}$) as follows:

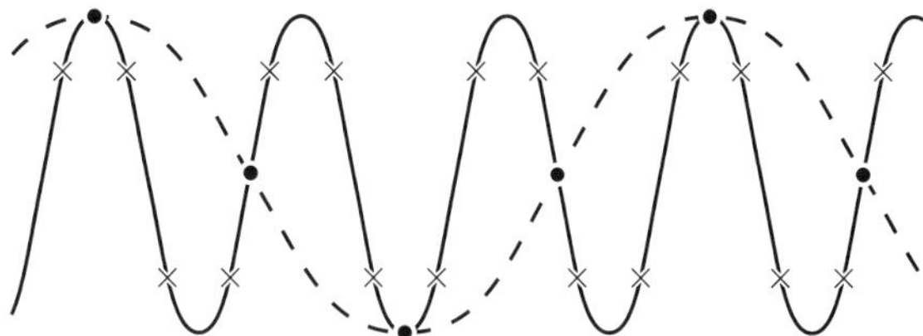

Figure 3.13 • Aliasing. The frequency of a simple sine wave (solid line) can be underestimated (dashed line) when the signal is sampled less than twice in a complete cycle.

$$f_{d\max} = \frac{PRF_{\max}}{2} = \frac{2V_{\max} f_t \cos\theta}{c} \quad (3.2)$$

This can be rewritten as:

$$V_{\max} = \frac{PRF_{\max} C}{4 f_t \cos\theta} \quad (3.3)$$

For a depth of interest, d, and speed of sound, c,

$$PRF_{\max} = \frac{c}{2d} \quad (3.4)$$

The 2 in the equation above arises from the fact that the pulse has to go to and return from the target. This gives:

$$V_{\max} = \frac{c^2}{8 d f_t \cos\theta} \quad (3.5)$$

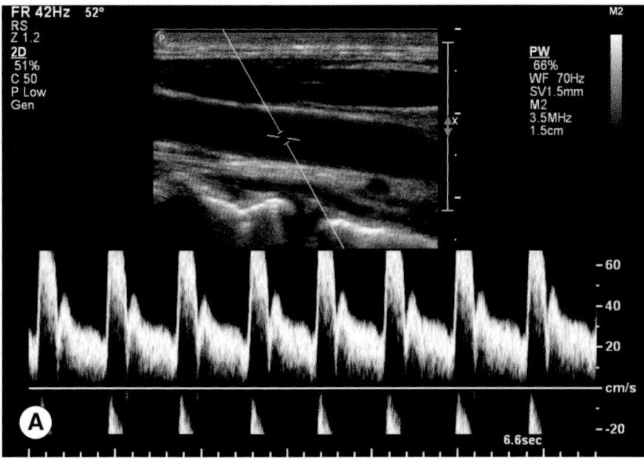

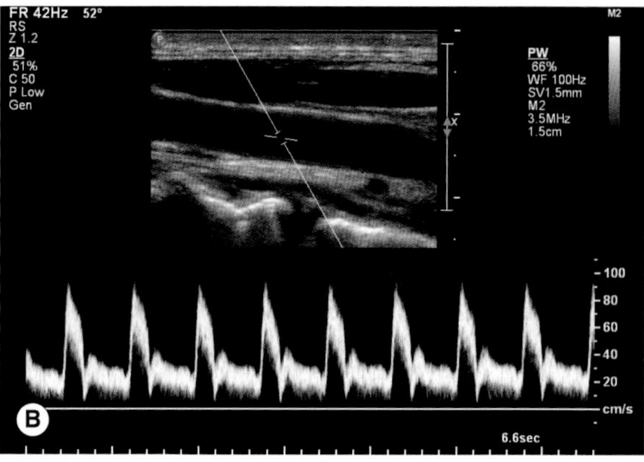

Figure 3.14 • (A) Aliasing leads to the high frequencies within the signal being underestimated and displayed below the baseline of the spectrum. (B) Aliasing can be overcome by increasing the pulse repetition frequency (shown as an increase in the upper limit of the velocity displayed on the velocity scale from 60 cm/s in A to100 cm/s in B).

The maximum velocity that can be detected without aliasing therefore depends on the depth of the vessel. When measuring very high blood flow velocities, especially at depth, some scanners will allow a "high PRF" mode to be selected. This allows more than one pulse to be in flight at a given time. The higher PRF allows higher velocities to be measured, but it also introduces range ambiguity (i.e., a loss of certainty as to the origin of the Doppler signal). In this mode, the scanner will typically show more than one sample volume displayed on the scan line. Using a lower transmitted frequency would produce a lower Doppler shift frequency. This lower frequency would not require as high a PRF to prevent aliasing. Therefore, reducing the transmit frequency would increase the maximum velocity that could be measured.

Limitations of CW versus pulsed Doppler

CW Doppler and pulsed Doppler have different limitations. There is no upper limit to the velocity of blood that can be detected by CW Doppler, but no information is available regarding the depth of the origin of the signal, and it is not always possible to detect arterial flow without the venous flow from a nearby vein also being detected. CW is most commonly used in simple hand-held systems to listen to blood flow, enabling ankle blood pressures to be measured (see Ch. 9), or for fetal heart detection. It can also be used in cardiology to allow high velocities to be measured through the heart valves. Pulsed Doppler provides information regarding the origin of the signal, enabling detailed studies of a specific vessel; however, this restricts the maximum velocity that can be detected. Pulsed Doppler is used in duplex systems both for spectral Doppler and color flow imaging.

DUPLEX ULTRASOUND

Duplex ultrasound systems, combining pulse echo imaging with Doppler ultrasound, have been commercially available for about 25 years. Combining the pulse echo imaging with Doppler ultrasound allows interrogation of a vessel in a known location and permits close investigation of the hemodynamics around areas of atheroma visualized on the image. Ideally, to produce a good image of a vessel wall, the vessel should be at right angles to the ultrasound beam. This is the case in the majority of peripheral vessels, as they mainly lie parallel to the skin. However, the Doppler equation shows that no Doppler signal will be obtained when the angle of insonation is at right angles to the direction of flow (as $\cos\theta = 0$). The greatest Doppler shift is detected when the beam is parallel to the direction of flow. Therefore, there is a conflict between the ideal angle of the beam used for imaging and that used for Doppler recordings. A compromise would involve the ability to steer or angle the Doppler beam independently of the imaging beam. Some early duplex systems did this by mounting a separate Doppler element, with an adjustable angle, next to the imaging element. Modern linear array and phased array transducers overcome this by producing a steered beam, as described in Chapter 2 (see Fig. 2.14). The transducer elements are most sensitive to the returning signals that are at right angles to the front face of the element. This means that, as the beam is steered, the sensitivity of the Doppler transducer will fall to some extent, and therefore the Doppler beam can only be steered by about 20° left and right of center. There is thus a compromise between the choice of Doppler angle and sensitivity.

Velocity measurements using duplex ultrasound

An important consequence of duplex ultrasound is that it allows the image of the vessel to be used to estimate the angle of insonation between the Doppler beam and the vessel. This enables the detected Doppler frequency to be converted into a velocity measurement using the Doppler equation (equation 3.1). Figure 3.15A demonstrates how the image of a vessel can be used to enable the angle of insonation to be measured by lining up an angle correction cursor with the vessel wall. In Figurc 3.15B the angle correction cursor has been lined up correctly with the cursor parallel to the vessel wall, but the angle of insonation is 70°, which is too large to make accurate measurements (see Ch. 6). The peak velocities seen in Figure 3.15B are higher than those seen in Figure 3.15A. The angle of insonation should be 60° or less to make velocity measurements. In Figure 3.15C the angle has been set to read an angle of insonation of 60° but the angle correction curor has not been set to be parallel to the vessel walls, therefore giving an incorrect angle of insonation leading to incorrect velocity measurements. Very large errors in velocity measurement can be generated by incorrect alignment of the angle correction cursor.

Although there are many potential sources of errors when using Doppler ultrasound to calculate

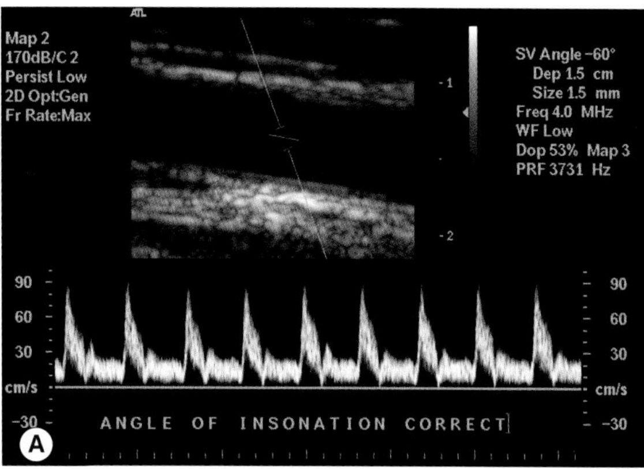

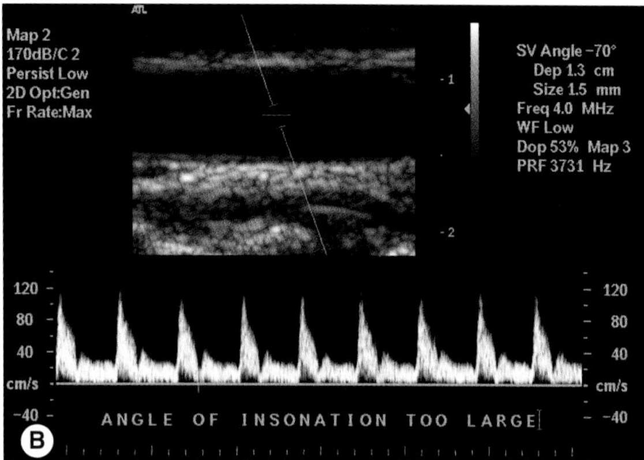

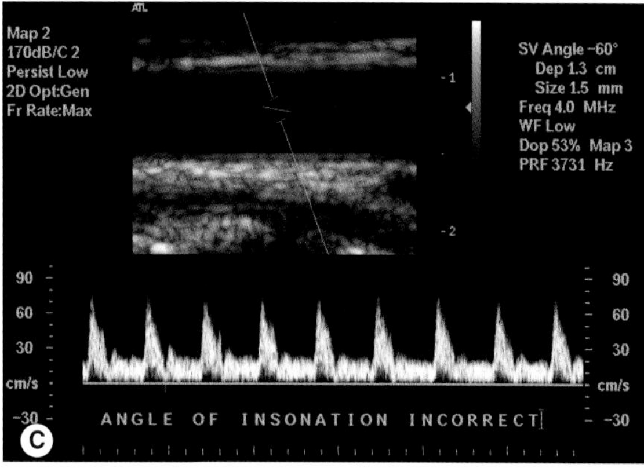

Figure 3.15 • (A) The image of a vessel can be used to enable the angle of insonation to be measured by lining up an angle correction cursor with the vessel wall. (B) The angle correction cursor has been lined up correctly with the cursor parallel to the vessel wall, but the angle of insonation is 70°, which is too large to make accurate measurements. (C) The angle has been set to read an angle of insonation of 60° but the angle correction cursor has not been set to be parallel to the vessel walls, therefore giving an incorrect angle of insonation, leading to incorrect velocity measurements.

blood flow velocity (see Ch. 6), it is a powerful technique for detecting and quantifying the degree of disease present in a vessel.

Reference

Fish P 1990 Physics and instrumentation of diagnostic medical ultrasound. Wiley, Chichester

Further reading

Evans D H, McDicken W N 2000 Doppler ultrasound: physics, instrumentation and signal processing. Wiley, Chichester

Zagzebski J A 1996 Essentials of ultrasound physics. Mosby, St Louis

Creation of a color flow image

4

CONTENTS

INTRODUCTION

Ultrasound scanners also use the detected blood velocity, with respect to the ultrasound beam, to form a color map of blood flow superimposed on to the anatomical map provided by pulse echo imaging. This map provides a means for rapid interrogation of a region of interest (ROI) and enables the operator to be selective in the points from which to obtain spectral Doppler information. The development of color flow imaging has greatly extended the capabilities of imaging small vessels and has also allowed for a reduction in investigation time, dramatically increasing the role of vascular ultrasound. The first real-time color flow images were produced in 1985 and were only possible due to the use of different mathematical methods to extract the mean velocity of flow relative to the beam (mean Doppler frequency). This made collection and analysis of the ultrasound echos fast enough to enable the production of color flow maps capable of displaying pulsatile blood flow in real time.

COLLECTION OF 2D DOPPLER INFORMATION

The two-dimensional (2D) color flow map is created by detecting the back-scattered signals from hundreds of sample volumes along each scan line and using over a hundred of scan lines to cover the ROI, as shown in Figure 4.1. The scanner divides the back-scattered signal into hundreds of samples along the scan line, each sample being at a different time delay after the transmitted pulse, and therefore returning from a slightly different depth in the tissue. The depth from which a signal has returned can be calculated from this time delay, using the speed of sound in tissue, in the

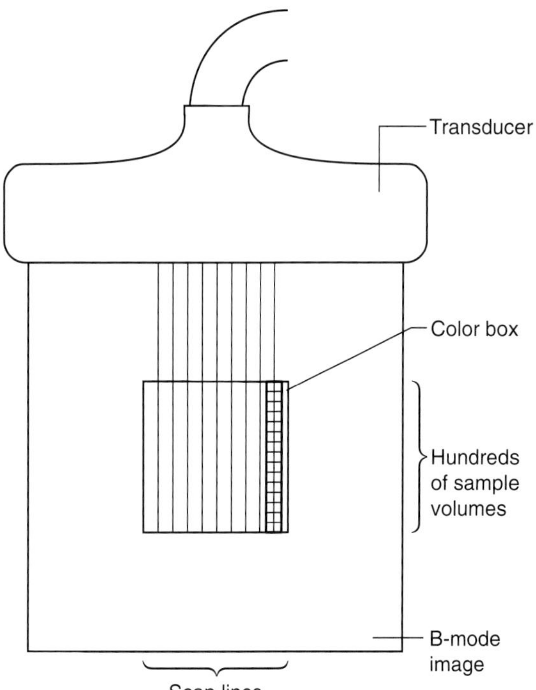

Figure 4.1 • The color flow image is created by detecting the back-scattered ultrasound from hundreds of sample volumes along over a hundred different scan lines.

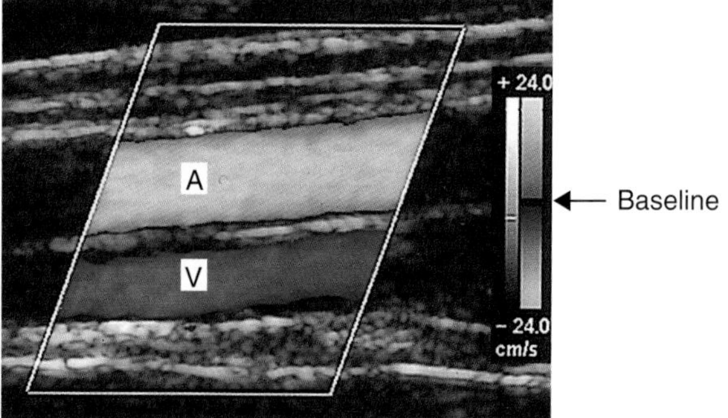

Figure 4.2 • The color flow image displays the mean velocity of the flow relative to the ultrasound beam (equivalent to Doppler frequency) detected within each sample volume. This image of an artery, A, overlying a vein, V, demonstrates the difference in the velocity and direction of the blood flow in the two vessels. In this image, the color scale shows that flow in the artery is toward the transducer and is displayed as red, whereas flow in the vein is away from the transducer and is displayed as blue.

same way as is used in pulse echo imaging. Several pulses must be transmitted and received along the scan line for the movement of the blood to be detected. Once sufficient samples have been detected from each sample volume to allow estimation of the blood velocity relative to the beam, a second scan line adjacent to the first can be produced. Hundreds of scan lines may be used to produce the 2D color flow image. The estimated mean relative velocity (equivalent to the Doppler frequency) from each sample volume within the tissue can be displayed in color, as shown in Figure 4.2. In this image of an artery lying next to a vein, the Doppler shift frequencies produced by flow toward the transducer are displayed in red, and those produced by flow away from the transducer are shown in blue. The higher relative velocities are shown as yellow and turquoise, whereas the lower relative velocities are displayed as deep red and deep blue.

METHODS OF ESTIMATING THE VELOCITY OF BLOOD

Spectral Doppler ultrasound uses fast Fourier transform (FFT) to provide detailed information on the frequency content of the Doppler signal. However, the time needed to collect sufficient data to perform an FFT on the signals obtained from several scan lines would be so great that it would take several seconds to produce each color image. This would not be a suitable method for imaging pulsatile blood flow. The FFT would also produce more information than could be easily displayed on the image, as each color pixel can only represent one value of velocity at any point in the color image, unlike the range of frequencies that can be displayed on the spectral display. Real-time color flow imaging has been made possible by the use of alternative techniques to estimate the mean velocity of blood relative to the beam. It requires only a few pulses to estimate the mean relative velocity, making the process faster to perform. The method used relies on the facts that the ultrasound is back-scattered from groups of blood cells that remain in the same formation during the time taken to perform the velocity estimate and that the echo intensity pattern is different for different groups of cells. This allows a group of cells to be

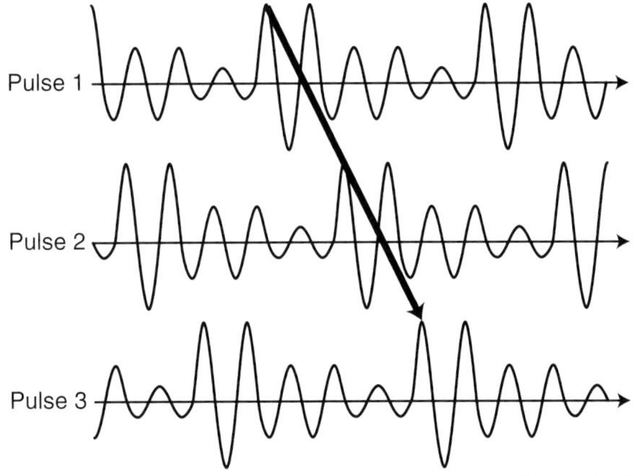

Figure 4.3 • Signals from three consecutive pulses returning from a given group of cells as they move farther away from the transducer. Note the short delay introduced. (Reprinted from Ultrasound in Medicine and Biology, 23/3, Ferrera & DeAngelis, Color Flow Mapping, 1997, with permission from Elsevier)

tracked as it moves through the sample volume. The velocity of the group of cells does not change significantly during the short time over which the blood flow velocity is being estimated.

Figure 4.3 shows the shapes of three consecutive returning pulses as a group of blood cells passes through the sample volume. A short delay is introduced into the signal returning from a given group of cells as they move farther away from the transducer between pulses. An estimate of the velocity can be made by detecting this delay in the echo complex. This shift in the waveform can be understood in two ways. First, it can be considered as a time delay introduced between returning pulses as the group of cells moves. Second, it can be considered as a phase shift of the signal between two pulses scattered from the same sample volume. To understand the concept of a phase shift, consider an example using two clocks. If both the clocks are set to read the same time, both minute hands will be moving at the same speed, giving a frequency of one complete revolution of the clock face an hour. Both clocks will also be in phase with each other (i.e., the minute hand will appear at the 12 on both clocks at the same time), giving a phase shift of zero. If, however, one clock has the minute hand set 30 min behind the other, the minute hands will still complete one revolution of the clock face an hour, but the two clocks will now be out of phase and the clock hands will appear at different places on the clock face. The time delay between the two clocks will be 30 min, or alternatively this delay could be measured as a phase shift, which in this case would be half a cycle of the clock face.

The delay between the returning ultrasound signals from the first and second pulses shown in Figure 4.3 can be measured in terms of a phase shift. We can see that the second signal is the same shape as the first but is delayed. This is analogous to the clock hands traveling at the same speed but with the second clock being half a cycle behind the first. A similar phase shift can be measured between signals 2 and 3. These phase shifts can be used to estimate the velocity of the blood. This method does not actually measure the Doppler shift frequency; however, the shape of the detected signal is similar to the Doppler shift that would be obtained from a continuous-wave system and therefore can be described by the Doppler equation.

Modern color flow imaging scanners use the phase shift approach, employing a process known as autocorrelation detection to estimate the mean velocity of the flow, relative to the beam. Autocorrelation compares two consecutive pulses returning from a given sample volume to produce an output that is dependent on the phase shift (i.e., dependent on the Doppler frequency). If the echoes are returning from stationary objects there will be no phase shift. The phase shifts between four or more pulses are used to estimate the mean velocity. The more pulses used, the more accurate is the result, as long as the time taken is not so great that the velocity of the blood cells has changed. This relatively small number of pulses required to estimate the mean relative velocity (Doppler shift frequency) enables several color images to be produced every second.

Another method, not currently used by ultrasound manufacturers, uses time domain processing, which employs time delay rather than phase shift to estimate the velocity of blood. From the operator's perspective, both the frequency and time domain processes produce similar color images.

ELEMENTS OF A COLOR FLOW SCANNER

Figure 4.4 shows the basic elements of a color flow scanner. Before any analysis of the returning echoes

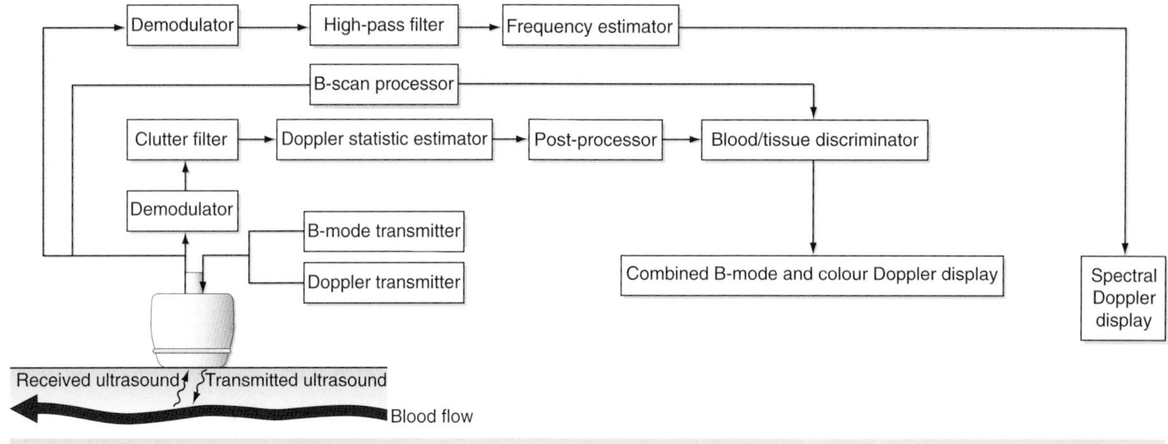

Figure 4.4 • The basic elements of a color flow scanner.

is carried out, the signal is filtered by the clutter filter to remove the high-amplitude signals returning from the surrounding stationary tissue and the slow-moving vessel walls, while preserving the low-amplitude signals from the blood. The filtered signal is then analyzed to obtain an estimate of the mean relative velocity (Doppler shift frequency) in each sample volume using the Doppler statistic estimator, as described earlier. Postprocessing is then used to smooth the data in order to produce a less noisy color image. This can be done by combining the data obtained from consecutive images, known as frame-averaging. As each point on the image can only be assigned either a specific color or level of gray, a decision has to be made as to whether to display the pulse echo information or any flow information detected. This involves the process known as blood–tissue discrimination.

Blood–tissue discrimination

Generally, the returning pulse echo signals from the vessel lumen are very low in amplitude compared with those from the vessel walls and surrounding tissue. In addition, larger Doppler frequencies are detected from the rapidly moving blood in comparison to the low Doppler frequencies obtained from the slow-moving vessel walls. No Doppler shift would be detected from stationary surrounding tissue. Ultrasound imaging systems are designed with an adjustable control called the 'color write enable' or 'color write priority' control. This control allows the operator to select the imaging signal intensity above which the gray-scale image is displayed rather than the color information. If a Doppler signal is obtained from an area in which the gray-scale signal is higher than the level set by the operator, the scanner assumes that the Doppler signal results from moving tissue and therefore does not display it. Below this level of gray, providing there is an adequate motion detected, it is assumed that any motion detected originates from blood, and color will overwrite the gray scale in areas where a Doppler signal is detected. If, for instance, the operator wishes to demonstrate flow in a small vessel that does not have an anechoic (echo-free) lumen on the image, the threshold for displaying gray-scale information will need to be increased, thus giving priority to writing color information.

Most systems also have a flash filter. This is designed to remove color flashes, known as flash artifacts, that are generated by rapid movement between the transducer and tissue, such as when the sonographer moves the transducer during scanning.

Color-coding the Doppler information

Having obtained a value of the mean Doppler frequency present in the multiple sample volumes, these data now have to be displayed on the image. This is done by color-coding the Doppler information. The color on the screen has three attributes:

luminosity, hue, and saturation. Luminosity is the degree of brightness or shade of the displayed color; hue is the wavelength (i.e., the actual color displayed, from violet through red), and saturation is the degree to which the color is mixed with white light (e.g., from red through light pink, producing up to 20 identifiable tints). These three attributes can be used to produce a variety of color scales, as shown in Figure 4.5, which can be displayed as a bar at the side of the image. The scale usually consists of a different color representing different flow directions, with red often used to show flow toward the transducer and blue depicting flow away from the transducer. Most scanners allow the operator to invert the color scale in order to display flow toward the transducer as blue and flow away as red. This is indicated by inverting the color scale displayed at the side of the image (Fig. 4.5E). It is essential for the operator to be aware of which colors represent which directions of flow within the image, otherwise serious diagnostic errors can occur. Ultrasound scanners provide a range of color scales, and certain scales are more appropriate in particular imaging situations. The various color scales may be selected to accentuate the different parts of the range of detected relative velocities seen in different clinical situations. For example, in an arterial scan, the color scale may accentuate the differences in the upper portion to highlight velocity changes in the higher range of velocities.

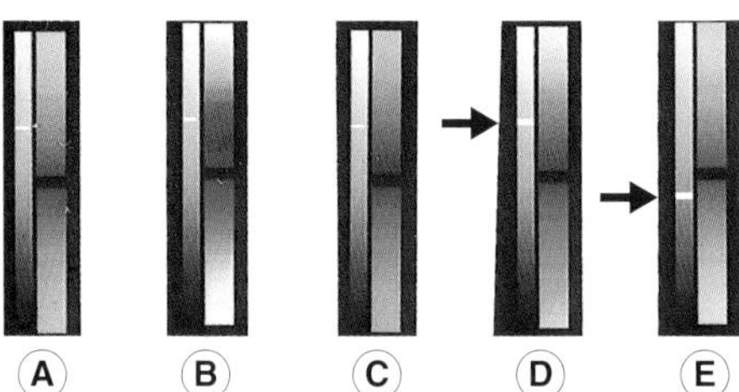

Figure 4.5 • (A–D) Examples of different color scales, used to accentuate different parts of the range of velocities detected in various clinical situations. (E) The inversion of the color scale shows that the image will now display flow toward the transducer as blue. The arrows on (D) and (E) show how the scanner displays the color write priority selected. The setting selected in (D) will display color in the presence of a brighter B-mode echo than the setting selected in (E).

The velocity estimator can calculate not only the mean relative velocity but also the variance. The variance is a measure of the range of velocities present within the sample volume and may relate to the presence of a flow disturbance. The variance can be displayed along with the mean frequency by using a red and blue scale with increasing amounts of yellow or green introduced as the variance increases, although this form of display is not widely used. Another form of color display uses increasing luminosity of orange to display the increasing back-scattered power detected. This is known as power Doppler and is discussed later in this chapter.

EFFECT OF ANGLE OF INSONATION ON THE COLOR FLOW IMAGE

As the detected velocity of the blood flow depends on the angle of insonation between the blood flow and the color Doppler beam (as seen in the Doppler effect), the appearance of the color image is very much dependent on the angle of insonation. Many of the peripheral vessels run parallel to the skin, perpendicular to the imaging beam. However, the color Doppler beam angle of insonation should ideally be less than 70° in order to obtain a Doppler signal. If the angle of insonation is near 90°, only a small Doppler shift will be detected; this will be removed by the high-pass filter, known as the clutter filter, and no signal will be displayed on the image.

When using a linear array transducer, it is possible to steer the beam, used to create the color image, from left or right, as described in Chapter 2 (see Fig. 2.14). The direction of the color Doppler beam runs parallel to the sides of the color box displayed on the image. Figure 4.6 demonstrates the change in the color image seen when the color box is steered in three different directions relative to the flow. The beam can only be steered either left or right by a maximum of 20–25° because the sensitivity of the transducer decreases as the beam is steered. There is thus a compromise between optimizing the angle of insonation and maintaining the sensitivity. This is not usually apparent when imaging large vessels with good flow but can become a problem when imaging smaller diseased vessels with low flow, as the intensity of the Doppler signal may be very low and the vessel may

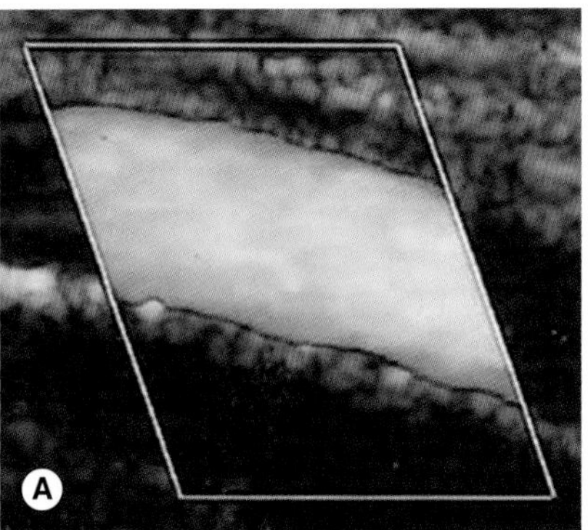

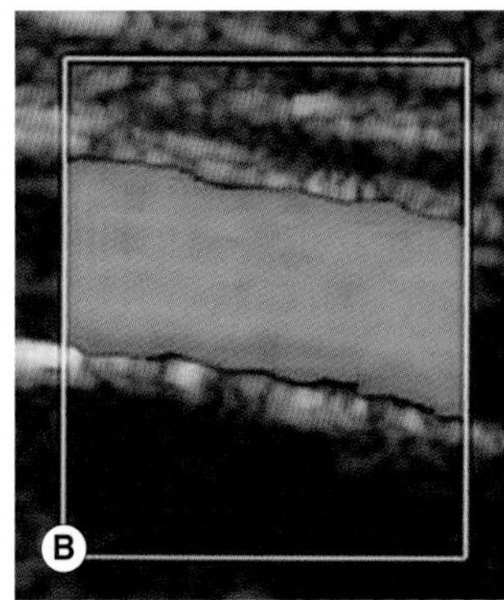

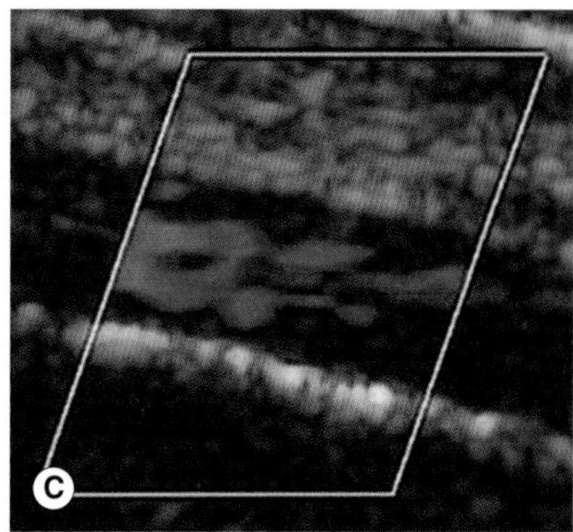

Figure 4.6 • Effect of changing the angle of insonation (shown on the image), by steering the color box, on the image produced. (A) A small angle gives a good image. (B) A moderate angle displays flow but is not optimal. (C) A large angle gives an unusable image.

have to be insonated at an angle above 70° to maintain transducer sensitivity. If demonstrating color filling of such a vessel proves difficult, it is worth changing the angle of insonation of the color beam to obtain the optimum compromise between the angle of insonation and sensitivity.

When imaging tortuous vessels, it is useful to obtain images with the color box steered in different directions to visualize the blood flow along the entire vessel. If the direction of the blood flow changes in relation to the beam, a different velocity will be detected and displayed due to the change in the angle of insonation, even though the actual blood velocity is the same. The color image will demonstrate a change of color within the vessel as the path of the vessel alters direction. Figure 4.7 shows an image of an internal carotid artery as its path dips deep into the neck. The arrows on the image show how the blood flow changes direction relative to the color Doppler beam, causing a change in the velocity (Doppler frequency) detected. This leads to a change in the color displayed, from red to orange and yellow then finally turquoise, due to aliasing, even though the velocity of the blood within the vessel has remained unchanged.

Curvilinear and phased array transducers produce scan lines that fan out over the sector image. These probes do not usually have the facility to steer the Doppler beam along a path independently of the direction of the imaging scan lines. If a straight vessel is imaged with a curvilinear or phased array transducer, there will be a change in the angle of insonation along the vessel, unless the vessel is parallel to the Doppler beam. This will lead to a change in the Doppler frequencies detected and therefore will affect the color displayed on the image, as shown in Figure 4.8. On the left of the image, Doppler shift frequencies are detected, as there is a suitable angle of insonation and flow is toward the probe. In the very center, the angle of insonation is approximately 90°, so low or no Doppler frequency is detected or displayed. On the right side of the image, the angle of insonation is now such that the flow is away from the transducer, and it is therefore displayed in red.

When interpreting a color image, it is important to remember that it is the velocity relative to the beam (the Doppler shift frequency) that is being displayed, and it is essential to consider the angle of insonation used to produce each point of the image. To be certain of the velocities present, spectral Doppler can be used as this has the facility to provide angle correction for velocity estimates. Diagnosis should be made using a combination of color and spectral Doppler investigations.

ALIASING IN COLOR FLOW IMAGING

The range of velocities displayed by the color scale is governed by the pulse repetition frequency (PRF, sometimes known as scale) used to obtain the

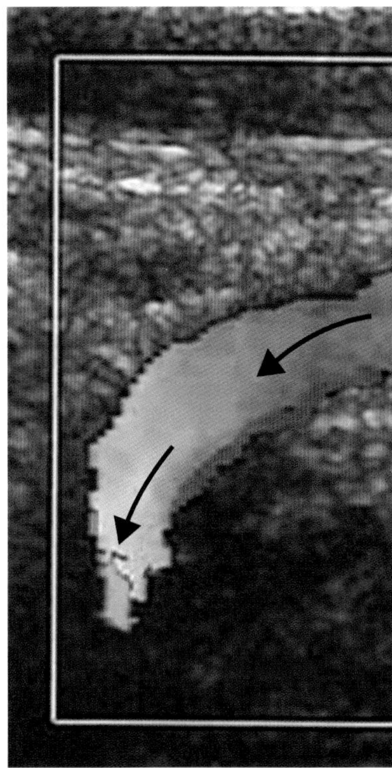

Figure 4.7 • An internal carotid artery as it dips deep in the neck. As the path of the artery changes relative to the Doppler beam (shown by the arrow), the relative velocity (Doppler frequency) detected will alter, leading to a change in the color displayed, despite the fact that the velocity of the blood flow has not changed.

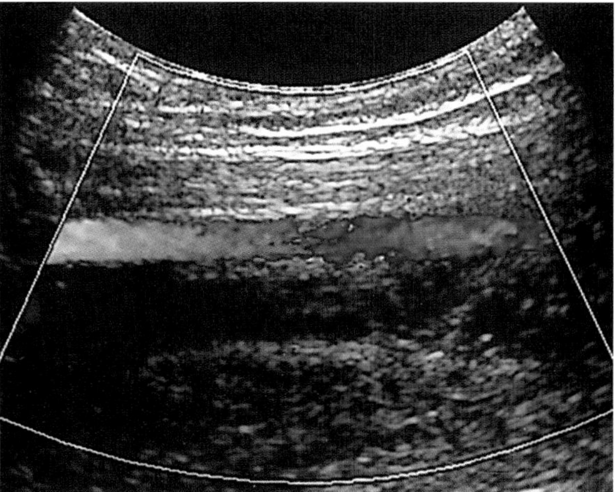

Figure 4.8 • As the scan lines of a curvilinear transducer diverge, the angle between the straight vessel and the beam will change. This will lead to a change in the detected velocity relative to the ultrasound beam (Doppler frequency), altering the color displayed. No flow is displayed in the center of the image, where the flow is at right angles to the beam.

blood flow information. The maximum frequency that can be detected with color flow imaging is limited by the sampling frequency in the same way as described for spectral Doppler (see Ch. 3). Aliasing due to undersampling will limit the maximum frequency that can be displayed correctly, causing frequencies beyond this limit to be displayed as flow on the opposite side of the baseline. An example of aliasing occurring in a color image is shown in Figure 4.9A. The highest velocities present are in the center of the vessel, but because of aliasing, these are displayed as turquoise (i.e., as high velocities in the opposite direction) instead of yellow (i.e., top of the color scale). If the PRF is increased, aliasing no longer occurs, and all the flow is displayed in the correct color (Fig. 4.9B). If the PRF is set too high, however, it may prevent low velocities, such as those near the vessel walls or during diastole, from being detected (Fig. 4.9C). One potential problem is differentiating aliasing from true flow reversal. True flow reversal, shown as a change in color within a vessel (i.e., from red to blue), can be seen where there is both forward and reverse flow present within a vessel due to a hemodynamic effect. Flow reversal is often seen in a normal carotid artery bulb, as described in Chapter 5. Apparent flow reversal can be due to an artifact and occurs when a vessel changes direction relative to the Doppler beam, although flow within the vessel has not changed direction.

Figure 4.10 shows an image of a slightly tortuous carotid artery, with flow away from the transducer on the right (shown in blue) and toward the transducer on the left (shown in red). The arrows marked on the image show how the direction of flow changes relative to the ultrasound beam. In the center of the image, where the direction of flow is close to being at right angles to the ultrasound beam, low frequencies are detected; these are

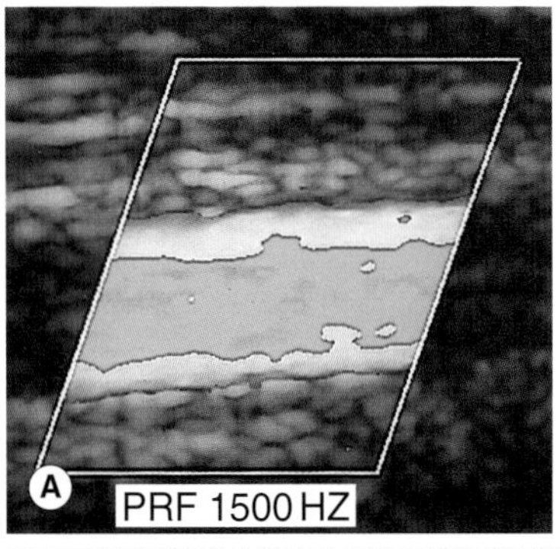

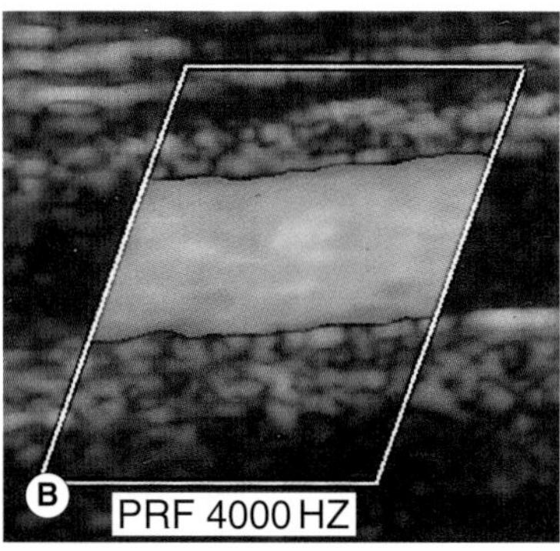

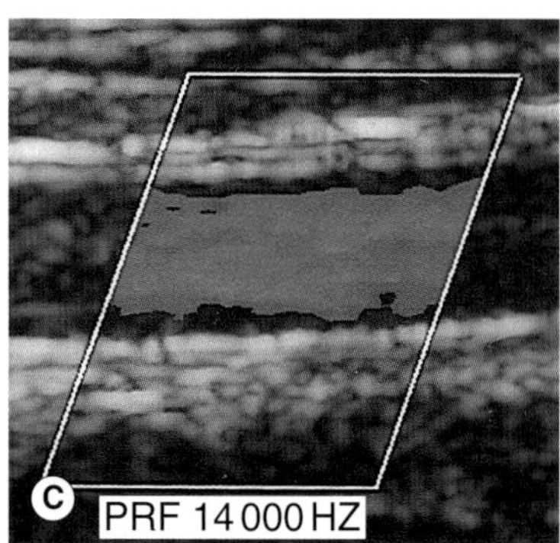

Figure 4.9 • Aliasing. (A) This will lead to the assignment of the incorrect color to represent the velocity present within the vessel, shown here in blue. (B) Increasing the pulse repetition frequency (PRF) may overcome aliasing. (C) If the PRF is set too high, it may prevent low velocities, present at the vessel walls, from being detected.

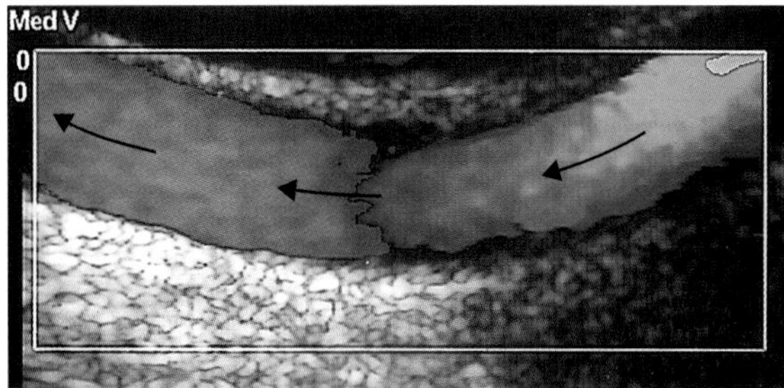

Figure 4.10 • Image of a bend in a carotid artery showing flow toward and away from the transducer in different colors. The path of the flow is shown by the arrows. Low flow or a thin black line is displayed in the center of the image, where the flow is at right angles to the beam.

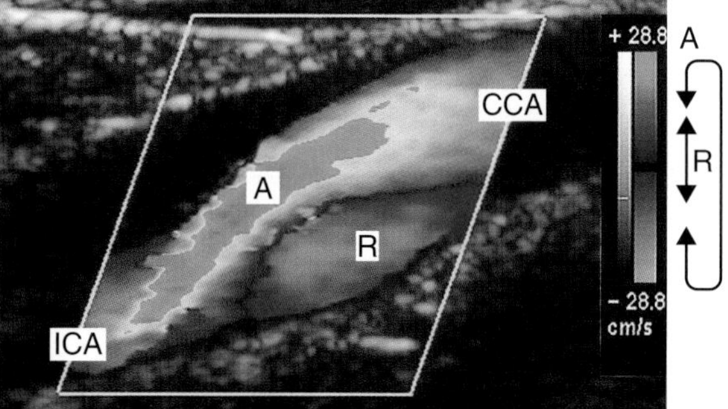

Figure 4.11 • Image demonstrating aliasing (A) and flow reversal (R) in an internal carotid artery (ICA). Aliasing can be recognized as a color change that wraps around from the top to the bottom of the color scale, or vice versa. A change in color due to a relative change in the direction of flow can be recognized as a change in color across the baseline, at the center of the color scale, passing through black (see color scale on right of image). CCA, common carotid artery.

removed from the signal by the high-pass filter and therefore low flow or a thin black line is displayed in this region.

It is possible to distinguish between aliasing and changes in the direction of flow relative to the transducer by the fact that the color transition seen in aliasing wraps around the farthest ends of the color scale. In contrast, the colors displayed when the flow changes direction are near the baseline and pass through black at the point where no or low flow has been detected. Figure 4.11 shows an image of a carotid artery that demonstrates both flow reversal and aliasing. The transitions in the colors displayed in both cases are shown on the color scales.

LOWER AND UPPER LIMITS TO THE VELOCITY DISPLAYED

The highest frequency that can be displayed without aliasing occurring is half the PRF, as with spectral Doppler. However, unlike spectral Doppler displays, aliasing does not necessarily make interpreting the image difficult and can sometimes be useful in highlighting sudden increases in velocity, as would be seen at a stenosis. This will be seen on images of stenosis in the chapters that follow. The aliasing artifact can be overcome, up to a limit, by increasing the PRF, using a larger angle of insonation or using a lower ultrasound transmitting frequency.

When investigating low-velocity flow, such as that seen in the venous system, the lower limit of the velocity that can be detected is governed by the length of time spent interrogating the flow. Suppose you wanted to estimate the speed at which the hands of a clock are moving. You would have to watch the clock for a much longer time to estimate the speed of the hour hand than to estimate the speed of the minute hand. The same is true of color Doppler (i.e., the lower the velocity flow that is to be detected, the longer the time that has to be spent measuring it). The length of time over which pulses are sent along a scan line in order to estimate the frequency is known as the dwell time (Fig. 4.12). If a low PRF is selected, the time taken for the 8–10 pulses to be transmitted along the scan line will be longer, and consequently the dwell time will be greater than that produced by a higher PRF. It is therefore very important to select the appropriate PRF for the flow conditions to be imaged. If a low PRF is selected to image high-velocity flow, aliasing will occur, and if a high PRF is selected to image low-velocity flow, the flow may not be detected at all, as the dwell time will be too short (Fig. 4.9C). Ideally, a PRF should be selected that displays the highest velocities present with the

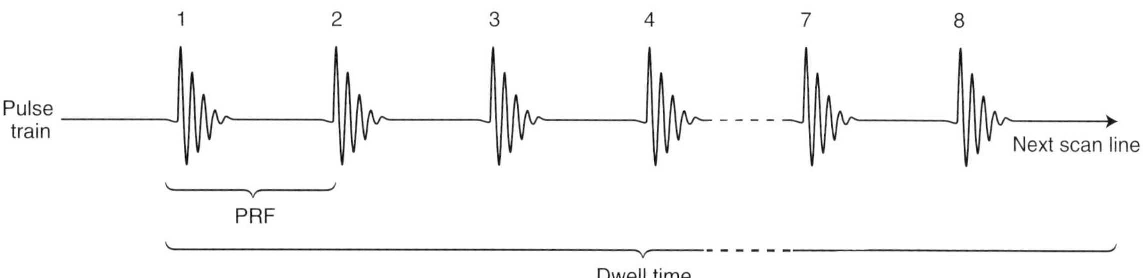

Figure 4.12 • The dwell time is the time the beam spends interrogating the blood flow to produce one scan line. This depends on the number of pulses, the ensemble length, used to perform the frequency estimate and the pulse repetition frequency (PRF) of the signal.

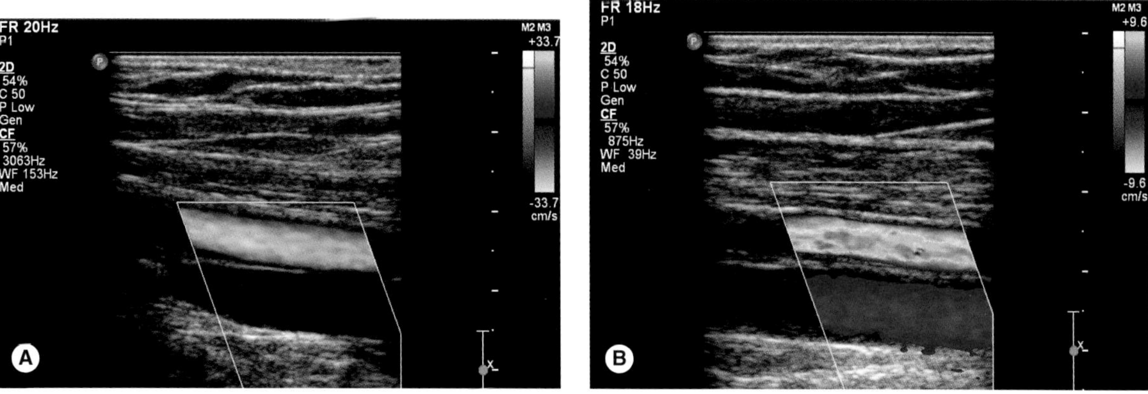

Figure 4.13 • Images of an artery overlying a vein. (A) The pulse repetition frequency (PRF) is set relatively high (3063 Hz) and no aliasing is seen within the artery; however no flow is detected in the vein as the scale has been set too high to detect the lower venous flow. (B) The PRF has been set lower (875 Hz) and now flow is detected in the vein but aliasing is seen in the artery. It is important that the appropriate PFR is selected depending on whether low- or high-velocity flow is being imaged to enable flow to be detected but without undesirable aliasing.

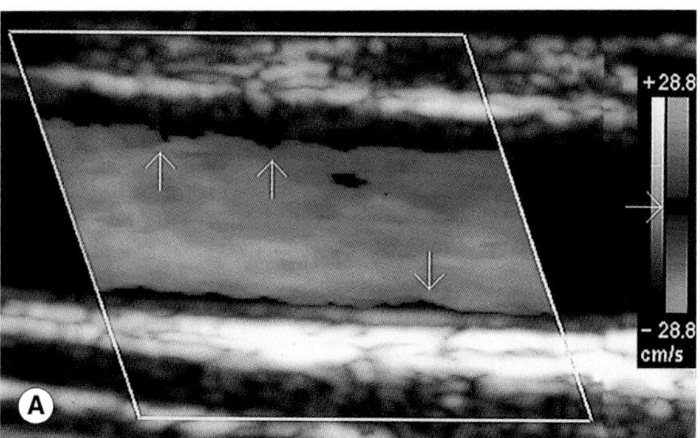

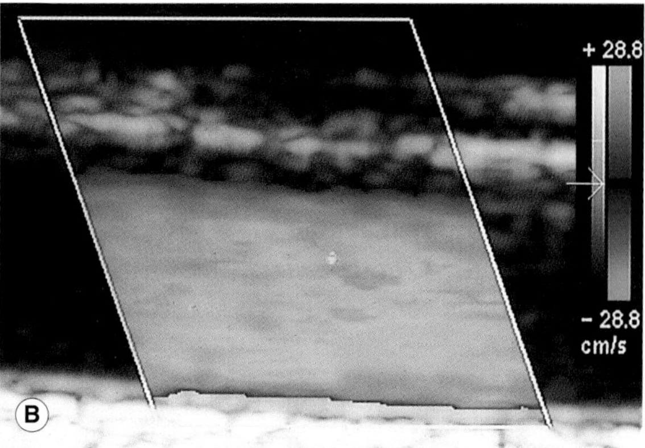

Figure 4.14 • Effect of using the filter. (A) The filter is set too high, removing the low-velocity flow near the vessel walls (vertical arrows). (B) The filter setting is reduced to display the low frequencies detected near the vessel walls. The filter setting may be indicated on the color scale (horizontal arrows).

colors near the top of the scale. Figure 4.13 shows two images of an artery overlying a vein. In Figure 4.13A the PRF is set high and no aliasing is seen within the artery; however no flow is detected in the vein as the scale has been set too high to detect the lower venous flow. In Figure 4.13B the PRF has be set lower and now flow is detected in the vein but aliasing is seen in the artery. It is important that the appropriate PFR is selected depending on whether low- or high-velocity flow is being imaged to enable flow to be detected but without undesirable aliasing.

The cut-off frequency of the high-pass clutter filter will also affect the lowest frequencies that can be displayed. The high-pass filter will only allow frequencies greater than the cut-off frequency to be displayed, so that if this is set too high, the Doppler frequencies detected from the lower-velocity blood flow will be removed. The level of the high-pass filter is usually displayed on the color scale (Fig. 4.14). Using the wrong filter setting has led to removal of the low velocities at the vessel walls or of low flow during diastole. The high-pass filter is linked to the PRF and therefore, as the PRF is increased, the high-pass filter is also automatically increased. However, some systems will allow the filter to be altered independently of the PRF, in which case the high-pass filter setting should be considered when the PRF is lower in order to image low-velocity flow.

FRAME RATE

The frame rate is the number of new images produced per second. For color flow imaging to be useful for visualizing pulsatile blood flow, a reasonably high frame rate is required. With pulse echo imaging alone, the frame rate can be greater than 50 images per second. However, the time required to produce a color flow image is much longer, as several pulses are require to produce each line of the color image, and therefore the frame rates are much lower. The frame rate is dependent on several factors when using color flow imaging (Fig. 4.15). The ROI refers to the color box, which can be placed anywhere within the image to examine blood flow. The size and position of the ROI have a significant effect on the frame rate. The width is especially important, as the wider the ROI, the more scan lines are required and therefore the longer it will take to collect the data for an image. The line density (the number of scan lines per centimeter across the image) also affects the time taken to produce the image as the pulses for each scan line have to return before the next line can be produced. The length of the color box is less important. This is because the scanner has to wait for all the returning echoes before sending the next pulse, even if the information is not used to produce the image, so as not to suffer from range ambiguity.

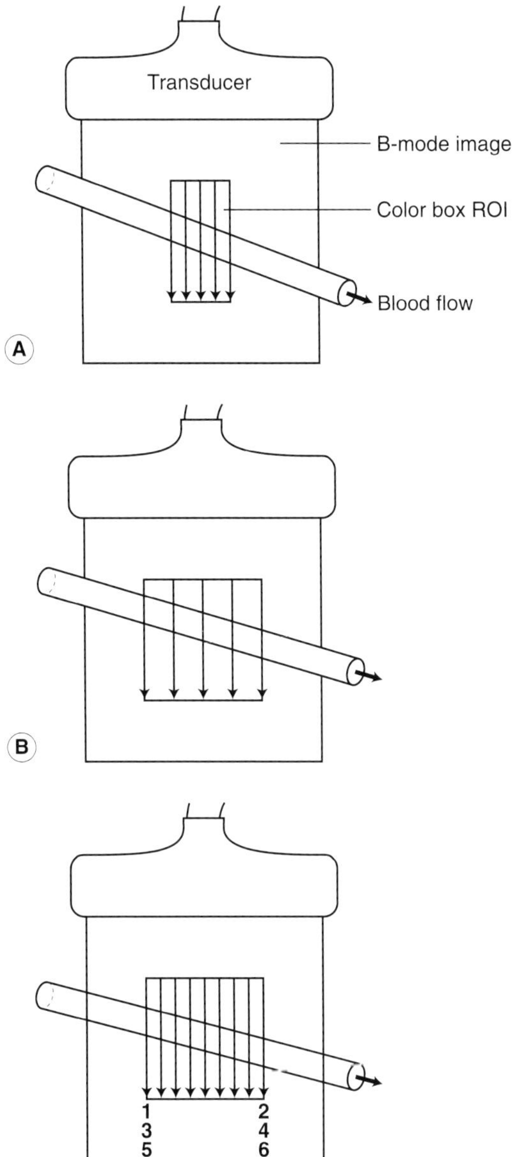

Figure 4.15 • The color image frame rate can be improved by (A) reducing the size of the color region of interest (ROI) or (B) reducing the density of the color scan lines. (C) The scanner may improve the frame rate by interleaving the acquisition of data from different parts of the ROI. (Reprinted from Ultrasound in Medicine and Biology, 23/3, Ferrera & DeAngelis, Color Flow Mapping, 1997, with permission from Elsevier)

The depth of the ROI is, however, an important factor. When the ROI is placed at depth the scanner will have to wait longer for the echoes to return from the greater depth and it will take longer to create each scan line, so reducing the frame rate. This is especially noticable when using a lower-frequency transducer, for improved penetration, e.g., when imaging the abdominal aorta in an obese patient.

Interleaving the acquisition from different scan lines that are a distance apart can enable more than one pulse to be transmitted at a time, allowing an improvement in the frequency estimate without a decrease in the frame rate. Figure 4.15C shows how the data from scan line 2 can be acquired while data from scan line 1 are being obtained, as scan line 1 will not detect pulses transmitted along scan line 2. The same is true for scan lines 3 and 4, and so forth. Extra lines of data can be created by averaging two adjacent lines to produce a scan line between them. As no new information is acquired to perform this, no change in the frame rate occurs.

The number of pulses used to produce each scan line of the color image is known as the ensemble length. Typically, an ensemble length of between 2 and 16 pulses is used to estimate the Doppler frequency. However, the more pulses that are used, the more accurate the estimate will be, and in situations in which the returning Doppler signal is poor, a high number of pulses is required. There is, therefore, a compromise between the accuracy of the frequency estimate and frame rate. The time taken for these 2–16 pulses to be transmitted and to return, the dwell time, depends on the rate at which the pulses are transmitted (i.e., the PRF). When a low PRF is used, it will take longer for the pulse ensemble to be transmitted, leading to a lower frame rate.

These various limitations require a compromise to be made between the area over which the color Doppler information is acquired, the accuracy of the Doppler frequency estimate, and the time it takes to acquire it. The selection of PRF, position of the ROI, and frequency of the transducer are governed by the region of the body being imaged and the type of blood flow in that region. However, the frame rate may be optimized by using as narrow an ROI as possible for the examination. The quality of the color image may be improved by averaging consecutive images, to reduce the

noise, and by displaying the image for a longer period of time. This control is sometimes known as the persistence.

RESOLUTION AND SENSITIVITY OF COLOR FLOW IMAGING

The spatial resolution of the color image can be considered in three planes, as described for B-mode imaging (see Fig. 2.20). However, as blood flow imaging is dynamic, the temporal resolution (i.e., the ability to display changes that occur during a short period of time) is also an important factor. The axial resolution of the color image is governed by the length of the individual sample volumes along each scan line. The lateral resolution of the color image depends on the width of the beam and the density of the scan lines across the field of view. The ability of the color image to follow the changes in flow over time accurately depends on the system having an adequate frame rate. Imaging arterial flow effectively usually requires a higher frame rate than does demonstrating venous flow, as changes in arterial flow occur much more rapidly.

The sensitivity of an ultrasound system to flow is another indication of the quality of the system and depends on many factors. First, the ultrasound frequency and output power must be appropriately selected to allow adequate penetration. Second, the time spent detecting the flow must be long enough to distinguish blood flow from stationary tissue. The filters used to remove wall thump and other tissue movement must be set so as not to remove signals from blood flow. The resolution and sensitivity of modern color flow systems have rapidly improved over the last decade, improving the range and quality of vascular examinations.

POWER DOPPLER IMAGING

So far, this chapter has described how the Doppler shift frequency can be displayed as a color map superimposed on to the gray-scale image. However, instead of displaying the detected velocity with respect to the beam (frequency shift) it is possible to display the back-scattered power of the Doppler signal. The color scale used shows increased luminosity with increased back-scattered power. This allows the scanner to display the presence of moving blood, but it does not indicate the relative velocity or direction of flow, as shown in Figure 4.16. This method of display has some advantages in that the power Doppler display is not dependent on the angle of insonation, and it has improved sensitivity compared with conventional Doppler frequency displays. Figure 4.17A shows how the beam used to produce the scan lines produces a range of angles of insonation within a vessel due to the range of elements used to form the beam. When the center of the beam is at an angle of 90° to the vessel, parts of the beam will produce an angle of insonation of less than 90°, and the blood flow will be toward part of the beam and away from other parts of the beam. Therefore, the range of frequencies detected will be as shown in Figure 4.17B, with the blood appearing to be traveling both toward the beam (producing a positive Doppler shift) and away from the beam (producing a negative Doppler shift). The mean of this range of Doppler frequency shifts is zero, and therefore no flow would be displayed with a color Doppler frequency map. If, however, the total power (i.e., the area under the curves in Fig. 4.17B) is displayed, this will be similar to a signal obtained at a smaller angle of insonation. The display of back-scattered power is therefore practically independent of the angle. As the frequency is not dis-

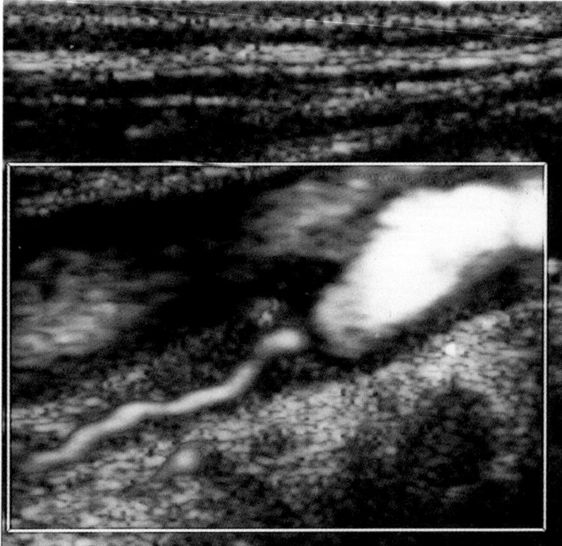

Figure 4.16 • Power Doppler image of a diseased internal carotid artery, showing a narrow-flow channel.

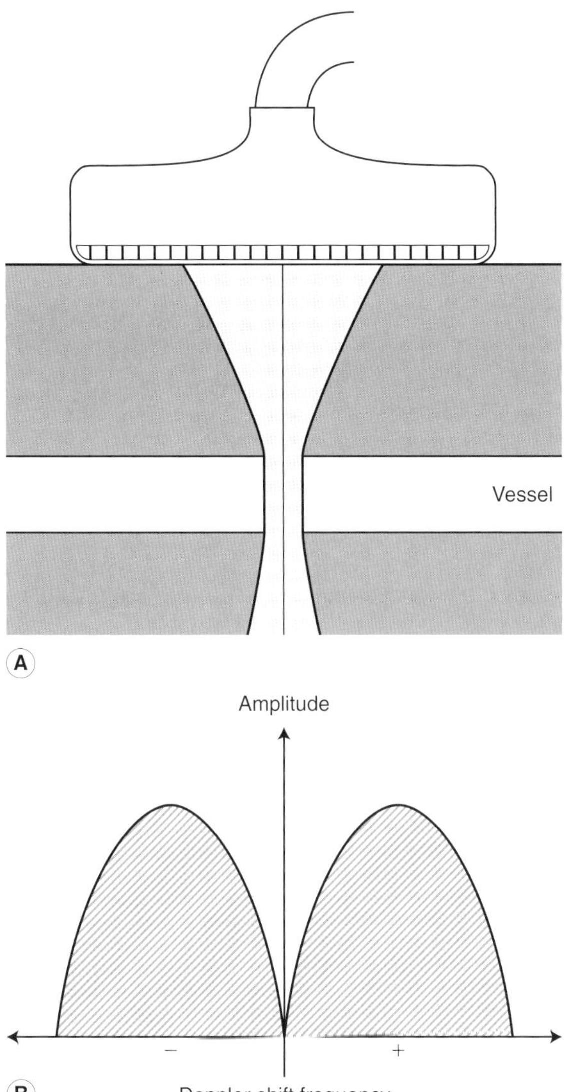

Figure 4.17 • (A) The beam used to detect the flow produces a range of angles of insonation. (B) When the beam is at right angles to the blood flow, this will result in both negative and positive Doppler shift frequencies within the signal.

played, power Doppler does not suffer from aliasing. The back-scattered power will, however, be affected by the attenuation of the tissue through which the ultrasound has traveled and will be lower for deep-lying vessels than for superficial vessels.

At the vessel walls, where the sample volume may be only partially filled by the vessel, the detected back-scattered power will be lower, and the power Doppler will be displayed by darker pixels than at the center of the vessel. Color Doppler imaging displays the mean frequency detected within a sample volume and therefore does not depend on whether the sample volume is totally or partially filled with the blood flow. Power Doppler is therefore able to provide better definition of the boundaries of the blood flow than color Doppler.

The improved sensitivity of the power Doppler is due to the relationship between the noise and the Doppler signal. If the color gain is increased to visualize the background noise, the operator will see the noise as a speckled pattern of all colors within the color box. This is because the noise generated within the scanner is a low-amplitude signal containing all frequencies. As the noise occurs in all frequencies, this noise is impossible to remove using the high-pass filter. As power Doppler displays power rather than frequency, it is less susceptible to this low-amplitude noise since it is displayed as a darker color or not displayed at all.

The main disadvantage with power Doppler is that in order to improve sensitivity, a high degree of frame-averaging is used, which means that the operator may have to keep the transducer still to obtain a good image. Therefore, this modality is less suitable for rapidly scanning along vessels. The lack of angle dependence makes power Doppler useful in imaging tortuous vessels. Power Doppler also provides improved edge definition (e.g., around plaque). Some ultrasound systems provide a color flow display that combines the power Doppler display with directional information. In this mode, the power of the signal is displayed as red for flow detected traveling toward the transducer, and the power of the signal detected from blood moving away from the transducer is displayed as blue. No velocity information is displayed in this mode.

ENHANCED FLOW IMAGING USING CONTRAST AGENTS AND HARMONIC IMAGING

A limiting factor in ultrasound imaging of flow is that the power of the ultrasound back-scattered from blood is much lower than that reflected from the surrounding tissue. The concept behind the use of contrast agents in ultrasound is to introduce a substance into the blood that provides a higher back-scattered power than is available from blood alone. This will increase the intensity of the Doppler signal detected from the blood flow.

Contrast agents used clinically at present consist of microparticles to which gas microbubbles adhere. It is these microbubbles that provide the increase in back-scattered power. Contrast agents are divided into two types: right heart and left heart agents. Right heart agents are destroyed as they pass through the lungs and, therefore, when injected intravenously, are only suitable for imaging the right side of the heart. Left heart, or transpulmonary, agents can pass through the lungs and can therefore be used to enhance the back-scattered signal from peripheral arteries. These agents effectively enhance the Doppler signal for approximately 5–10 min, so are only really suitable for investigations that do not take longer than this to perform.

Bubbles insonated with ultrasound will oscillate and will back-scatter ultrasound both at the frequency at which they were insonated and at higher frequencies. These higher frequencies are harmonics of the original frequency (i.e., they are multiples of the fundamental frequency) (see Ch. 2). If, for example, a broad-band transducer is used to insonate the contrast agent at a frequency of 3 MHz, the scanner will be able to detect a back-scattered signal from the microbubbles at a frequency of 6 MHz. The surrounding tissue, however, does not oscillate to the same extent and will therefore not produce as big a back-scattered signal at the higher harmonic frequency. Contrast agents can be used in conjunction with harmonic imaging by imaging an increase in image brightness on B-mode representing the presence of the contrast medium which will have been introduced to the scanned region by the presence of blood flow. One of the negative aspects of the use of contrast agents is that the ultrasound examination becomes an invasive procedure.

Reference

Ferrara K, DeAngelis G 1997 Color flow mapping. Ultrasound in Medicine and Biology 23: 321–345

Further reading

Evans D H, McDicken W N 2000 Doppler ultrasound: physics, instrumentation and signal processing. Wiley, Chichester

Hoskins P R, Thrush A, Martin K et al. (eds) 2003 Diagnostic ultrasound: physics and equipment. Greenwich Medical Media, London

Zagzebski J A 1996 Essentials of ultrasound physics. Mosby, St Louis

Blood flow and its appearance on color flow imaging

5

CONTENTS

INTRODUCTION

Arterial blood flow is complex and consists of pulsatile flow of an inhomogeneous fluid through viscoelastic arteries that branch, curve, and taper. However, a useful understanding of hemodynamics can be gained by first considering simple models, such as steady flow in a rigid tube. Factors affecting venous flow will also be considered. This will allow us to interpret spectral Doppler and color Doppler images of blood flow more easily. However, when interpreting color flow images it is important to remember that the color represents the mean velocity of flow obtained from the sample volumes and that this will depend on the angle between the ultrasound beam and blood flow. The pulse repetition frequency (PRF) and filter setting used and the length of time over which the image is created may also affect the appearance of the image. Artifactual effects also have to be considered carefully before drawing conclusions about the blood flow.

STRUCTURE OF VESSEL WALLS

The arterial and venous systems are often thought of as a series of tubes that transport blood to and from organs and tissues. In reality, blood vessels are highly complex structures that respond to nervous stimulation and interact with chemicals in the blood stream to regulate the flow of blood throughout the body. Changes in cardiac output and the tone of the smooth-muscle cells in the arterial walls are crucial factors that affect blood flow. The structure of a blood vessel wall varies considerably depending on its position within the vascular system.

Arteries and veins are composed of three layers of tissue, with veins having thinner walls than arteries. The outer layer is called the adventitia and is predominantly composed of connective tissue with collagen and elastin. The middle layer, the media, is the thickest layer and is composed of smooth-muscle fibers and elastic tissue. The intima is the inner layer and consists of a thin layer of endothelium overlying an elastic membrane. The capillaries, by contrast, consist of a single layer of endothelium, which allows for the exchange of molecules through the capillary wall. It is possible to image the structure of larger vessel walls using ultrasound and to identify the early stages of arterial disease, such as intimal thickening.

The arterial tree consists of elastic arteries, muscular arteries, and arterioles. The aorta and subclavian arteries are examples of elastic or conducting arteries and contain elastic fibers and a large amount of collagen fibers to limit the degree of stretch. Elastic arteries function as a pressure reservoir, as the elastic tissue in the vessel wall is able to absorb a proportion of the large amount of energy generated by the heart during systole. This maintains the end-diastolic pressure and decreases the load on the left side of the heart. Muscular or distributing arteries, such as the radial artery, contain a large proportion of smooth-muscle cells in the media. These arteries are innervated by nerves and can dilate or constrict. The muscular arteries are responsible for regional distribution of blood flow. Arterioles are the smallest arteries, and their media is composed almost entirely of smooth-muscle cells. Arterioles have an important role in controlling blood pressure and flow, and they can constrict or dilate after sympathetic nerve or chemical stimulation. The arterioles distribute blood to specific capillary beds and can dilate or constrict selectively around the body depending on the requirements of organs or tissues.

WHY DOES BLOOD FLOW?

Energy created by the contraction of the heart forces blood around the body. Blood flow in the arteries depends on two factors: (1) the energy available to drive the blood flow, and (2) the resistance to flow presented by the vascular system.

A scientist named Daniel Bernoulli (1700–1782) showed that the total fluid energy, which gives rise to the flow, is made up of three parts:

- Pressure energy (p) – this is the pressure in the fluid, which, in the case of blood flow, varies due to the contraction of the heart and the distension of the aorta.
- Kinetic energy (KE) – this is due to the fact that the fluid is a moving mass. Kinetic energy is dependent on the density (ρ) and velocity (V) of the fluid:

$$KE = \frac{1}{2}\rho V^2 \qquad (5.1)$$

- Gravitational potential energy – this is the ability of a volume of blood to do work due to the effect of gravity (g) on the column of fluid with density (ρ) because of its height (h) above a reference point, typically the heart.

Gravitational potential energy (ρgh) is equivalent to hydrostatic pressure but has an opposite sign (i.e.$-\rho gh$). For example, when a person is standing, there is a column of blood – the height of the heart above the feet – resting on the blood in the vessels in the foot (Fig. 5.1A) causing a higher pressure, due to the hydrostatic pressure, than that seen when the person is lying down (Fig. 5.1B). As the heart is taken as the reference point, and the feet are below the heart, the hydrostatic pressure is positive. If the arm is raised so that it is above the heart, the hydrostatic pressure is negative, causing the veins to collapse and the pressure in the arteries in the arm to be lower than the pressure at the level of the heart. The total fluid energy is given by:

$$\text{Total fluid energy} = \text{pressure energy} + \text{gravitational energy} + \text{kinetic energy}$$

$$E_{tot} = p + (-\rho gh) + \frac{1}{2}\rho V^2 \qquad (5.2)$$

Figure 5.2 gives a graphical display of how the total energy, kinetic energy, and pressure alter with continuous flow through an idealized narrowing. Usually the kinetic energy component of the total energy is small compared with the pressure energy. When fluid flows through a tube with a narrowing, the fluid travels faster as it passes through the narrowed section. As the velocity of the fluid increases in a narrowed portion of the vessel, the kinetic energy increases and the potential energy (i.e., the pressure) falls. The pressure within the narrowing is therefore lower than the pressure in the portion

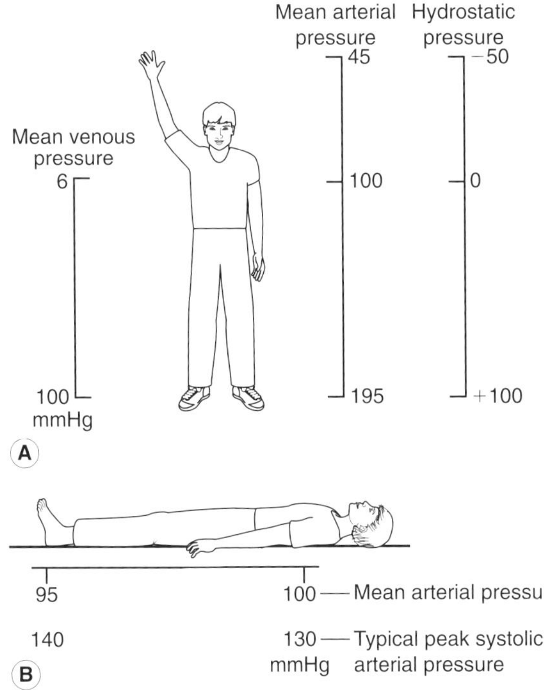

Figure 5.1 • Schematic diagram showing typical pressures in arteries and veins with the subject standing (A) and lying (B). The component due to hydrostatic pressure when the subject is vertical is shown alongside A.

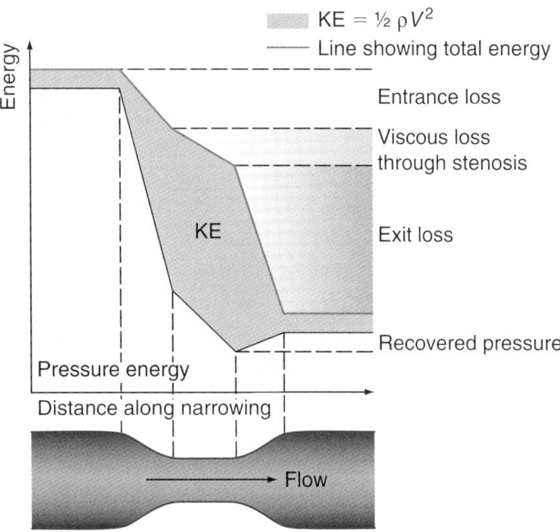

Figure 5.2 • Diagram showing how energy losses can occur across a narrowing. KE, kinetic energy. (Oates (ed), Cardiovascular Haemodynamics and Doppler Waveforms Explained. 2008. Cambridge University Press)

of the vessel before the narrowing. As the fluid passes beyond the narrowing, the velocity drops again and the kinetic energy is converted back to potential energy (the pressure), which increases. Energy is lost as the fluid passes through the narrowing (Fig. 5.2), with the extent of the entrance and exit losses depending on the geometry and degree of the narrowing (Oates 2008). In normal arteries, very little energy is lost as the blood flows away from the heart toward the limbs and organs, and the mean pressure in the small distal vessels is only slightly lower than in the aorta. However, in the presence of significant arterial disease, energy may be lost from the blood as it passes through tight narrowings or small collateral vessels around occlusions, leading to a drop in the pressure greater than that which would be expected in a normal artery; this can lead to reduced blood flow and tissue perfusion distally. Because the entrance and exit losses account for a large proportion of the pressure loss, it is likely that two adjacent stenoses will have a more significant effect than one long one (Oates 2008).

RESISTANCE TO FLOW

In 1840, a physician named Poiseuille established a relationship between flow, the pressure gradient along a tube, and the dimensions of a tube. The relationship can simply be understood as:

$$\text{Pressure drop} = \text{flow} \times \text{resistance} \quad (5.3)$$

where the resistance to flow is given by:

$$R = \frac{\text{viscosity} \times \text{length} \times 8}{\pi \times r^4} \quad (5.4)$$

where r is the radius.

Viscosity causes friction between the moving layers of the fluid. Treacle, for example, is a highly viscous fluid, whereas water has a low viscosity and therefore offers less resistance to flow when traveling through a small tube. Poiseuille's law shows that the resistance to flow is highly dependent on changes in the radius (r^4). In the normal circulation, the greatest proportion of the resistance is thought to occur at the arteriole level. Tissue perfusion is controlled by changes in the diameter of the arterioles. The presence of arterial disease in the arteries, such as stenoses or occlusions, can significantly alter the resistance to flow, with the reduction in vessel diameter having a major effect on the change in resistance seen. In severe disease, the arterioles distal to the disease may become maximally dilated in order to reduce the peripheral resistance, thus increasing blood flow in an attempt to maintain tissue perfusion. Poiseuille described nonpulsatile flow in a rigid tube, so his equation does not completely represent arterial blood flow; however, it gives us some understanding of the relationship between pressure drop, resistance, and flow.

VELOCITY CHANGES WITHIN STENOSES

We have already seen that fluid travels faster through a narrowed section of tube. The theory to determine these changes in velocity is described below. The volume flow through the tube is given by:

Flow = velocity of the fluid × cross-sectional area

$$Q = V \times A \qquad (5.5)$$

where V is the mean velocity across the whole of the vessel, averaged over time, and A is the cross-sectional area of the tube. If the tube has no outlets or branches through which fluid can be lost, the flow along the tube remains constant. Therefore, the velocity at any point along the tube depends on the cross-sectional area of the tube. Figure 5.3 shows a tube of changing cross-sectional area (A_1, A_2); now, as the flow (Q) along the tube is constant:

$$Q = V_1 \times A_1 = V_2 \times A_2 \qquad (5.6)$$

This equation can be rearranged to show that the change in the velocities is related to the change in the cross-sectional area, as follows:

$$\frac{V_2}{V_1} = \frac{A_1}{A_2} \qquad (5.7)$$

As the cross-sectional area depends on the radius r of the tube ($A = \pi r^2$), we have:

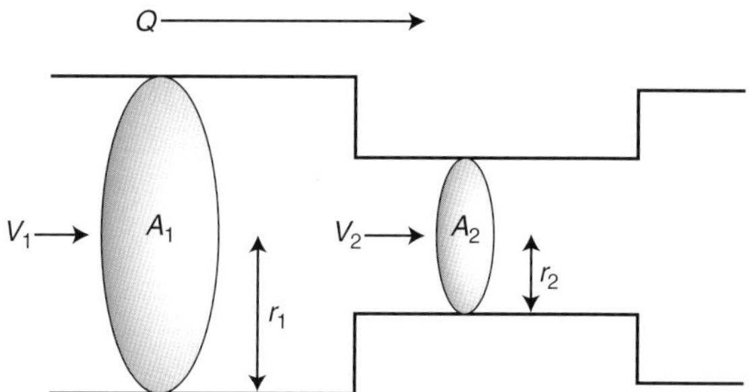

Figure 5.3 • Change in cross-sectional area. As the flow is constant through the tube, the velocity of the fluid increases from V_1 to V_2 as the cross-sectional area decreases from A_1 to A_2.

$$\frac{V_2}{V_1} = \frac{A_1}{A_2} = \frac{r_1^2}{r_2^2} \qquad (5.8)$$

This relationship describes steady flow in a rigid tube, but it does give us an indication as to how the velocity will change across a stenosis in an artery.

Figure 5.4 shows how the flow and velocity within an idealized stenosis vary with the degree of diameter reduction caused by the stenosis, based on the predictions from a simplified theoretical model. On the right-hand side of the graph, where the diameter reduction is less than 70–80%, the flow remains relatively unchanged as the diameter of the vessel is reduced. This is because the proportion of the resistance to flow due to the stenosis is small compared with the overall resistance of the vascular bed that the vessel is supplying. However, as the diameter reduces farther, the resistance offered by the stenosis becomes a significant proportion of the total resistance, and the stenosis begins to limit the flow. This is known as a hemodynamically significant stenosis. At this point, the flow decreases quickly as the diameter is reduced.

The graph also predicts the behavior of the velocity as the vessel diameter is reduced and shows that the velocity increases with diameter reduction. Noticeable changes in velocity begin to occur at much smaller diameter reductions than would produce a flow reduction. Therefore, measurement of velocity changes is a more sensitive method of detecting small-vessel lumen reductions than measurement of flow. Measurements of

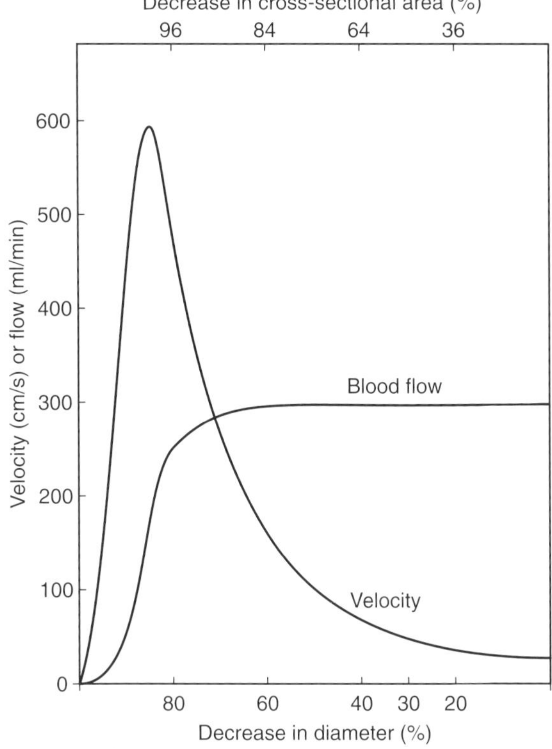

Figure 5.4 • Changes in flow and velocity as the degree of stenosis alters, predicted by a simple theoretical model of a smooth, symmetrical stenosis. (Spencer & Reid, Quantitation of carotid stenosis with continuous-wave (C-W), Doppler Ultrasound. Stroke 10:326-330, 1979)

velocity made using Doppler ultrasound are also more accurate than measurement of flow, as will be discussed later (see Ch. 6). Therefore, it is usually the change in velocity of blood within a diseased artery that is used to quantify the degree of narrowing. Eventually, there comes a point at which the resistance to flow produced by the narrowing is so great that the flow drops to such an extent that the velocity begins to decrease, as shown on the left side of the graph. This is seen as 'trickle flow' within the vessel. It is especially important to be able to identify trickle flow within a stenosis as the peak velocities seen may be similar to those seen in healthy vessels, but the color image and waveform shapes will not appear normal.

As blood flow is pulsatile and arteries are non-rigid vessels, it is difficult to predict theoretically the velocity increase that would be seen for a particular diameter reduction. Instead, velocity criteria used to quantify the degree of narrowing are produced by comparing Doppler velocity measurements with arteriogram results, as arteriography has been considered to be the 'gold standard' for the diagnosis of arterial disease.

FLOW PROFILES IN NORMAL ARTERIES

There are three types of flow observed in arteries:
1. laminar
2. disturbed
3. turbulent.

The term laminar flow refers to the fact that the blood cells move in layers, one layer sliding over another, with the different layers being able to move at different velocities. In laminar flow, the blood cells remain in their layers. Turbulent flow occurs when laminar flow breaks down, which is unusual in normal healthy arteries but can be seen in the presence of high-velocity flow caused by stenoses, as discussed later in this chapter.

Figure 5.5 is a schematic diagram showing how the flow profile is expected to change as fluid enters a vessel. When flow enters a vessel from a reservoir (in the case of blood flow, this is the heart), all the fluid is moving at the same velocity, producing a flat velocity profile. This means that the velocity of the fluid close to the vessel wall is similar to that at the center of the vessel. As the fluid flows along the vessel, viscous drag exerted by the walls causes the fluid at the vessel wall to remain motionless, producing a gradient between the velocity in the center of the vessel and that at the walls. As the total flow has to remain constant (as there are no branches in our imaginary tube), the velocity at the center of the vessel will increase to compensate for the low velocity at the vessel wall. This leads to a change in the velocity profile

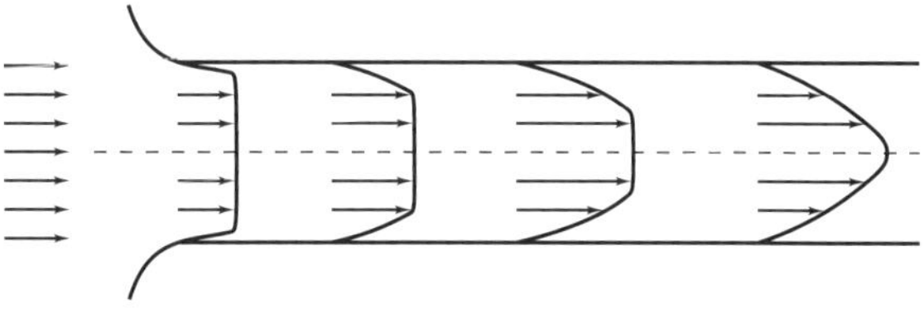

Figure 5.5 • The change in velocity profile with distance along a vessel from a blunt to a parabolic. (After Caro et al. 1978, with permission.)

from the initial blunt flow profile to a parabolic flow profile. This is often known as an entrance effect. The distance required for the flow profile to develop from the blunt to the parabolic profile depends on vessel diameter and velocity, but it is usually several times the vessel diameter. With blood flow, the velocity profiles are complicated by the pulsatile nature of the flow.

A color flow image obtained from the superficial femoral artery, during systole, is shown in Figure 5.6. This image shows high velocities in the center of the mid superficial femoral artery and lower velocities near the artery wall.

Pulsatile flow

The flow profiles considered in Figure 5.5 describe steady flow, but clearly arterial flow is pulsatile. So how will this affect the velocity profile across the vessel? The mean velocity profile of the pulsatile flow will develop as described for steady-state flow but will have a pulsatile component superimposed upon it. The flow direction and velocity are governed by the pressure gradient along the vessel. The pressure pulse generated by the heart is transmitted down the arterial tree and is altered by pressure waves reflected from the distal vascular bed. Figure 5.7A shows the pressure waveforms, typical of those seen in the femoral arteries, from two different points along the vessel, 'a' and 'b'. The pressure difference between these two points is given by a – b, as shown in Figure 5.7B, such that a negative pressure gradient is produced at periods during the cardiac cycle. This leads to periods of reverse flow, as seen in a typical Doppler waveform obtained from a normal superficial femoral artery (Fig. 5.8). If we consider a slowly oscillating pressure gradient applied to the flow, this will slow down, stop, and then reverse the direction of flow. If this oscillation is gradual, the parabolic velocity profile will be maintained, but if the pressure gradient is cycled more frequently, the velocity profile will become increasingly complex.

As the laminae of flowing blood near the vessel wall tend to have a lower velocity (due to the effect of viscosity), and hence lower momentum, they will reverse more easily when the pressure gradient along the vessel reverses. This can lead to a situation in which flow near the vessel wall is in a different direction to flow at the center of the vessel. Figure 5.9 shows a color image obtained from a normal superficial femoral artery during diastole. The image shows forward flow near the vessel wall, while flow in the center of the vessel is reversed.

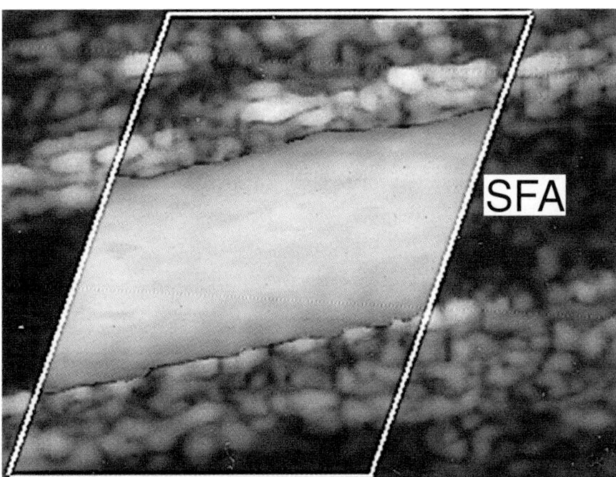

Figure 5.6 • Color flow image showing high velocities (shown as yellow) in the center of a normal superficial femoral artery, with lower velocities (shown as red) nearer the vessel wall.

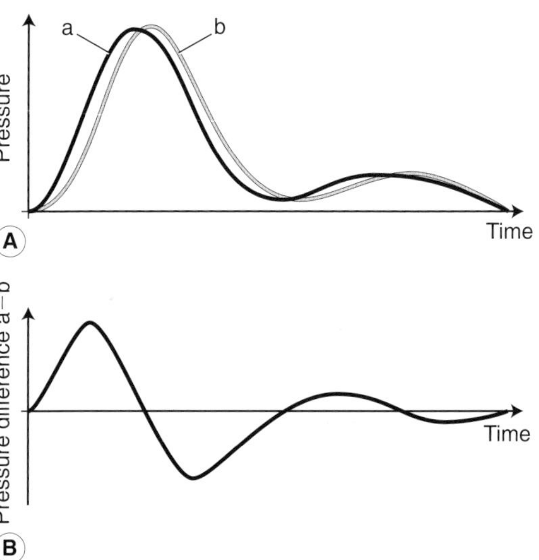

Figure 5.7 • (A) Idealized pressure waveforms obtained from two sites (a and b) along the femoral artery. (B) The direction of blood flow between 'a' and 'b' will be governed by the pressure difference, given by 'a – b'. (Nichols & O'Rourke, McDonald's Blood Flow in Arteries (Hodder Arnold, 1990). Reprinted by permission of Edward Arnold (Publishers) Ltd)

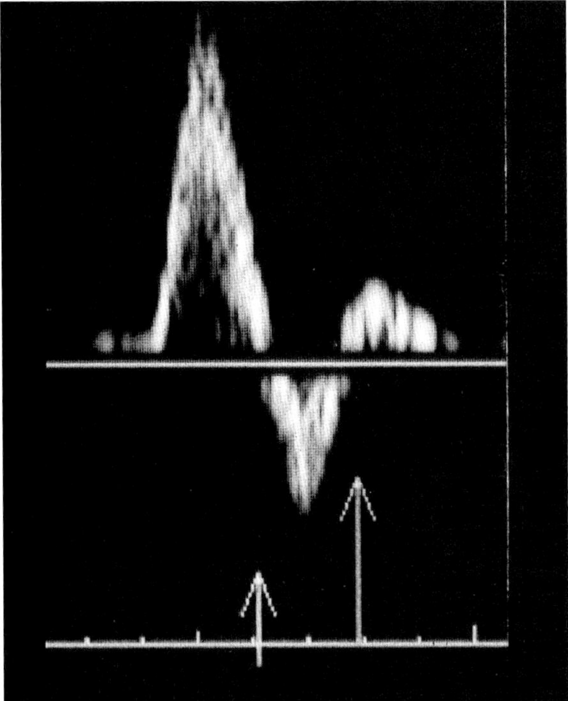

Figure 5.8 • Velocity waveform in a normal superficial femoral artery. The arrows represent points in the cardiac cycle where both forward and reverse flows are seen simultaneously.

This would occur at the point in the cardiac cycle marked by the long arrow in Figure 5.8. The short arrow shows another point at which both forward and reverse flow may occur simultaneously. Figure 5.10 shows velocity profiles, as they vary over the cardiac cycle, for the common femoral artery (Fig. 5.10A) and the common carotid artery (Fig. 5.10B) that have been calculated from mean velocity waveforms. They show that reversal of flow is seen in the common femoral artery, but that, although the flow is pulsatile, reverse flow is not seen in the normal common carotid artery. Reversal of flow will only be seen if the reverse pulsatile flow component is greater than the steady flow component upon which it is superimposed. This greatly depends on the distal vascular bed. Total reversal of flow is rarely seen in normal renal or internal carotid arteries, both of which supply highly vascular beds with low resistance. However, there are hemodynamic effects at bifurcations and branches that may cause areas of localized flow reversal. There is a different appearance between waveform shapes obtained from vessels supplying

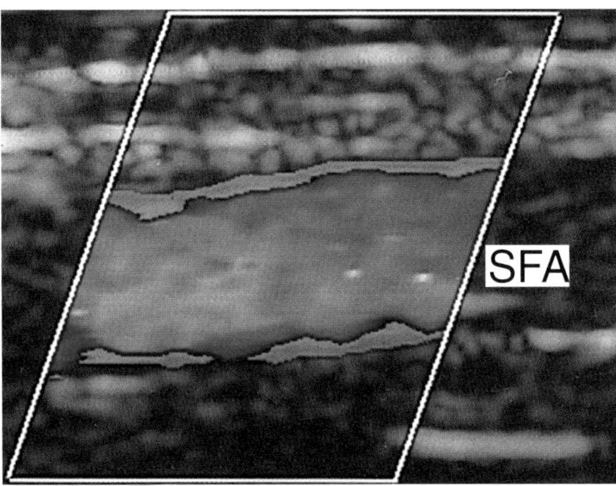

Figure 5.9 • Color flow image showing forward and reverse flow simultaneously in a normal superficial femoral artery. The red represents forward flow near the vessel wall whereas the blue represents reverse flow in the center of the vessel.

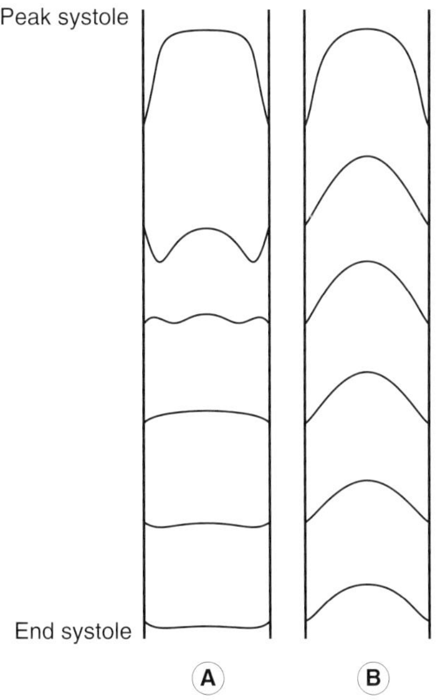

Figure 5.10 • Velocity profiles from a common femoral artery (A) and a common carotid artery (B), calculated from the mean velocity waveforms. (After Evans & McDicken 1999, with permission.)

a low-resistance vascular bed (i.e., organs such as the brain and kidney) and those obtained from peripheral vessels in the arms and legs, which supply high-resistance vascular beds.

Changes in peripheral resistance will change the flow pattern. For example, the waveform in the dorsalis pedis artery in the foot changes from bi-directional flow at rest (Fig. 5.11A) to hyperemic monophasic flow (i.e., flow that is always in the same direction; Fig. 5.11B) following exercise. Hyperemic flow can also be induced by temporary occlusion of the calf arteries using a blood pressure cuff. The lack of blood flow during the arterial occlusion with the cuff, or the increase in demand during exercise, causes the distal vessels to dilate in order to reduce peripheral resistance and maximize blood flow, and this is reflected in the change in shape of the waveform seen directly after cuff release. The hyperemic flow soon returns to bi-directional flow once adequate perfusion has occurred. This change in shape can also be seen when hyperemic flow is induced by infection. Monophasic flow is also seen in the lower limb, distal to severe stenoses or occlusions (Fig. 5.11C). This waveform shape is also due to distal vasodilatation, in an attempt to maximize flow distal to the diseased vessel, but this can usually be distinguished from hyperemic flow as the velocity of the flow is low and the systolic rise time may be longer. The systolic rise time is the time between the beginning of systole and peak systole.

An occlusion or severe stenosis distal to the site at which a Doppler waveform has been obtained may also cause a change in the waveform shape due to an increase in the resistance to flow. Figure 5.12A shows a Doppler spectum obtained from a superficial femoral artery proximal to a normal popliteal artery and demonstrates a normal triphasic waveform shape. Figure 5.12B shows the Doppler spectrum obtained from the superficial femoral artery in the other leg of the same individual but this time the popliteal artery is occluded. Although the waveform shape in Figure 5.12B still appears triphasic, a ledge can be seen on the downward slope of the systolic peak and this is caused by the presence of the distal occlusion. This change in appearance of the waveform shape is due to changes in the reflected pressure wave (see Fig. 5.7) and can be used as an indication that there may be

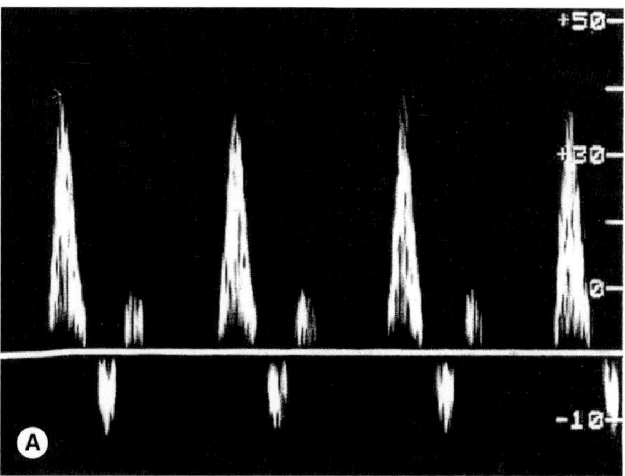

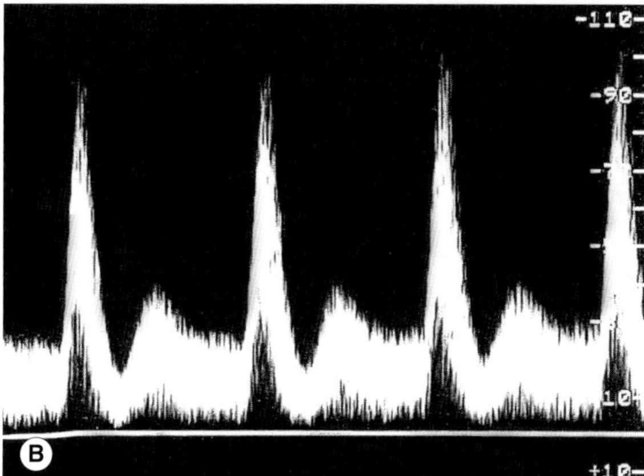

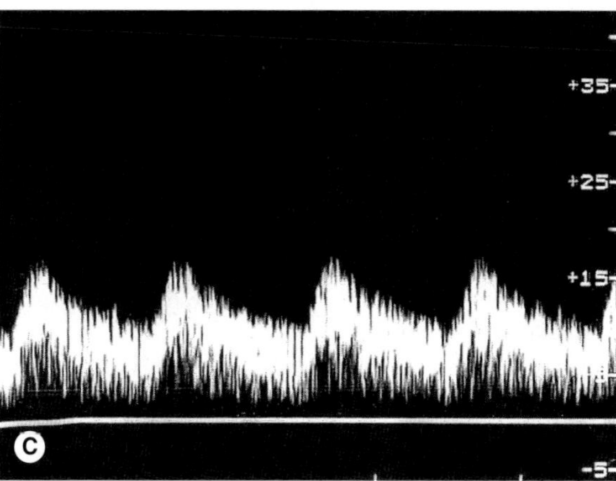

Figure 5.11 • Doppler spectra obtained from a normal dorsalis pedis artery in the foot showing bi-directional flow at rest (A) and monophasic hyperemic flow following exercise (B). Low-volume monophasic flow is seen in the foot distal to an occlusion (C).

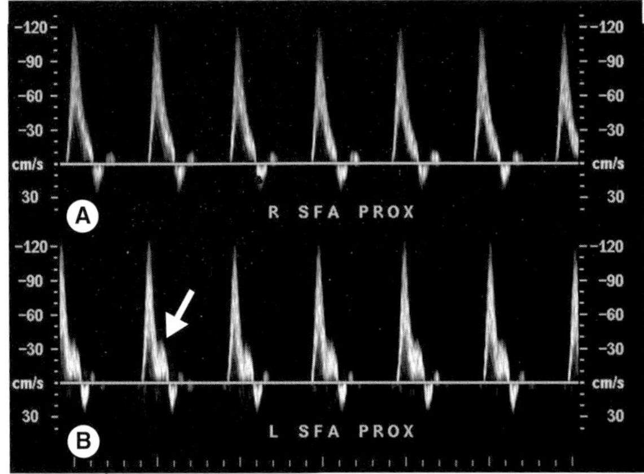

Figure 5.12 • Doppler spectrum obtained from a superficial femoral artery (A) proximal to normal popliteal artery and (B) proximal to an occluded popliteal artery. The ledge seen (arrow) on the downward slope of the systolic peak is an indication of the distal disease.

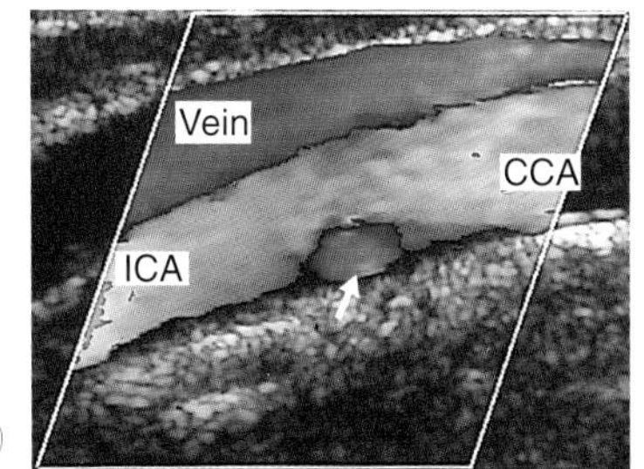

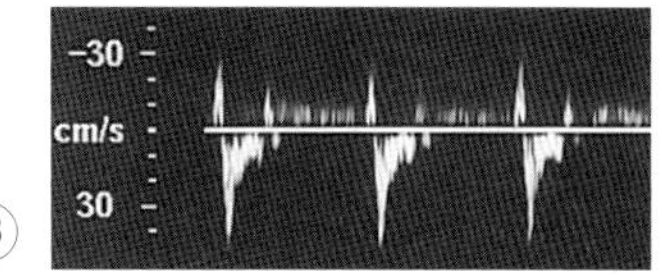

Figure 5.13 • (A) Colour flow image showing reverse flow in the origin of a normal internal carotid artery. (B) Spectral Doppler waveform obtained from the area of flow separation shown by the arrow in (A).

significant disease distal to the site of measurement that would require futher investigation.

Flow at bifurcations and branches

The arterial tree divides many times, and each branch will affect the velocity profiles seen. The hemodynamics of the carotid bifurcation has been extensively investigated using multigate pulsed Doppler systems, and color Doppler systems, and these investigations show that localized reversed flow is seen at the carotid bifurcation in normal subjects. Figure 5.13A shows reversal of flow, due to flow separation, at the origin of a healthy internal carotid artery. Figure 5.14 indicates how the asymmetric flow profile in a normal proximal internal carotid artery develops, with the high-velocity flow occurring toward the flow divider and the reverse flow occurring near the wall away from the origin of the external carotid artery. The effect is primarily due to a combination of the pulsatile flow, the relative dimensions of the vessels, the angle of the bifurcation, and the curvature of the vessel walls, making it difficult to predict these profiles. Figure 5.13B is a spectral Doppler signal obtained from the area of flow separation shown by an arrow in Figure 5.13, illustrating reverse flow during systole in that part of the vessel. This normal finding could potentially be misleading if the whole bifurcation is not observed and, typically, spectral Doppler recordings are made beyond the bifurcation unless the presence of disease indicates otherwise (see Ch. 8).

Flow reversal can also occur when a daughter vessel branches at right angles from the parent vessel. Figure 5.15 is a schematic diagram of the results obtained with dye in steadily flowing water in a tube with a right-angled branch and shows how the flow is divided between the main vessel and its branch. The flow is seen to separate from the inner wall of the junction and a region of reverse flow develops, primarily due to the sharp bend.

Flow around curves in a vessel

Curvature of vessels can also have an effect on the velocity profile. When a fluid flows along a curved tube, it experiences a centrifugal force, as well as the viscous forces at the vessel wall, and the combination of these forces results in secondary flow, in the form of two helical vortices (Oates 2008). In the case of parabolic flow, the fluid in the center of the vessel has the highest velocity and will thus experience the greatest force. These vortices will cause the high-velocity flow to move toward the outside wall of the vessel, as seen in Figure 5.16.

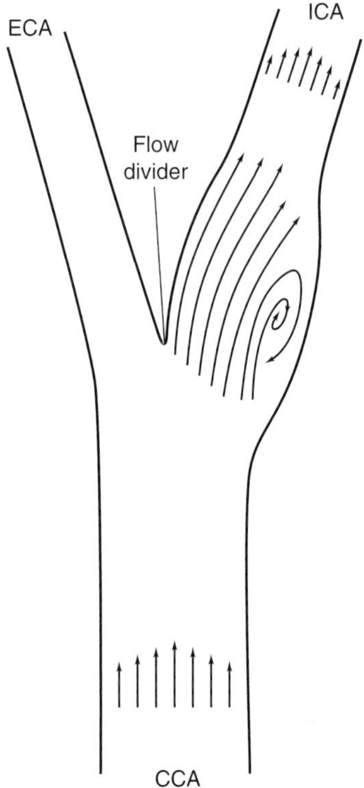

Figure 5.14 • Schematic diagram of the velocity patterns commonly observed in the normal carotid bifurcation. The velocity profile is flat and symmetric in the common carotid artery (CCA) and flat but slightly asymmetric in the internal carotid artery (ICA). In the carotid bulb the velocities are highest near the flow divider. Flow separation with flow reversal is observed on the opposite side to the flow divider. ECA, external carotid artery. (From Reneman et al. 1985, with permission.)

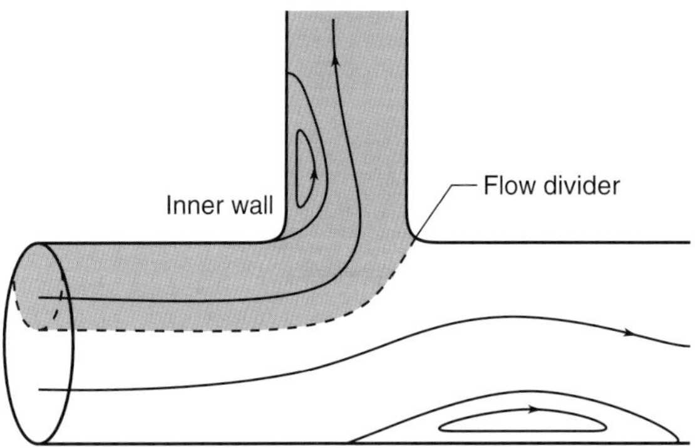

Figure 5.15 • Flow in a right-angle junction. The dashed line shows the surface that divides fluid flowing into the side branch from that continuing down the parent vessel. (After Caro et al. 1978, with permission.)

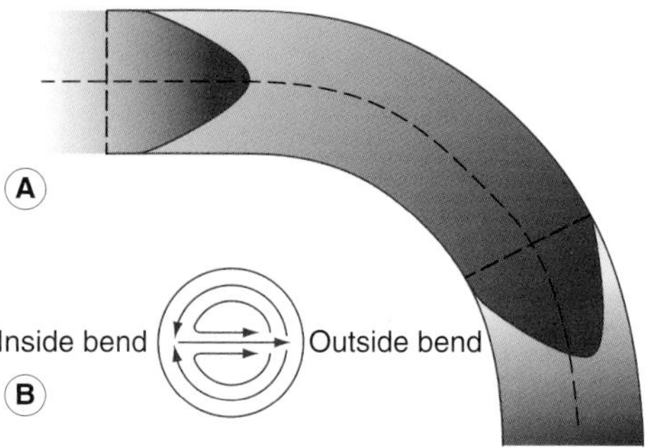

Figure 5.16 • (A) Distortion of parabolic flow caused by tube curvature. (B) Secondary flow, in the form of two helical vortices. (After Caro et al. 1978, with permission.)

Figure 5.17 shows a color flow image obtained from a tortuous internal carotid artery, with flow going from right to left. The image shows the highest velocities beyond the bend (left), represented in orange due to aliasing, skewed toward the outside of the bend. This is confirmed by spectral Doppler recordings showing that the peak velocity recorded on the outside of the bend (Fig. 5.17B) measures 70 cm/s compared to the peak velocity on the inside of the bend (Fig. 5.17C), which measures 55 cm/s. If the flow profile is blunt when it enters a bend in the vessel (as seen in the ascending aorta), the profile becomes skewed in the opposite direction (i.e., toward the inner wall of the curve). Secondary helical flow also occurs at bifurcations, as the daughter vessels bend away from the path of the parent vessel, leading to skewed velocity profiles in the daughter vessels (Fig. 5.14).

FLOW THROUGH STENOSES

Flow separation leading to flow reversal can also be seen in diseased arteries. At an arterial stenosis, the velocity of the blood has to increase because the same volume of blood needs to pass through a smaller cross-sectional area. If the vessel lumen rapidly returns to its normal diameter following the narrowing, flow separation can occur. Whereas the velocity increases as the blood passes through the constriction, the pressure within the stenosis falls, but the pressure rises again just distal to the stenosis as the lumen expands, having the effect of

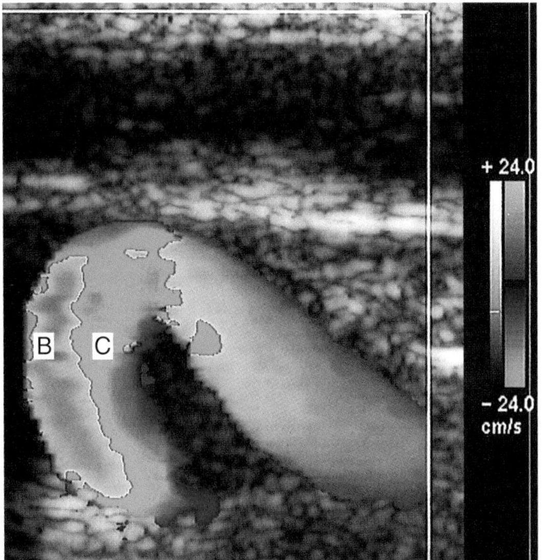

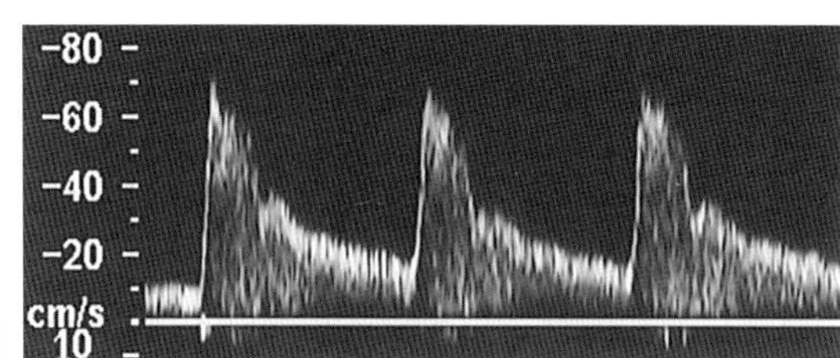

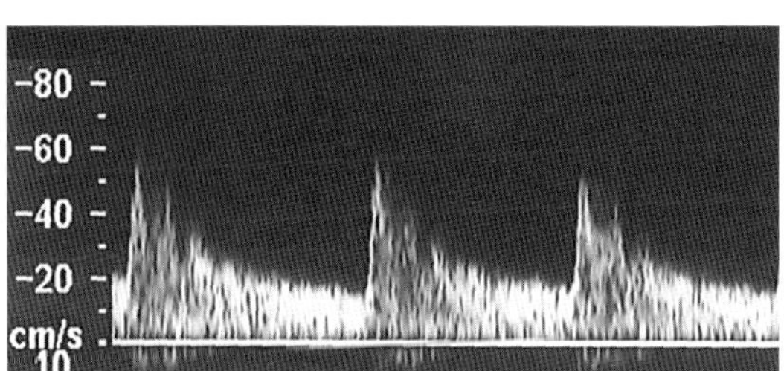

Figure 5.17 • (A) Color flow image from a tortuous internal carotid artery, with flow going from right to left, shows the highest velocities beyond the bend (left), represented in orange due to aliasing, skewed toward the outside of the bend. Spectral Doppler recordings showing that the peak velocity recorded on the outside of the bend (B) measure 70 cm/s compared to the peak velocity on the inside of the bend (C), which measures 55 cm/s.

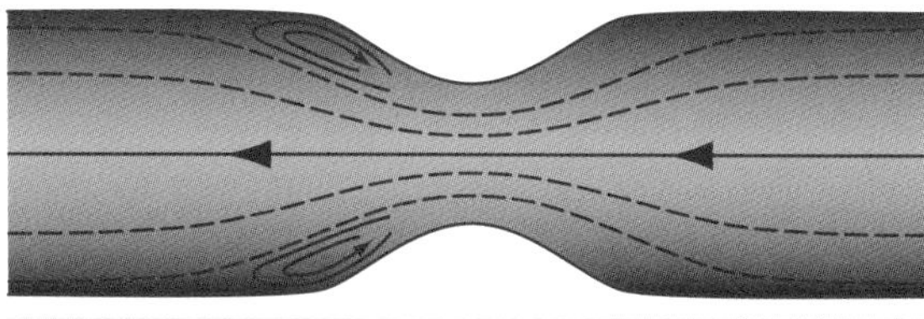

Figure 5.18 • Schematic diagram of flow through a constriction followed by a rapid expansion downstream, showing the regions of flow reversal. The velocity increases as the blood flows through a stenosis (from right to left) followed by an area of flow reversal beyond the narrowing. (After Caro et al. 1978, with permission.)

Figure 5.19 • The increase in velocity as the blood flows from right to left through a stenosis (arrow) produces the color change from red to turquoise (due to aliasing). Beyond the stenosis, flow reversal occurs along the posterior wall, represented by the deep blue, as the vessel lumen returns to its normal diameter. ICA, internal carotid artery; CCA, common carotid artery.

retarding the flow. As the flow near the vessel wall has a lower velocity, and therefore lower inertia, it will reverse, while the higher-velocity flow in the center of the vessel is reduced but not reversed. A schematic diagram of this effect is shown in Figure 5.18. The color image in Figure 5.19 demonstrates the increase in velocity as the blood flows through a stenosis, with flow reversal occurring along the distal wall beyond the stenosis as the vessel lumen returns to its normal diameter.

The geometry of stenoses is very variable, and these narrowings are often not symmetrical, sometimes producing eccentric jets, so it is impossible to predict the typical velocity profiles. As the degree of narrowing increases, the velocity within the vessel will increase, making the breakdown of laminar flow to turbulent flow more likely. Turbulent flow can withstand more acute geometric changes than laminar flow, so flow separation is less likely to be seen beyond a stenosis that has produced turbulent flow.

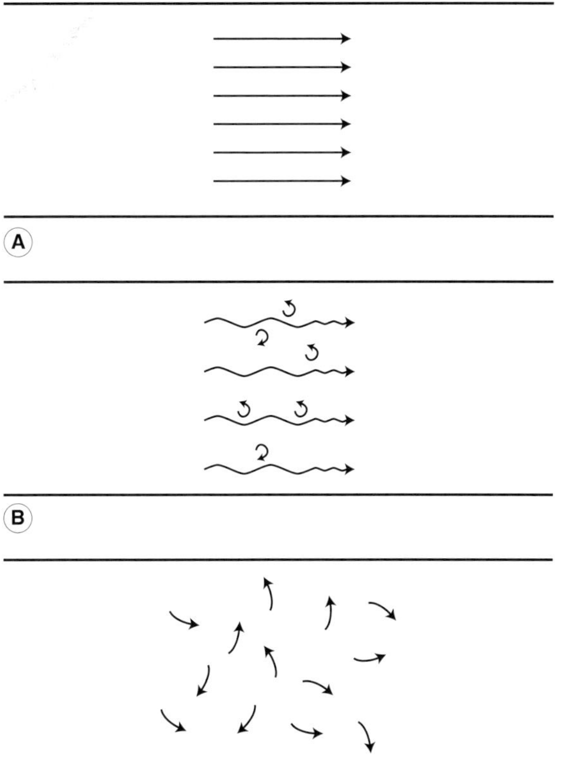

Figure 5.20 • (A) Laminar flow. (B) Disturbed flow. (C) Turbulent flow. (After Taylor et al. 1995, with permission.)

ARTERY	REYNOLDS NUMBER
Ascending aorta	1500
Abdominal aorta	640
Common carotid	217*
Superficial femoral	200
Posterior tibial	35*

*Estimated values.

Table 5.1 Typical values of the Reynolds number in various arteries in the body (after Evans & McDicken 1999, with permission)

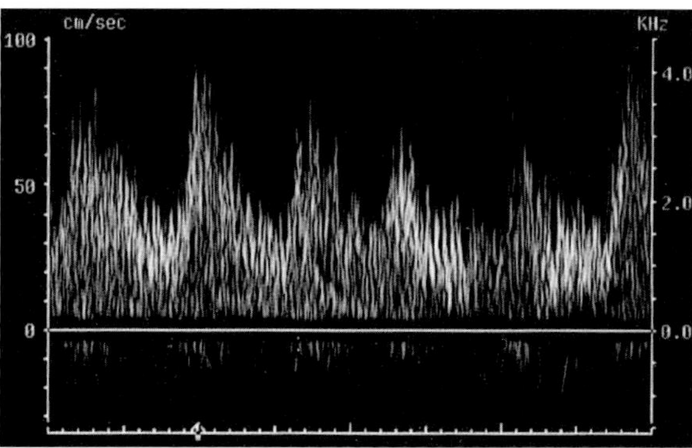

Figure 5.21 • Doppler waveform demonstrating turbulent flow.

Transition from laminar to turbulent flow

Turbulent flow occurs when laminar flow breaks down and the particles in the fluid move randomly in all directions with variable speeds. The transition from laminar flow to disturbed and then to turbulent flow is shown in Figure 5.20. Turbulent flow is more likely to occur at high velocities (V), and the critical velocity at which flow becomes turbulent depends on the viscosity (μ) and the density (ρ) of the fluid and the diameter of the vessel (d). Reynolds described this relationship, which defines a value called the Reynolds number (Re):

$$R_e = \frac{dV\rho}{\mu} \qquad (5.9)$$

Once the Reynolds number has exceeded the critical value of approximately 2000, turbulent flow will occur. Table 5.1 gives typical values of the Reynolds number in various arteries in the body and shows that in normal vessels the velocity of blood is such that turbulent flow does not occur, with the exception of the proximal aortic flow during heavy exercise, for which cardiac output is increased. The presence of an increase in the blood velocity, due to arterial disease, can cause turbulent flow. Figure 5.21 is a Doppler waveform demonstrating turbulent flow. In the presence of turbulence, not all the blood is traveling in the same direction, resulting in the angle of insonation being smaller for some parts of the blood flow. This results in turbulent spikes seen on the Doppler spectrum. It is possible for turbulent flow to occur only during the systolic phase of the cardiac cycle, when the systolic flow exceeds the critical velocity and the diastolic flow does not.

The presence of turbulent flow causes energy to be lost, leading to an increased pressure drop across the stenosis. It is thought that bruits in the tissue near a stenosis may be due to perivascular tissue vibration caused by turbulence, and this may also lead to poststenotic dilatation of the vessel. Vortices or irregular movement of a large portion of the fluid are more correctly referred to as disturbed flow rather than turbulent flow.

VENOUS FLOW

The venous system acts as a low-resistance pathway for blood to be returned to the heart. Veins are collapsible, thin-walled vessels capable of distending to a larger cross-sectional area than their corresponding arteries, so acting as a blood volume storage system that is important in the regulation of cardiac output. In addition, they also have a thermoregulation role in which blood is diverted to the superficial veins to reduce body temperature. The venous system can be divided into the central system (within the thorax and abdomen), the deep peripheral system, and the superficial peripheral veins.

An important structural feature of the vein is the presence of very thin, but strong, bicuspid valves which prevent retrograde flow away from the heart. The vena cava and common iliac veins are valveless. Valves are found in the external iliac or common femoral veins in a proportion of the population. Generally, the more distal the vein, the greater the number of valves.

Venous flow back to the heart is influenced by respiration, the cardiac cycle, and changes in posture.

Changes in flow due to the cardiac cycle

The central veins include the thoracic and abdominal veins, which drain to the right side of the heart via the inferior and superior venae cavae. The flow pattern and pressure in the central venous system are affected by changes in the volume of the right atrium that occur during the cardiac cycle. Reverse flow occurs in the thoracic veins when the right atrium contracts, as there is no valve in the vena cava. This flow reversal can also be seen in the proximal veins of the arm and neck (Fig. 5.22) due to their proximity to the chest. During ventricular contraction, the atrium expands, increasing venous flow into the right atrium, and then flow gradually falls during diastole, only increasing briefly as the tricuspid valve opens. Flow patterns in the lower-limb veins and peripheral arm veins are not significantly affected by the cardiac cycle due to vein compliance (which allows damping of the pressure changes), the presence of valves, and changes in intra-abdominal pressure during respiration.

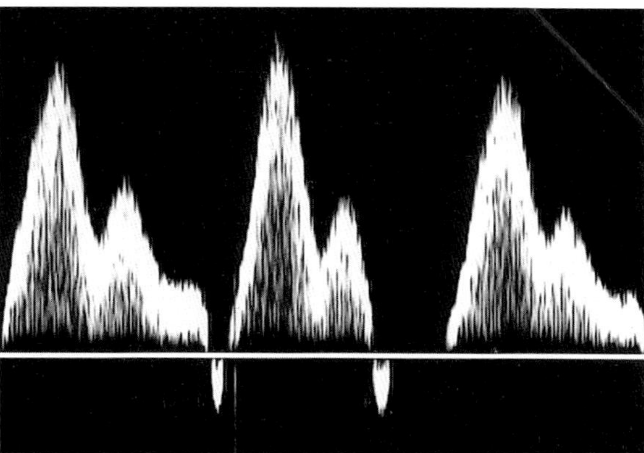

Figure 5.22 • Doppler waveform showing the effect of changes in the pressure in the right atrium on blood flow in the jugular vein.

Effects of respiration on venous flow

Respiration has an important effect on venous pressure and flow because of changes in the volume of the thorax brought about by movement of the diaphragm and ribs. Inspiration during calm breathing expands the thorax, leading to an increase in the volume of the veins in the chest, which in turn causes a reduction in the pressure in the intrathoracic veins. This creates a pressure gradient between the veins in the upper limb and head and those in the thorax, producing an increase in flow into the chest. Flow is decreased during expiration as the volume of the thorax decreases, leading to an increase in central pressure.

The reverse situation is seen in the abdomen as the diaphragm descends during inspiration, increasing intra-abdominal pressure. This leads to a decrease in the pressure gradient between the peripheral veins and the abdominal veins, thus

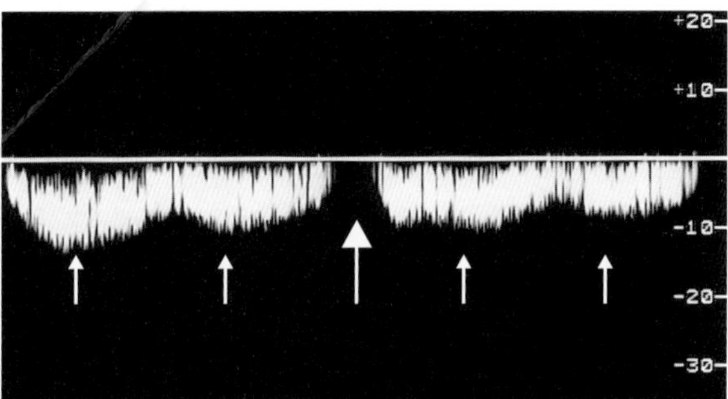

Figure 5.23 • Doppler waveform demonstrating the effect of respiration on the blood flow in the common femoral vein. The large arrow indicates the cessation of flow during inspiration and the small arrows show small changes in flow due to the cardiac cycle, which may not always be seen in the common femoral vein.

reducing flow. During expiration the diaphragm rises, producing a reduction in intra-abdominal pressure, and the pressure gradient between the abdominal veins and peripheral veins increases, causing increased blood flow back to the heart. The effects of respiration are observed as phasic changes in flow in proximal deep peripheral veins (Fig. 5.23). Breathing maneuvers are often used to augment flow when investigating venous disorders (see Ch. 13).

Changes in venous blood pressure due to posture and the calf muscle pump

Large pressure changes occur in the venous system, due to the effects of hydrostatic pressure generated by posture (Fig. 5.1). If an individual is lying supine, for example, there is a relatively small pressure difference between the venous pressures at the ankle and right atrium. However, when an individual is standing, there is a column of blood between the right atrium and the veins at the ankle. If the hydrostatic pressure is assumed to be zero in the right atrium, the hydrostatic pressure at the ankle will be equal to the distance between the two, which is dependent on the person's height, but is usually between 80 and 100 mmHg. Therefore, in a standing position, there is a significant pressure gradient to overcome in order for blood to be returned to the heart; this is achieved by the calf muscle pump mechanism assisted by the presence of the venous valves.

The muscle compartments in the calf contain the deep veins and venous sinuses, which act as blood reservoirs. Regular small contractions occur in the deep muscles of the calf, causing compression of the veins, thereby propelling blood flow out of the leg, with the venous valves preventing the blood refluxing back down. This also generates a pressure gradient between the superficial and deep veins in the calf, and blood drains through the perforating veins and major junctions from the superficial to the deep venous system. The valves in the perforators prevent blood flowing from the deep to the superficial veins. During more active exercise, such as walking or running, the calf muscle pump mechanism is able to produce a significant pressure reduction in the deep and superficial venous systems to approximately 30 mmHg. The pressure change that occurs during exercise is called the ambulatory venous pressure. At rest, because the hydrostatic pressure is the same on both the arterial and venous sides, the pressure drop across the capillary bed is the same whether the person is standing or lying down. However, after exercise the pressure on the venous side of the capillary bed will drop, but the pressure on the arterial side will remain the same, creating a pressure drop across the capillary bed and aiding the return of blood to the heart. Once the muscle contraction stops, the venous pressure in the lower leg will begin to rise due to filling of the venous system from the arterial system via the capillaries.

It is possible to measure the ambulatory venous pressure by inserting a small cannula into a dorsal foot vein, which is then connected to a pressure transducer and recorder. The pressure in the vein is first recorded with the patient standing. The patient is asked to perform 10 tiptoe maneuvers and then to stand still. The pressure recording demonstrates the pressure reduction during the exercise, and the venous refilling time can also be calculated. With normal veins, the refilling of the venous system occurs gradually by capillary inflow and takes 18 s or more to return to pre-exercise pressures (Fig. 5.24A). If there is significant failure of the venous valves in either the superficial or the deep venous system, reflux will occur, leading to a shorter refilling time and a higher postexercise pressure (Fig. 5.24B). Reflux in the deep or superficial venous systems, or in both, can lead to chronic venous hypertension in the lower leg and may result in the development of venous ulcers. Failure of the calf muscle pump due to poor flexion of the ankle and poor contraction of the calf muscle can lead to a reduction in the volume of blood ejected from the calf. This results in an inability to lower venous pressure adequately and can cause chronic venous hypertension. Patients at greatest risk due to poor calf muscle pump mechanism include those with limited ankle flexion due to chronic injury, osteoarthritis, or rheumatoid arthritis.

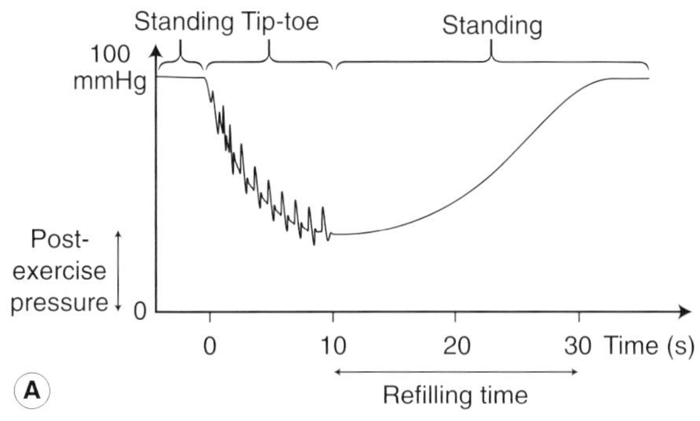

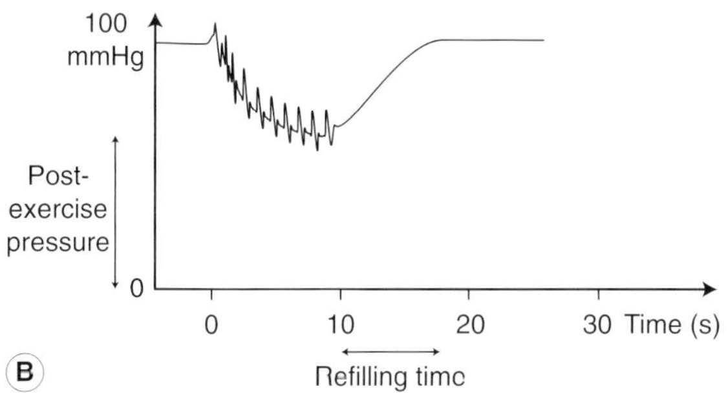

Figure 5.24 • Typical ambulatory venous pressure recordings. (A) Normal venous refilling. (B) Incompetent veins leading to a shorter refilling time.

Abnormal venous flow

Venous disease can dramatically alter the flow patterns seen in the veins. Valve incompetence allows retrograde flow in the veins, which can easily be demonstrated with color flow imaging and spectral Doppler. Venous outflow obstruction results in the loss of the spontaneous phasic flow generated by respiration seen in normal veins. Congestive heart failure may lead to increased pulsatility of the flow in the femoral and iliac veins. Ultrasound now plays an important role in the diagnosis of venous disease, which is discussed further in Chapters 13 and 14.

References

Caro C G, Pedley T J, Schroter R C et al. 1978 The mechanics of the circulation. Oxford University Press, Oxford

Evans D H, McDicken W N 1999 Doppler ultrasound: physics, instrumentation, and signal processing. Wiley, Chichester

Nichols W N, O'Rourke M F 1990 McDonald's blood flow in arteries. Edward Arnold, London

Oates C P (ed) 2008 Cardiovascular haemodynamics and Doppler waveforms explained. Cambridge University Press, Cambridge

Reneman R S, van Merode T, Hick P et al. 1985 Flow velocity patterns in and distensibility of the carotid artery bulb in subjects of various ages. Circulation 71: 500–509

Spencer M P, Reid J M 1979 Quantitation of carotid stenosis with continuous-wave (C-W) Doppler ultrasound. Stroke 10: 326–330

Taylor K J W, Burns P N, Wells P N T 1995 Clinical applications of Doppler ultrasound. Raven Press, New York

Factors that influence the Doppler spectrum

CONTENTS

INTRODUCTION

The shape of the Doppler spectrum can provide much useful information about the presence of disease and enables the sonographer to make measurements to quantify the degree of vessel narrowing. However, the shape of the spectrum will also depend on other factors, such as the velocity profile of the blood flow being interrogated and how evenly the ultrasound beam insonates the vessel. Factors that relate to the equipment rather than the blood flow can also affect the shape of the waveform. It is important to understand how these factors influence the waveform shape in order to be able to interpret the Doppler waveform. The sonographer should also be aware of potential errors involved in any measurements made.

FACTORS THAT INFLUENCE THE DOPPLER SPECTRUM

Blood flow profile

The Doppler spectrum displays the frequency content of the signal along the vertical axis, with the relative brightness of the display relating to the proportion of back-scattered power at each frequency, and the time along the horizontal axis. The velocity profiles seen within arteries can be quite complex and will vary over time, as discussed in Chapter 5. The frequency content displayed in the Doppler spectrum will depend on the velocities of the cells present within the blood. If we assume that the vessel is uniformly insonated by the Doppler beam, all the different velocities of blood present within the vessel will be detected and displayed on the spectrum. If blood is traveling with a blunt flow profile, most of the blood cells will be moving with the same velocity, and the spectrum will show only a small range of frequencies (Fig. 6.1A–C). If, however, the blood is traveling

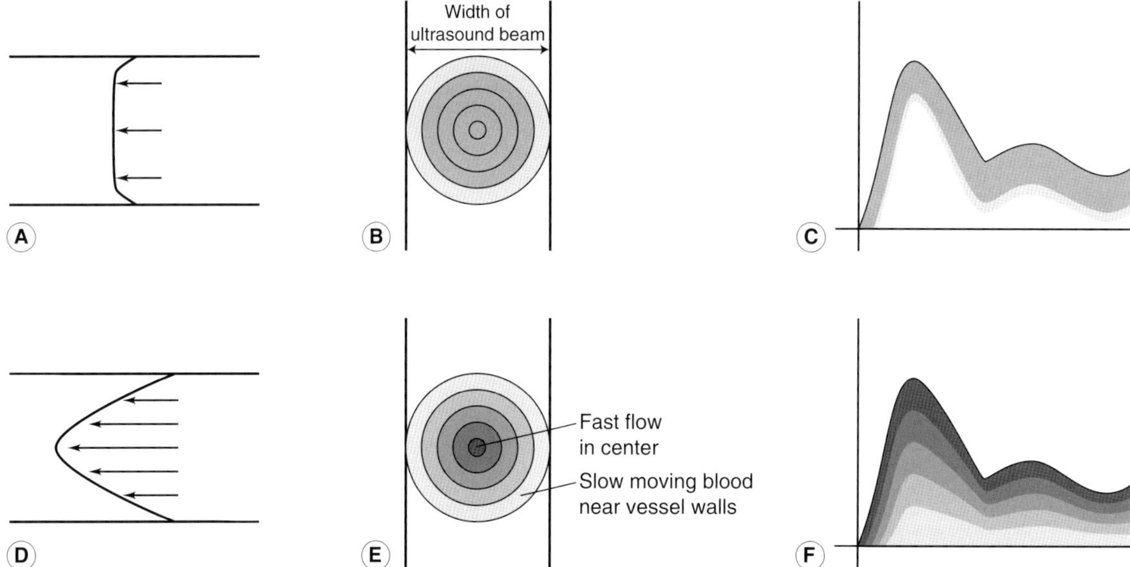

Figure 6.1 • (A, D) Velocity profiles for blunt flow and parabolic flow, respectively. (B, E) If a wide ultrasound beam is used to insonate the vessel, all the velocities present will be detected. (C, F) Idealized Doppler spectra that would be obtained from complete insonation of blunt flow and parabolic flow, respectively.

with a parabolic flow profile, then the blood in the center of the vessel will be traveling faster than that near the vessel walls and therefore the Doppler spectrum will display a wide range of frequencies (Fig. 6.1D–F).

The spread of frequencies present within the spectrum at a given point in time is known as the degree of spectral broadening. Figure 6.1 shows the way in which the degree of spectral broadening depends on the velocity profile of the flow being interrogated, with greater spectral broadening seen in Figure 6.1F than in Figure 6.1C. The presence of turbulent flow (e.g., as a result of a stenosis) will increase spectral broadening, as the blood cells will be traveling with different velocities in random directions (see Fig. 5.21). Therefore, increased spectral broadening may indicate the presence of disease. However, the degree of spectral broadening can also be influenced by Doppler instrumentation, and this is known as intrinsic spectral broadening (ISB: discussed later in this chapter).

Nonuniform insonation of the vessel

The examples of idealized spectra given in Figure 6.1 assume that the beam evenly insonates the whole cross-section of the blood vessel in order to detect the correct proportions of all the blood velocities present. This is, however, an unrealistic situation as the Doppler beam can be quite narrow (of the order of 1–2 mm wide) and therefore may insonate only part of the artery or vein. If the beam passes through the center of the vessel (Fig. 6.2A), only part of the flow near the vessel walls (i.e., near the anterior and posterior walls) will be detected. The blood flow along the lateral walls will not be detected as it is not insonated by the Doppler beam. Therefore, in the presence of parabolic flow, the low-velocity flow near the walls will only be partially detected and the Doppler spectrum will no longer truly represent the low-velocity flow present within the vessel.

Sample volume size

The size and position of the sample volume, which can be controlled by the operator, will also affect the proportion of the vessel insonated. A small sample volume placed in the center of a large vessel may not detect any of the flow near the vessel wall (Fig. 6.2D–F). However, a larger sample volume, which could cover the whole depth of

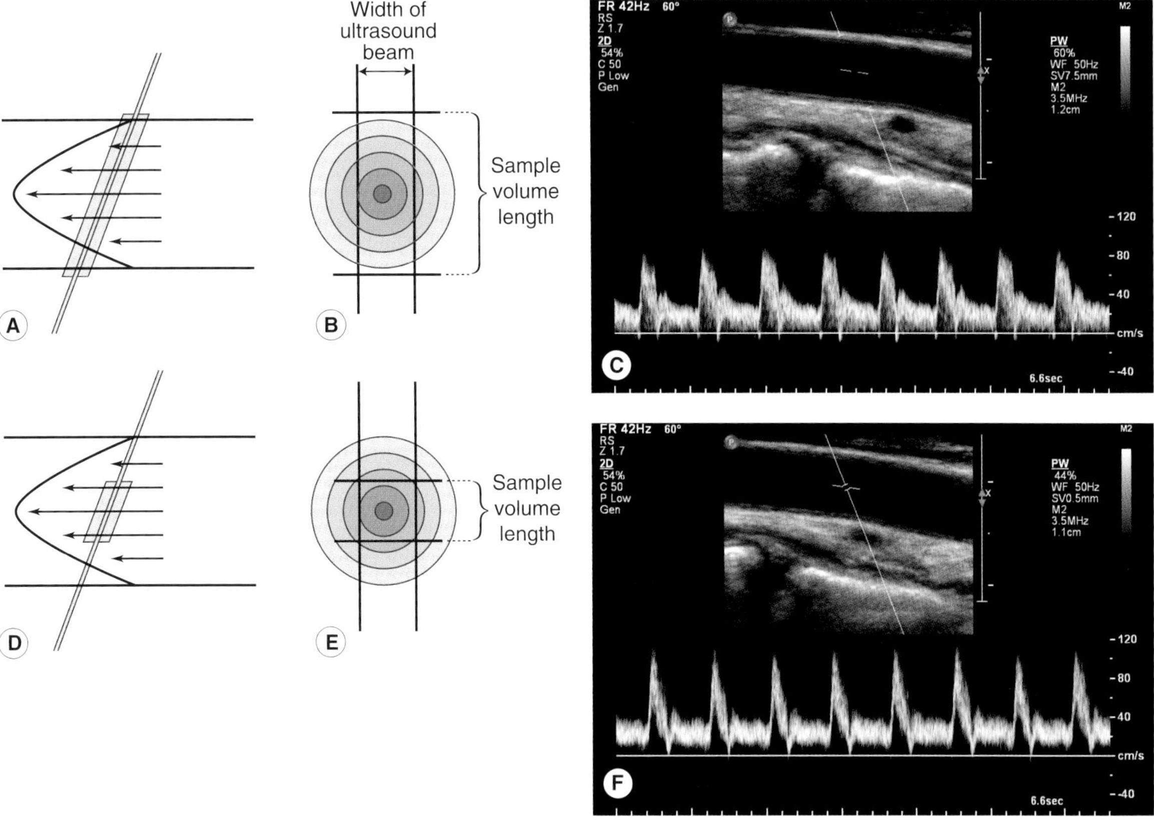

Figure 6.2 • Incomplete insonation of the vessel will occur when a narrow beam is used. The area within the vessel where flow is detected is shown when a large sample volume length (A and B) and a small sample volume length are used (D, E) along with typical Doppler spectra that may be obtained (C and F). Note the absence of low-velocity flow in (F) compared with (C) creating a window under the spectrum.

the vessel (Fig. 6.2A–C), would detect the flow near the anterior and posterior walls but not the lateral walls. The size of the sample volume (i.e., the sensitive region of the beam) will therefore affect the range of Doppler frequencies detected and should be taken into account when interpreting the degree of spectral broadening. The Doppler spectrum obtained with the large sample volume in Figure 6.2C displays low-velocity flow near the baseline, detected from near the vessel walls, and demontrates spectral broadening. The spectrum obtained with a small sample volume, placed in the center of the vessel, shows none of the low flow but has a clear window beneath the detected velocities. A narrow Doppler beam with a small sample volume placed in the center of the vessel may detect only the fast-moving blood and therefore, in normal circumstances, would not demonstrate much spectral broadening. However, in the presence of disease, increased spectral broadening may be seen due to the presence of turbulent flow.

Pulse repetition frequency, high-pass filter and gain

The high frequencies present in the Doppler signal will be incorrectly displayed on the Doppler spectrum if aliasing has occurred as a result of a low pulse repetition frequency (PRF). This results in misleading waveform shapes and errors in velocity measurement. The effect of aliasing is easily visualized, as the Doppler waveform appears to 'wrap around' from the top of the spectrum to the

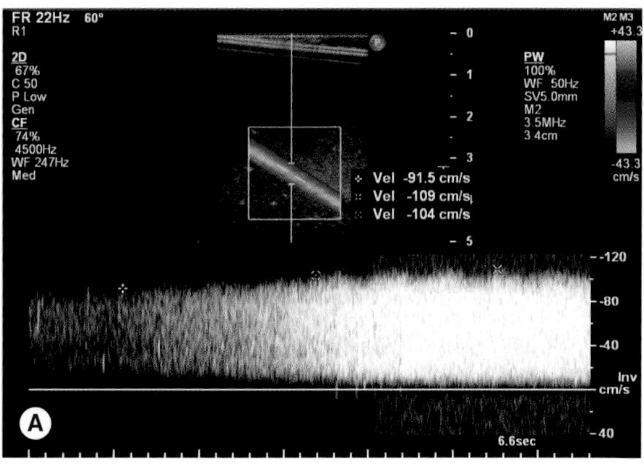

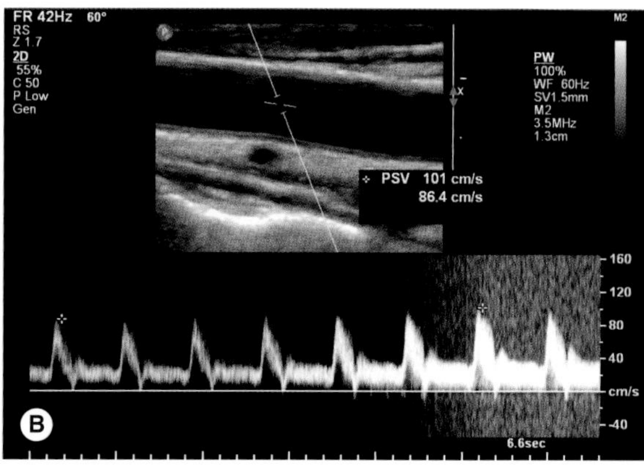

Figure 6.3 • Doppler spectrum detected from a flow phantom (A) with constant flow, and a normal carotid artery (B) obtained as the Doppler gain is increased from left to right. On the left, the gain is too low and the signal is barely detected. On the right, the gain is set too high, leading to saturation of the signal and increased spectral broadening that may lead to an overestimate of the peak velocity. The measured peak velocity can also be seen to change as the gain is increased (from 86 cm/s right side B to 101 cm/s left sibe B).

bottom. Aliasing can be corrected by increasing the PRF.

The shape of the Doppler spectrum can also be altered if the high-pass filter is set too high, removing important information from the spectrum, such as the presence of low-velocity diastolic flow. The gain used to amplify the Doppler signal may also alter the appearance of the spectrum. If the gain is set too low, flow may not be detected. Increasing the gain can increase the appearance of spectral broadening, as shown in Figure 6.3, and may also lead to errors in velocity measurements. An inappropriately high gain can also lead to overloading of the instrument, causing poor direction discrimination, and this may result in a mirror image of the spectrum appearing in the reverse direction on the display (Fig. 6.4). The gain should be set so that the signal is detected but saturation, i.e., complete whitening of the signal, as seen on the right-hand side of the signal in Figure 6.3A&B, does not occur.

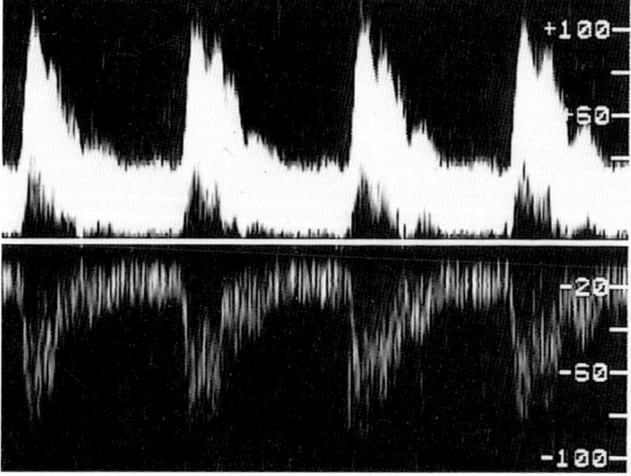

Figure 6.4 • Doppler spectrum demonstrating the appearance of a mirror image below the baseline that may occur when the scanner's Doppler gain control is set too high.

Intrinsic spectral broadening

ISB is broadening of the Doppler spectrum that is an artifact, related to the scanner rather than the blood flow interrogated. Linear and curvilinear array transducers use several elements to form the beam (see Ch. 2). Figure 6.5 shows how the ultrasound beam from a linear array transducer can produce a range of angles of insonation, with the Doppler signals being detected at many angles. As the Doppler shift frequency detected is proportional to the cosine of the angle of insonation, θ, this will lead to a range of frequencies being detected even in the presence of a single target. A test object constructed of a string driven at a

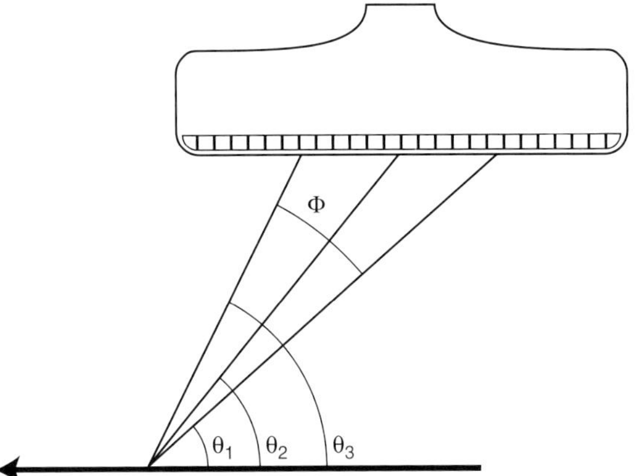

Figure 6.5 • A schematic diagram showing the range of angles of insonation produced by a linear array transducer when making blood velocity measurements. θ_1 and θ_3 represent the smallest and largest angles of insonation generated by the array, respectively, and θ_2 represents the angle produced by the midpoint of the active elements. Φ is the angle produced by the aperture of the active elements generating the Doppler beam. The arrow represents the direction of the blood flow. (Reprinted from Journal of Vascular Investigation, 1:187–192, Thrush and Evans, Intrinsic spectral broadening: a potential cause of misdiagnosis of carotid artery disease, 1995, with permission from Elsevier)

constant speed by a motor can be used to investigate this effect (Fig. 6.6A). The spectrum obtained from the moving string shows that a large range of Doppler shift frequencies have been detected despite the fact that the target is a single object moving at a constant velocity (Fig. 6.6B). This is due to the range of angles of insonation produced from different elements within the active portion of the probe and is the effect known as ISB. The degree of ISB depends on the range of angles over which back-scattered ultrasound is received by the transducer (Φ in Fig. 6.5) – i.e., it depends on the aperture of the transducer – and on the angle of insonation of the beam (θ).

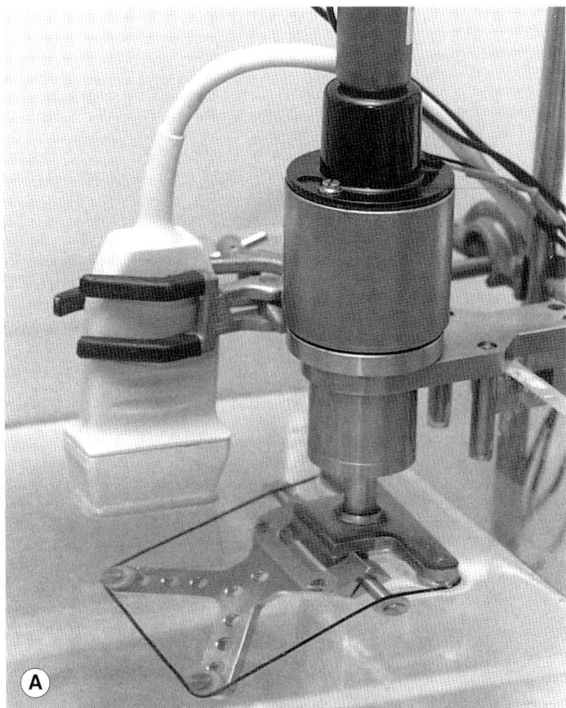

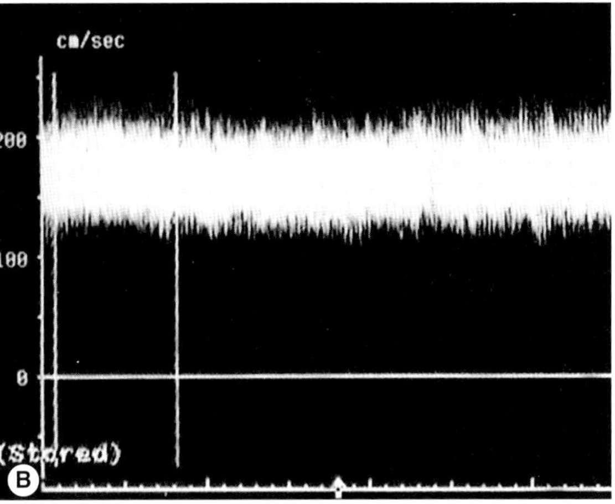

Figure 6.6 • (A) The moving-string test object mounted in a water tank at 45° to the ultrasound transducer. (B) A typical spectrum obtained from the moving string, showing the spread of frequencies detected. (Reprinted from Journal of Vascular Investigation, 1:187–192, Thrush and Evans, Intrinsic spectral broadening: a potential cause of misdiagnosis of carotid artery disease, 1995, with permission from Elsevier)

VELOCITY MEASUREMENTS

Converting Doppler shift frequencies to velocity measurements

The combination of imaging and spectral Doppler ultrasound allows an estimate of the angle of insonation (θ) between the Doppler ultrasound beam and the blood flow. The angle of insonation is measured by lining up the angle correction cursor with the estimated direction of flow.

The Doppler equation (equation 3.1) can be used to estimate the velocity of the blood (V) from the measured Doppler shift frequency (f_d), as the transmitted frequency of the Doppler beam (f_t) is known and the speed of sound in tissue (c) is assumed to be constant (1540 m/s). As the velocity of the blood usually varies across the vessel, a range of velocities will be recorded at any given point in time. The velocity of blood also varies with time, due to the pumping action of the heart. This means that the velocity of the blood is not actually a single value. A choice has to be made as to which value to use to represent the velocity of the blood. The value most commonly used in vascular ultrasound is maximum peak systolic velocity. This is the maximum velocity recorded within the spectrum at the point in time that represents peak systolic flow, as shown on the sonogram in Figure 6.7A. This velocity represents the fastest-moving blood in the vessel. The maximum velocity can similarly be measured at end diastole. These measurements do not take into account the slower-moving blood near the vessel walls.

An alternative is to measure mean velocity at any point in time. This can be calculated by the scanner by finding the average of all the velocities recorded at an instant in time, as shown as a black line superimposed on the Doppler spectrum in Figure 6.7B. As with maximum velocity, the mean velocity will change during the cardiac cycle. If the mean velocity for each line of the sonogram is averaged over a complete cardiac cycle, this will give the value known as the time-averaged velocity (TAV). This can be used to estimate volume flow (discussed later in this chapter).

Many diagnostic criteria are based on velocity ratios rather than on absolute velocity measurements. For example, stenoses may be categorized by the velocity ratio of the maximum peak systolic

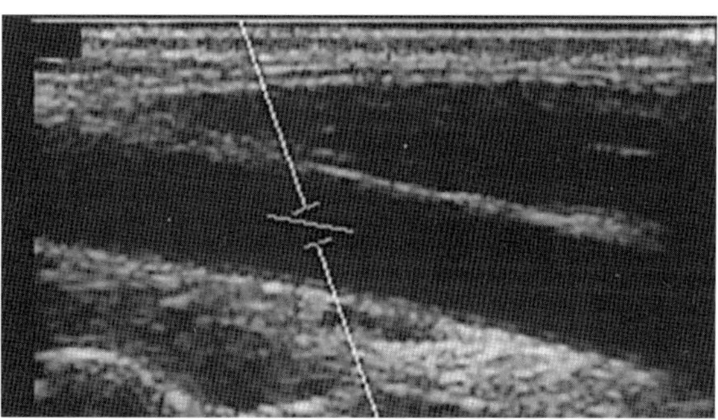

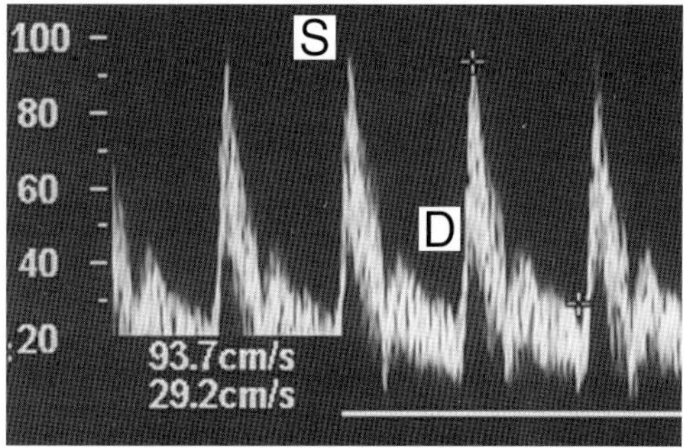

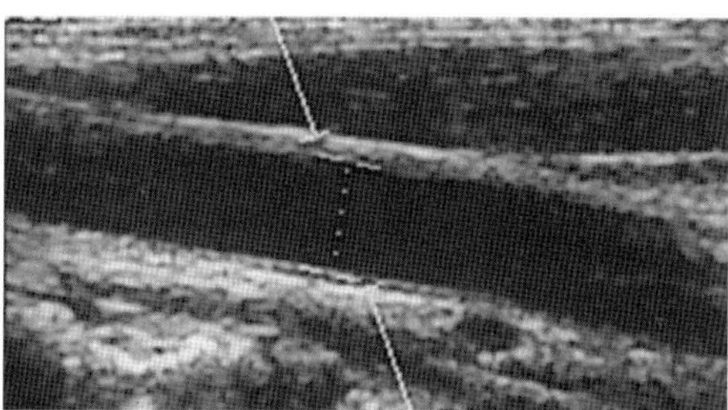

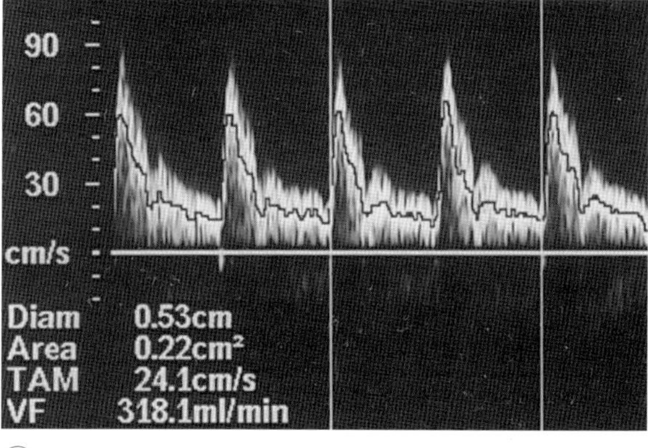

Figure 6.7 • (A) Doppler spectrum showing the measurement of maximum peak systolic velocity, *S*, and maximum end-diastolic velocity, *D*. (B) The mean velocity can be calculated from the Doppler spectrum, displayed by the black line. A large sample volume will allow the blood velocity at the anterior and posterior walls, as well as in the center of the vessel, to be estimated but may not detect the flow along the lateral wall. The time-averaged mean velocity, TAM, can be found by averaging the mean velocity over one or more complete cardiac cycles. Volume flow can be calculated by multiplying the TAM measurement by the cross-sectional area of the vessel (displayed bottom left).

velocity within the stenosis, V_{sten}, divided by the maximum peak systolic velocity in the normal proximal vessel, V_{prox}:

$$\text{Velocity ratio} = \frac{V_{sten}}{V_{prox}} \tag{6.1}$$

Errors in maximum velocity measurements relating to the angle of insonation

An estimate of the angle of insonation is required to convert the detected Doppler shift frequency into a velocity measurement. Any inaccuracy in placing the angle correction cursor parallel to the direction of flow will lead to an error in the estimated angle of insonation. This in turn will lead to an error in the velocity measurement. The velocity calculation depends on the cosθ term, so the error created will be greater for larger angles of insonation. Figure 6.8 shows the relationship between the percentage error in the velocity measurement as the angle of insonation increases where there is a 5° error in the placement of the angle correction cursor. For example, Figure 6.8 shows that this 5° error in cursor placement causes an error in velocity measurement of 23% when the angle of insonation is 65°. In order to minimize this error, angles of insonation of greater than 60% should not be used. However, estimating the angle of insonation is not always straightforward, especially in the presence of disease. Some of the limitations are listed below.

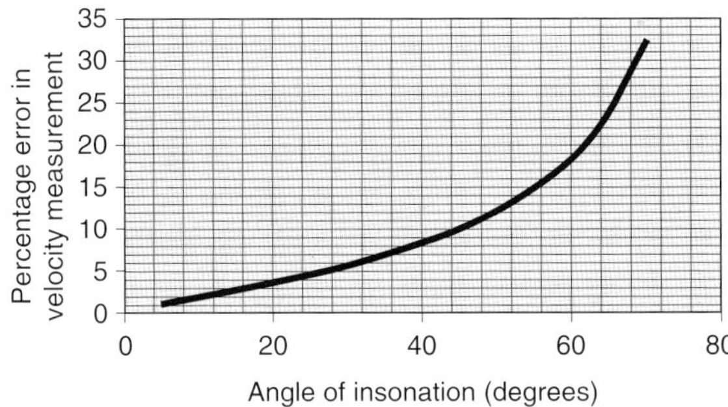

Figure 6.8 • Graph showing the relationship between the percentage error in the velocity measurements as the angle of insonation increases, for a 5° error in the placement of the angle correction cursor. (After Evans D H & McDicken W N 2000 Doppler ultrasound: physics, instrumentation, and signal processing. © John Wiley & Sons Limited, with permission.)

Errors relating to the direction of flow relative to the vessel walls

The direction of the blood flow may not be parallel to the vessel wall, especially in the presence of a stenosis, vortices, or helical flow. Therefore, in these cases aligning the angle correction cursor parallel to the walls may lead to large errors. If there is a clear image of the flow channel through a narrowing it may be possible to line up the angle cursor with the flow channel. However, the maximum velocity may be just beyond the stenosis, and the direction of flow may be less obvious at that point. The color image may be used to identify the site of maximum velocity, although this can be misleading as the color image displays mean velocity of the blood in relation to the direction of the beam, so is dependent on the angle of insonation. What appears to be the maximum velocity on the image may instead be the site at which the angle between the Doppler beam and the direction of the blood flow is smallest. It is important to consider this when estimating the site of maximum velocity and the direction of flow from the color image. The blood velocity may need to be measured at a few points through and beyond a stenosis to ensure the highest velocity has been obtained.

Errors relating to the out-of-imaging plane angle of insonation

It is important to remember that the interception of the ultrasound beam with the blood flow occurs in a three-dimensional space and not just in the two-dimensional plane shown on the image. An underestimate of the true velocity will be obtained if the out-of-imaging plane angle of insonation is not close to 0°. Therefore, the transducer should be aligned with a reasonable length of the vessel, as seen on the image, to ensure a minimal error.

Creation of a range of insonation angles by the Doppler ultrasound beam aperture

The large aperture used by linear and curvilinear array transducers not only results in ISB but also leads to another problem. For velocity to be calculated from the Doppler shift frequency, the cosθ term is required, but clearly only a single value for the angle can be used. Substituting the two extreme angles shown in Figure 6.5 (θ_1 and θ_3) into the Doppler equation would give different values for the velocity. A decision has to be made as to which angle is most suitable for use in converting the detected Doppler frequency into velocity. Typically, ultrasound scanners use the angle between the center of the active elements and the direction of flow (i.e., angle θ_2). This would be an appropriate angle to select for estimation of the mean velocity, but it leads to an overestimation of the calculated maximum velocity. In fact, in order to obtain a correct value for the peak velocity from the frequency spectrum, the smallest angle of insonation present (i.e., θ_1) should be used; however, this is not under the sonographer's control.

Figure 6.9 gives an example of the possible errors in peak velocity measurements on a typical ultrasound scanner caused by ISB. The graphs show that the larger the angle of insonation, the greater the potential source of error in velocity measurement. It is therefore important not to use a Doppler angle greater than 60°. These overestimates in peak velocity measurements could lead to an overestimate in the degree of narrowing unless the ISB produced by a given scanner is taken into account when developing velocity criteria for the quantification of disease. Early duplex scanners, before the development of linear array transducers, used single-element Doppler probes that produce low ISB. The velocity measurements made using these older ultrasound scanners were not prone to ISB errors, and therefore the velocity criteria produced using them may differ from those produced using linear array transducers. The error produced due to spectral broadening can vary with changes in the active aperture that accompany changes in the sample volume depth or changes in position of the Doppler beam in relation to the transducer face, i.e., center, left, or right. The error also varies among manufacturers. It is therefore recommended that departments compare their ultrasound results with those obtained from angiography or other imaging techniques.

Diagnosis of vascular disease often depends on velocity ratio measurements, and these are not affected by the errors produced by ISB as long as both measurements used to calculate the ratio are made with a similar angle of insonation. If the velocity ratios are calculated using two velocity measurements made with significantly different angles of insonation, significant errors may be introduced.

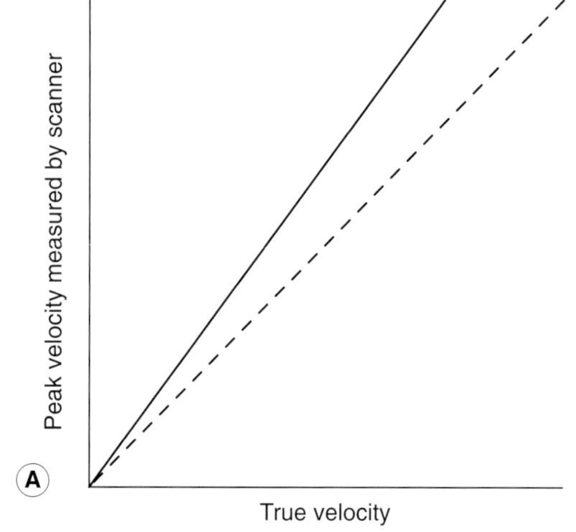

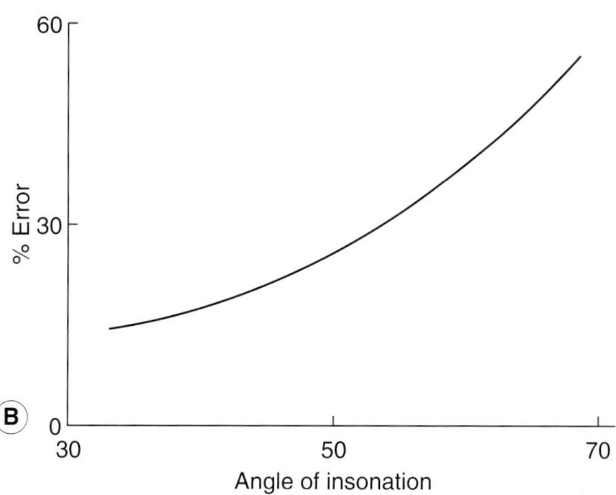

Figure 6.9 • (A) Graph showing an example of the overestimation of peak velocity measured at a given angle of insonation by a typical linear array transducer due to intrinsic spectral broadening (solid line). Dashed line shows correct value of velocity. (B) Graph showing an example of how the error in peak velocity measurements may increase with an increase in the angle of insonation.

Optimizing the angle of insonation

Ideally, the angle of insonation for estimating velocity measurement should be zero to minimize errors; however, as peripheral vessels often lie parallel to the skin, this is not possible. No single choice of angle of insonation is completely reliable, especially when comparisons between velocity measurements are being made. The possibilities are discussed below.

Velocity ratio measurements

Ideally the angle of insonation used to make the velocity measurement proximal to and at the stenosis should be similar. This will result in the two velocities having similar systematic errors that will cancel out when calculating the ratio.

Absolute velocity measurements

There are two schools of thought about selecting the angle of insonation when making absolute velocity measurements:

1. Always set the angle of insonation to 60°.

This ensures that any error in alignment of the angle correction cursor only leads to a moderate error in the velocity estimate (Fig. 6.9) and that the errors caused by ISB are kept similar between measurements. However, it can be difficult to insonate all vessels at a fixed 60° angle.

2. Always select as small an angle of insonation as possible.

This ensures that any error in the alignment of the angle correction cursor produces as small an error in velocity estimation as possible. The error due to ISB will also be minimized. However, this error will be different for measurements made at different angles of insonation. This may make comparisons between measurements made at different angles less meaningful.

A possible solution is to make velocity measurements at an angle approching 60°, allowing some flexibility in the angle of insonation used whilst minimizing errors due to measurements being made with widely varing angles of insonation. Doppler criteria developed over the years may not have been produced with a full understanding of all these possible sources of error. Different models of ultrasound system may produce different results for the same blood flow. However, despite these sources of error, velocity measurements have been successfully used to quantify vascular disease for the past three decades. A greater understanding of the sources of error in velocity measurement may lead to improvements in accuracy.

Other potential sources of error in maximum-velocity measurements

Figure 3.7 has shown how high-pass filters can be used to remove unwanted signals. The high-pass filter setting will not affect the peak systolic velocity measurements, but the shape of the peak velocity envelope (the outline of the spectrum) may be affected if the filter is set so high that it removes the diastolic flow. This would lead to an incorrect finding that the end-diastolic velocity is zero. Figure 3.14 shows how aliasing will lead to an underestimation in the mean velocity and the maximum velocity due to the incorrect estimation of the high frequencies present within the signal. Noise may be introduced into the Doppler signal, especially if the signal is recorded at depth, requiring significant amplification. The maximum Doppler frequency may be difficult to define in the presence of high levels of noise.

MEASUREMENT OF VOLUME FLOW

Volume flow is a potentially useful physiological parameter (see Fig. 5.4) that can be measured using ultrasound, although it involves several possible sources of error (Evans & McDicken 2000). An estimation of the volume flow of blood can be made if the cross-sectional area of the vessel and the velocity of the blood through the vessel are known. Ultrasound scanners usually have the facility to perform volume flow measurements by enabling the sonographer to measure diameter or cross-sectional area from the image and then to measure the TAV from the Doppler spectrum, calculating the flow as follows:

$$\text{Flow} = \text{cross-sectional area} \times \text{TAV} \qquad (6.2)$$

The most straightforward method of obtaining the vessel cross-sectional area is to measure the vessel diameter (d) and calculate the area as follows:

$$A = \frac{\pi d^2}{4} \qquad (6.3)$$

Some scanners also allow the sonographer to outline the circumference of the vessel, imaged in transverse section, using a cursor. This method tends to be less reliable as it requires a steady hand and a good image of the lateral walls of the vessel. The cross-sectional area can then be multiplied by the TAV to give the flow, as shown in Figure 6.7B.

Sources of error in vessel diameter measurement

Errors in either the velocity measurement or the diameter measurement will introduce errors into the estimation of volume flow. As flow is proportional to the cross-sectional area of the vessel, which in turn depends on the square of the radius, any error in the diameter will produce a fractional error in the flow measurement that is double the fractional error in the radius. The possible sources of error in vessel diameter measurement are discussed below.

Image resolution

The ability to image an object is dependent on the resolution of the scanner, as described in Chapter 2. The resolution along the axis of the beam is better than that across the image (i.e., the lateral resolution). The axial resolution is of the order of the wavelength of the ultrasound. For example, the wavelength of a 3 MHz transducer is 0.5 mm, whereas the wavelength of a 10 MHz transducer is 0.15 mm, the latter therefore providing more accurate distance measurements. Lateral measurements are much less accurate, as a result of the poorer image resolution and reduced image quality due to the beam being parallel to the vessel wall. The vessel diameter is especially difficult to measure in the presence of disease.

Calliper velocity calibration

Accurate diameter measurements rely on correct calliper velocity calibration. Most scanners assume the mean sound velocity in tissue to be 1540 m/s; however, the velocity of sound in blood is actually 1580 m/s. This results in a systematic underestimate of the order of 2.6% in diameter measurement, leading to a 5% error in cross-sectional area.

Variable vessel diameter

The arterial diameter is not, in fact, constant but varies during the cardiac cycle due to the changing pressure within the vessel. This means that a single measurement of the diameter may not be representative of the mean diameter. It has been shown that vessel wall pulsatility may result in up to a 10% change in vessel diameter between systole and diastole. This cyclical variation in diameter will lead to errors in volume flow estimation, but it may be reduced by taking several diameter measurements and finding a mean value. Ideally, an instantaneous diameter measurement should be multiplied by the instantaneous mean velocity to obtain a more accurate volume flow measurement, but this technique is not currently available on commercial ultrasound scanners.

Noncircularity of the vessel lumen

The calculation of cross-sectional area from the diameter measurement assumes that the vessel lumen is circular, which may not be the case, especially in the presence of disease.

Errors in measuring TAV

Incomplete insonation of the vessel will lead to an underestimation of the proportion of slower-moving blood at the vessel wall, which in turn will lead to errors in the mean velocity measurements. For example, if a Doppler recording is obtained from a vessel with parabolic flow using a narrow beam (as shown in Fig. 6.2A and B), the high-velocity flow in the center of the vessel will be adequately sampled, but a large proportion of the slower-moving blood at the vessel wall will not be detected. When the mean velocity is calculated from the spectra, this will be an overestimate of the true mean velocity due to the undersampling of the flow at the lateral edges of the vessel. This is true even if the sample volume is set to cover the near and far walls of the vessel as the out-of-imaging plane flow will not be sampled. Incomplete insonation of the vessel can lead to errors of up to 30% in the TAV (Evans & McDicken 2000).

Alternatively, the mean TAV can be estimated from the maximum TAV if the flow is measured at an adequate distance from geometric changes (e.g., bifurcations or stenosis) and the shape of the flow profile in the vessel is known. If there is a blunt flow, the maximum velocity will be equal to the mean velocity across the vessel. However, if the velocity is parabolic then the maximum velocity will be twice the value of the mean. One advantage of the maximum velocity measurement is that it is not affected by the width of the beam, provided the beam passes through the center of the vessel.

If the wall thump filter is set too high, the low-frequency signals from the slower moving flow will be removed, and this would lead to an overestimate in the mean velocity. Aliasing would lead to underestimation of the mean velocity due to the incorrect estimation of the high frequencies present within the signal. The presence of high-amplitude noise will bias the estimate of the mean velocity, as the Doppler system is unable to differentiate between the noise and the Doppler signals.

WAVEFORM ANALYSIS

As well as the blood velocity and flow changing with the presence of significant disease, the shape of the waveform will also be altered (as discussed in Ch. 5). The waveform may indicate whether the disease is proximal or distal to the site at which the Doppler signal is obtained. Over the years, several researchers have attempted to quantify these changes in waveform shape by defining various indices, and many modern scanners incorporate facilities to calculate such quantities, some of which are listed below.

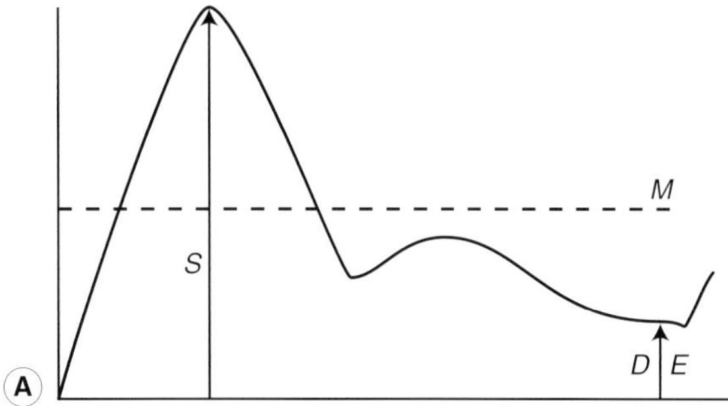

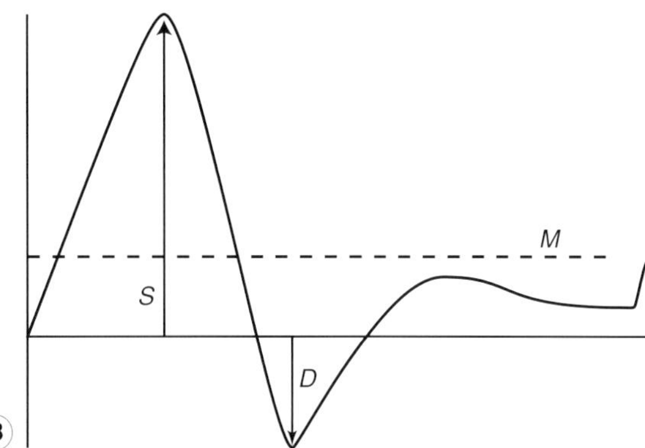

Figure 6.10 • Pulsatility index (A and B) and resistance index (A) can be calculated from the peak systolic, *S*, minimum diastolic, *D*, end-diastolic, *E*, and mean velocity (or frequency), *M*, shown here on two different waveforms.

Pulsatility index

The pulsatility index (PI) is probably the most commonly used of all the indices. It can be used to quantify the degree of pulse wave damping at different measurement sites. It is defined as the maximum height of the waveform, *S*, minus the minimum diastolic, *D* (which may be negative), divided by the mean height, *M*, as shown in Figure 6.10:

$$PI = \frac{S - D}{M} \tag{6.4}$$

Damped flow beyond significant disease will have a lower PI value than a normal pulsatile waveform.

Pourcelot's resistance index

The resistance index (RI) was first used on common carotid waveforms as an indicator of the peripheral resistance and has also been used to study neonatal cerebral hemodynamics. It is defined as follows (Fig. 6.10A):

$$RI = \frac{S - E}{S} \tag{6.5}$$

where *E* is end-diastolic velocity. The value of RI can be calculated by the scanner and displayed on the screen.

Spectral broadening

There have been several definitions of spectral broadening (SB) described over the years in an attempt to quantify the spread of frequencies present within a spectrum. One such definition is as follows:

$$SB = \frac{f_{max} - f_{min}}{f_{max}} \tag{6.6}$$

Increased spectral broadening indicates the presence of arterial disease but can, to some extent, also be introduced by the scanner itself, as in ISB (described above).

Pulse wave velocity

The pressure pulse and the associated velocity wave travel along the vessel at a different speed from the flowing blood. The speed at which the pulse is transmitted along the vessel depends on the elasticity of the vessel wall. For example, the pulse will travel much faster down the stiff-walled artery of a diabetic patient than down the normal artery of a younger person. The pulse wave velocity of a pulse can be measured using two Doppler transducers to detect the transit time of the pulse along a known length of vessel. The transit time is given by the delay in the beginning of the pulse detected distally compared with that detected by the proximally positioned transducer (Fig. 6.11). The pulse wave velocity is given by the distance along the vessel between the two transducers divided by the transit time. Measurement of the pulse wave velocity has been used by researchers to study vessel wall elasticity changes (e.g., with age or diabetes).

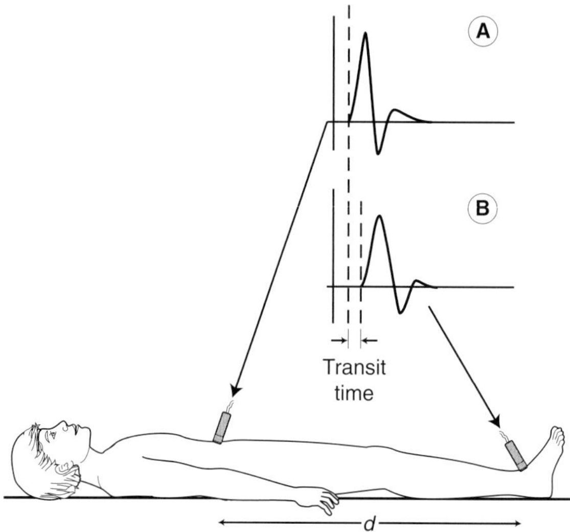

Figure 6.11 • The pulse wave velocity can be calculated using two transducers at a distance d apart along the vessel and measuring the transit time of the pulse.

Subjective interpretation

Subjective interpretation of the Doppler spectrum can give many clues as to the level and extent of any disease. For example, changes in the pulsatility of the waveform shape can help to identify disease. The systolic rise time of the waveform is influenced by changes in the cardiac impulse and circulation proximal to the measurement site, whereas the decay of the velocity tends to relate to the distal circulation. Even if these various indices are not quantified, understanding the concept behind them can help when interpreting waveform shapes.

References

Evans D H, McDicken W N 2000 Doppler ultrasound: physics, instrumentation, and signal processing. Wiley, Chichester

Thrush A J, Evans D H 1995 Intrinsic spectral broadening: a potential cause of misdiagnosis of carotid artery disease. Journal of Vascular Investigation 1: 187–192

Optimizing the scan

CONTENTS

INTRODUCTION

The preceding chapters have covered some of the basic scientific principles behind ultrasound, the Doppler effect, and hemodynamics. The sonographer should now have a clearer understanding of how a B-mode image is created and how color flow imaging can be used to interrogate blood flow in vessels rapidly, allowing the blood flow in selected areas to be assessed with spectral Doppler. This has made duplex scanning a powerful technique for the investigation of patients with vascular diseases, and many vascular surgeons are making clinical decisions on the basis of duplex scanning alone. It is therefore vitally important that the operator understands the use of the scanner controls and the limitations of the technique. Some manufacturers have introduced auto-optimization controls, but there are still many situations in which the controls will need to be adjusted manually. Manufacturers often use different names or terms for the same scanner control or function, such as power imaging and color angiography, both of which relate to power Doppler imaging. Another interchangeable control used by manufacturers is pulse repetition frequency (PRF) and scale. It is important to consult the operator's manual or ask the manufacturer if the function of any control is not clear.

Ultrasound scanners have a range of examination-specific presets that optimize the system for a particular examination and it is important to start the scan with the appropriate preset selected. However, in many instances the scanner controls need adjusting, or optimizing, to demonstrate pathology. In addition, a number of imaging and Doppler artifacts may be confused or misinterpreted as significant disease, leading to serious diagnostic errors. The aim of this chapter is to introduce the sonographer to the practical aspects of scanning, covering the basic use of scanner controls and reiterating some of the principles discussed in the preceding chapters. Imaging artifacts will also be discussed to assist the sonographer in the interpretation of images. It is likewise essential that the sonographer has a good understanding of the principles relating to ultrasound safety in order to minimize any exposure risks to the patient.

THE PATIENT

It is an ironic fact that a sonographer may use a state-of-the-art duplex scanner but fail to obtain any useful diagnostic information because of an inadequate approach to the examination and the patient. For example, an introduction and simple explanation of the test may put patients more at ease and willing to cooperate, especially if they are nervous or in some discomfort. Local protocols that are rigid and do not allow any flexibility can also lead to problems. For example, a protocol that requires that patients always be completely flat with the head fully extended during carotid scans may lead to severe discomfort for patients with breathing difficulties, dizziness, angina, or spondylosis of the neck. It is possible they will not be able to tolerate the examination at all. An alternative would be to perform the scan with the patient sitting up on a low chair. It is still possible to obtain good images from this scanning position. Most problems can be solved with a little careful thought and the occasional inventive approach.

STARTING THE SCAN

Advice

In most circumstances, start the scan with a cross-sectional survey of the region of interest before a longitudinal scan, as this helps to relate structures to each other and makes the anatomy easier to identify. For instance, the position of carotid bifurcation is easier to locate in cross-section by sweeping the transducer up the neck.

Image orientation

CROSS-SECTION

The general covention is to orient the image as if you are looking at the patient. For instance, the right saphenofemoral junction will appear on the right-hand side of the screen and the left saphenofemoral junction on the left side of the screen.

LONGITUDINAL OR SAGITTAL

The general convention is to have the direction of the patient's head on the left side of the screen and the foot direction towards the right side of the screen.

The scan should be carried out in a dimly lit room to optimize visualization of the black and white image. The transducer selected should be of the highest frequency that allows adequate penetration to the area to be examined. When scanning, it is important to adopt a logical approach. Using a systematic technique cuts down on examination time and ensures that pathology is less likely to be missed. The scan is best started by examining the region of interest with B-mode imaging alone, to identify relevant structures. Avoid switching on the color flow or spectral Doppler straight away, unless they are essential for identifying vessels, as the imaging frame rate will be reduced and the display may be confusing if anatomy has not been clearly identified.

B-MODE CONTROLS

Always set the focal zones at the depth of interest on the scan image. B-mode frame rates of modern scanners are generally high even when multiple focus zones have been selected. If the region of interest in the B-mode image is very small, or very deep, consider using the write zoom control to magnify the area. This will improve the frame rate and allow closer inspection of the anatomy. Many vascular sonographers prefer B-mode images with a reasonable degree of contrast using a lower dynamic range. Duplex systems have examination-specific presets that are optimized to produce the best images of vascular structures. It is also worthwhile experimenting with different pre- and postprocessing controls in order to understand the function of these controls. Try this when imaging a carotid plaque and note the difference in the appearance of the image. Optimize the total gain and depth gain compensation sliders so that the returning echoes are of relatively uniform intensity throughout the image. In general, the gain should be set so that the lumen of any large nondiseased vessel appears clear or black but any further increase in gain would introduce noise or speckle. Harmonic imaging can be especially useful in the abdomen and may produce clearer and less noisy images. The use of compound imaging, may also improve the overall image.

IMAGING ARTIFACTS

An imaging artifact is a feature on the image that does not relate exactly to a structure within the tissue being investigated. This can be due to a feature being misplaced on the image, a feature appearing that is not present within the tissue, or an existing structure that is absent from the image. The creation of an image relies on the assumption that the ultrasound beam travels in a straight path between the transducer and the structures within the tissue and returns along the same path once reflected. It is also assumed that the attenuation of tissue is constant. Any process that alters this situation can lead to the misplacement or absence of information. This can be caused by the following:

- Multiple reflections can lead to reverberation artifacts, seen as several equidistant echoes that reduce in brightness with depth. This is due to multiple reflections, along the same path, between the transducer and a strongly reflecting boundary (Fig. 7.1A) or between two parallel, strongly reflecting surfaces (Fig. 7.1B). If the

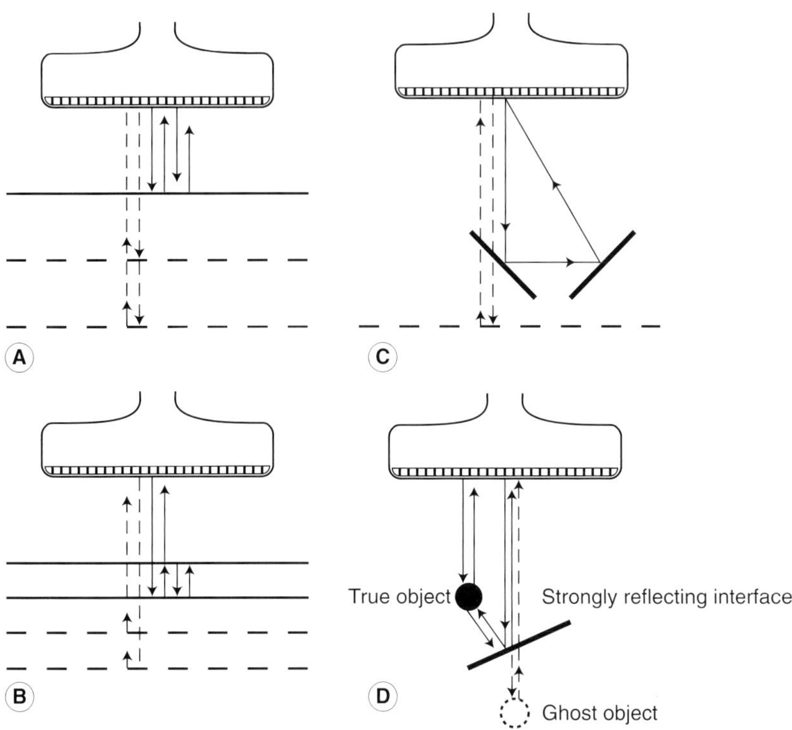

Figure 7.1 • Imaging artifacts can be produced by multiple reflections from strongly reflecting surfaces. The solid line shows the true path of the ultrasound beam. The dashed lines show the path of the beam assumed by the ultrasound scanner and the assumed interfaces displayed on the ultrasound images. (A) Multiple reflections between the transducer and a strongly reflecting boundary. (B) Multiple reflections between two parallel, strongly reflecting surfaces. (C) Multiple reflections not returning along the same path. (D) Mirror image produced in the presence of a strongly reflecting surface.

multiple reflections do not return along the same path, the structure may be misplaced on the image (Fig. 7.1C).

- A mirror image of a structure can be produced in the presence of a strongly reflecting surface. Figure 7.1D shows how the true position of a structure is displayed, with a second ghost image also displayed. The ghost image has been created by an ultrasound beam that has undergone multiple reflections from the strongly reflecting surface.
- Refraction can lead to bending of the path of the ultrasound when the beam passes through an interface between two media in which the speed of sound is significantly different (see Fig. 2.7).
- Range ambiguity can occur if an echo from the previously transmitted pulse is received back from a distant boundary after the current ultrasound pulse has been transmitted. The scanner will assume that the echo is from the current pulse and place it nearer to the top of the image rather than at its true depth.
- Grating lobes are areas of lower-intensity ultrasound outside the main beam and are produced as a function of the multi-element structure of array transducers. These grating lobes can lead to strongly reflecting surfaces outside the main beam being displayed in the image.

The image in Figure 7.2 shows how an artifact, created by multiple reflections from a strongly reflecting surface such as the vein wall or a muscle boundary, can give the appearance of a dissection, or tear, of the carotid artery wall. If an artifact is suspected, the vessel should be imaged in different planes or from different angles by tilting the transducer. The artifact may then appear in a different position relative to the vessel or may not appear at all, confirming that it is not a true structure that has been visualized. It is usually easier to identify artifacts in real-time imaging than on a frozen image. If there is a significant difference in the attenuation seen by different scan lines, the tissue at depth may appear as different levels of gray, despite having similar back-scatter properties (Fig. 7.3). For example, the tissue beneath a low-attenuation, anechoic region, may appear brighter than adjacent areas (see Fig. 13.32B). Highly attenuating tissue, however, such as calcified plaque, can cause loss of ultrasound information beneath the region, leading to a shadow (Fig. 8.27).

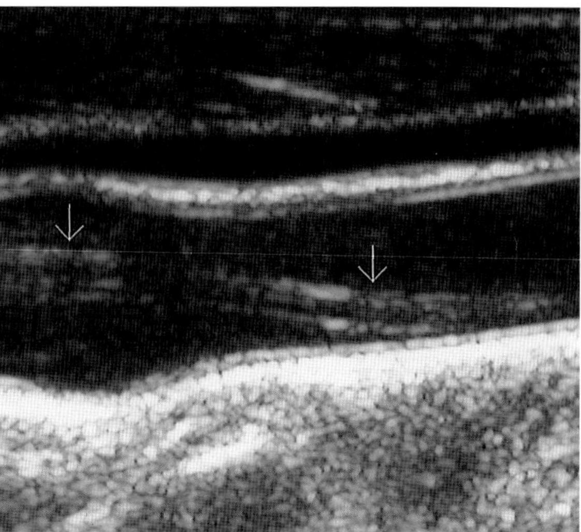

Figure 7.2 • An image showing how an artifact (arrow) can give the impression of a dissection, or tear, of the carotid artery wall.

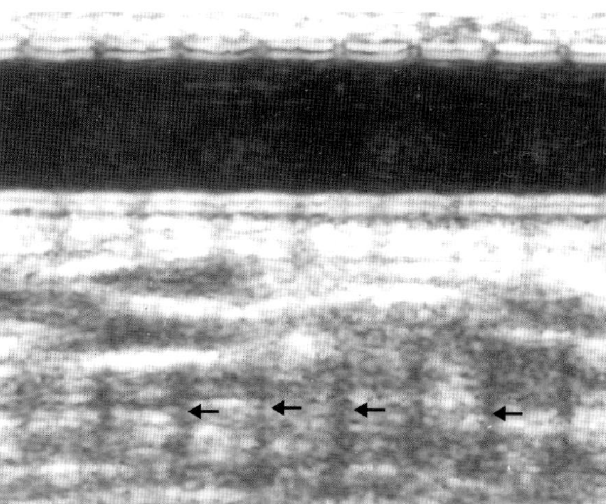

Figure 7.3 • Differences in attenuation can be observed in this image of a synthetic bypass graft. The graft has spaced external supporting rings that are causing increased attenuation in the tissue lying below the rings (arrows).

COLOR DOPPLER CONTROLS

Color pulse repetition frequency

PRF, sometimes called scale, on scanner controls should be adjusted to optimize the image of the blood flow in the vessel under examination. Many duplex systems display the value of the PRF in hertz. However, some systems only indicate the PRF as a mean velocity on the color bar, in centimeters per second, or specify the sampling rate as high-, medium-, or low-velocity flow. The examination preset selects a nominal PRF to start a specific examination. The PRF is generally set moderately high for sampling normal arterial flow, typically a PRF of 3000 Hz, so that the peak systolic phase of the cardiac cycle appears in the upper portion of the color scale without aliasing, as demonstrated in Figure 4.9B. If the PRF is set too low, aliasing will be demonstrated in a normal vessel during the peak systolic phase, making it more difficult to identify areas of true flow disturbance. If the PRF is set too high, the peak systolic phase of the cardiac cycle will appear in the lower region of the color scale, flow changes will be less well differentiated on the image, and minor flow disturbances could be overlooked. Low-velocity flow in diastole may also go undetected.

In situations in which there is significant pathology, the flow velocities may be much lower than normal. For example, the flow velocities in a calf artery distal to a long superficial femoral and popliteal artery occlusion may be very low. Using a default PRF setting of 3000 Hz may not adequately demonstrate the low-velocity flow in the patent calf artery because the sampling rate is too high (Fig. 7.4). The PRF should be lowered to demonstrate the low-velocity flow, showing the systolic phase in the upper part of the color scale (Fig. 7.4C). By optimizing the PRF for the flow velocities present in a vessel, it is possible to investigate longer segments of an artery using color flow imaging, reducing the amount of time spent taking spectral Doppler measurements, provided that the color display does not indicate any changes in velocity. Color aliasing is an artifact rather than the representation of a true change in flow direction. If a vessel changes direction it can result in a change in insonation angle (and thus to detected velocity), leading to a change in color. In this situation, angle-corrected spectral Doppler should be used to record the flow velocities in the vessel, to confirm the absence of a stenosis, as the peak systolic velocity should remain the same despite the change in vessel direction.

The flow velocities recorded in the venous system are lower than those recorded in the arterial system and therefore the PRF will have to be lowered. A PRF setting of 1000 Hz is a typical starting value for many venous examinations. Most ultrasound systems link the high-pass filter to the PRF, and in most examinations there may be little need to make any adjustments to the filter setting. However, in situations in which there may be very low-velocity flow, such as that found in a suboccluded internal carotid artery, the filter should be lowered as far as possible to avoid missing the flow. Conversely, the color filter can be increased to cut out the low-frequency noise, such as that produced by bowel movement seen when scan-

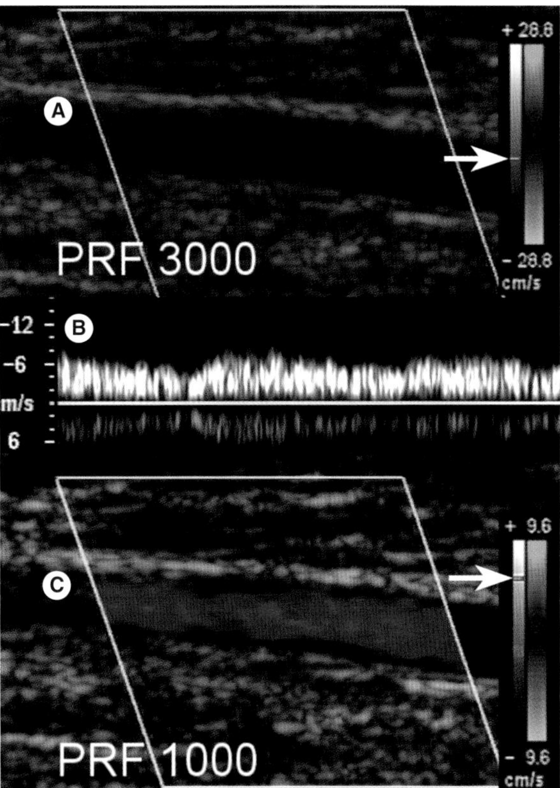

Figure 7.4 • (A) Poor color filling is seen in the posterior tibial artery distal to a long arterial occlusion because the pulse repetition frequency (PRF) is set too high at 3000 Hz, and the color controls have not been optimized. (B) The Doppler waveform confirms low-velocity damped flow with a peak systolic velocity of 8 cm/s. (C) In order to improve the color flow display, the PRF has been lowered to 1000 Hz, the color write priority increased (arrow), and the color sensitivity control (number of pulses sent per scan line) increased. Note that only 79% color gain is needed in image C, compared to 85% in image A.

ning the iliac arteries. In practice, many experienced sonographers can cope with additional color noise in the image.

Color box angle and size

When using linear array transducers it is possible to steer the color box to the left or right by 20° to 25° depending on the system. It is therefore possible to optimize the color box angle to the flow direction in order to obtain the highest velocities. Inexperienced sonographers often find this one of the most confusing aspects of duplex scanning when learning color Doppler techniques, and it may be a case of trial and error to get used to optimizing the color image. Areas of poor filling in the image may be caused by a poor angle of insonation, preventing the signal from being detected. It may be necessary to image a vessel with the color box steered in more than one direction in order to demonstrate flow in all parts of the vessel (Fig. 7.5). For curvilinear array transducers, it is necessary to optimize the transducer position and the position of the color box in the sector display to obtain suitable Doppler angles.

It is important to keep the color box size reasonably small and to keep the area of interest within it by adjusting the color box or transducer position. Increasing the color box width means that more time is spent producing the color flow image, and consequently the imaging frame rate will decrease; however this is less of a problem in modern duplex systems. Many systems have a control for increasing the color sensitivity, which increases the number of pulses sent down each scan line. This can improve the color image but decreases the overall frame rate. In certain situations, pulsatile low-volume flow in a vessel may be seen as a brief flash of color on the image, and it may be difficult to follow the vessel. Increasing the color persistence will display the color in the vessel for a longer period of time and can make the vessel easier to follow. The color write priority control can be adjusted to write color on an image where a high B-mode gain is necessary (see below).

COLOR IMAGING ARTIFACTS

Color flow imaging artifacts can lead to failure to display flow when, in fact, it is present, as shown in Figure 7.5. A bright black and white imaging artifact (as seen in Fig. 7.2) may be displayed in preference to the color flow information, and this may give the appearance of a structure within the vessel lumen, around which the flow is displayed. If the color write priority is set too low in the presence of a noisy black and white image, flow detected may not be displayed due to the lack of a clear vessel lumen. Giving priority to the color flow imaging means that the B-mode image can be reasonably bright without losing color information on the screen (see Ch. 4).

A strongly reflective or absorbing structure can lead to the loss of ultrasound signals beyond the interface. For example, calcification within the vessel wall or the presence of bowel gas can produce

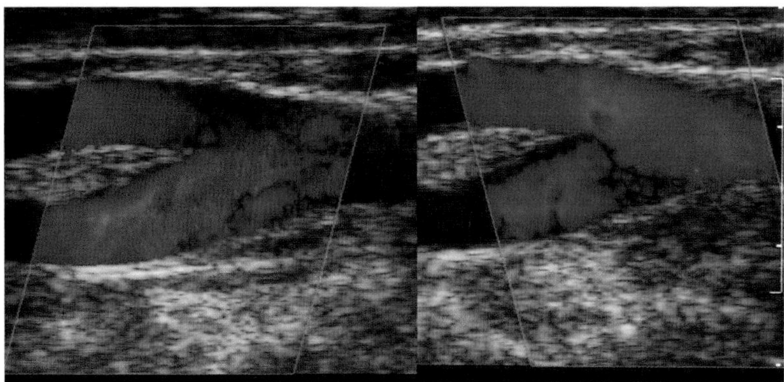

Figure 7.5 • Images of a carotid artery showing how a vessel may need to be imaged with the color box steered in more than one direction to demonstrate flow in the whole vessel.

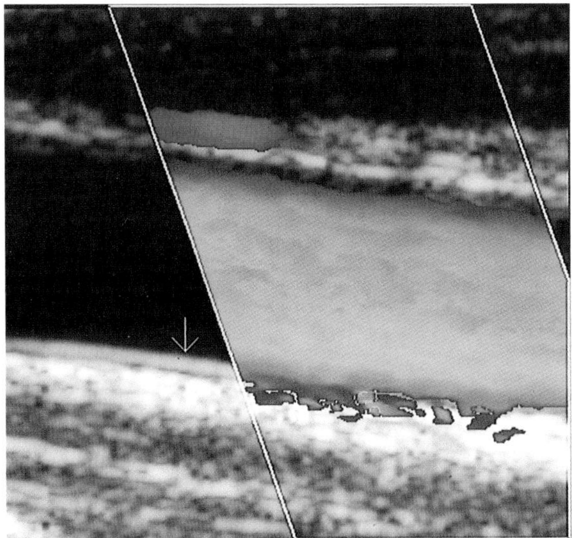

Figure 7.6 • The color flow image may give the impression of flow 'bleeding' out of the vessel if the color gain is set too high (arrow shows position of posterior artery wall).

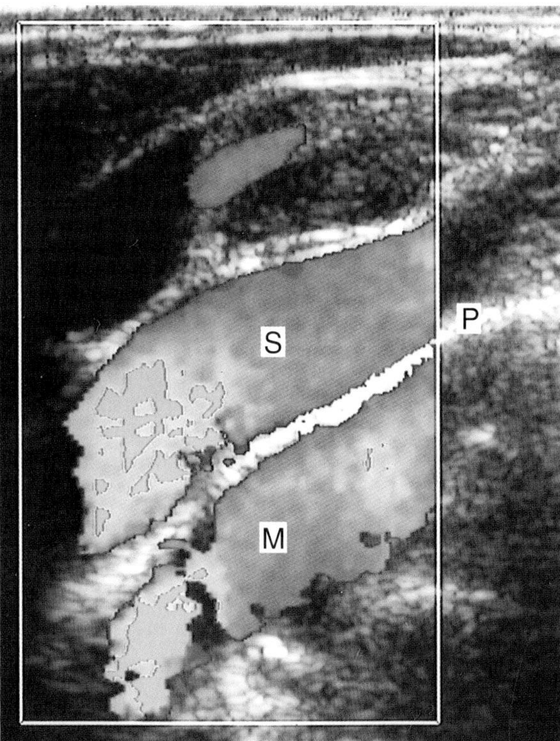

Figure 7.7 • Color image of the subclavian artery (S) with a mirror image (M) below the pleura (P).

shadowing on both the black and white image and color flow image and will prevent spectral Doppler recordings (see Fig. 8.27).

Artifacts can also be introduced into the color image, whereby color is displayed when blood flow is not present. This can occur when the color gain is set too high, giving the appearance of the color 'bleeding' out of the vessel (Fig. 7.6). Alternatively, anechoic areas can be filled with speckled color due to noise, if the gain is set high or if there is low-velocity tissue motion present (e.g., due to respiration). Tissue bruits (e.g., near a stenosis) may result in color appearing outside the vessel wall.

Multiple reflections can produce color image artifacts. Figure 7.7 shows a mirror image of the subclavian artery produced by multiple reflections from the pleura overlying the lung. This mirror image artifact can be seen where a vessel overlies a strongly reflecting surface, such as the tissue–air interface present at the pleura. The tibial vessels or bypass grafts may also suffer from this artifact when lying above bone. The path of the reflected ultrasound that has undergone multiple reflections is different from that of the ultrasound back-scattered directly from the blood to the transducer. Therefore, the Doppler shift frequency detected and displayed for the mirror image may not be the same as for the vessel itself. The artifactual Doppler signal displayed on the color image can also be detected with spectral Doppler, if the sample volume is placed over the mirror image.

The color image may not give a true representation of the relative blood velocities within the vessel. Changes in the angle of insonation, owing to changes in vessel direction, can lead to color imaging artifacts, giving the false impression of changes in blood velocity (see Fig. 4.7). Aliasing artifacts will also change the appearance of the color image (see Figs 4.9A and 4.11).

SPECTRAL DOPPLER OPTIMIZATION

The spectral Doppler PRF should be set to avoid aliasing and the high-pass filter should be set to remove wall thump but not useful Doppler signals. The spectral Doppler PRF may be referred to as 'scale' or 'flow rate' on some systems. The selection of the size of the sample volume is an important consideration. If detailed investigation of flow within a stenosis is to be performed, a small sample volume is required. The sample volume should be placed in the center of the vessel or at the point of maximum velocity indicated by the color image. However, if the presence of flow within a vein is to be detected, a large sample volume may be more appropriate. The issue of spectral Doppler angle correction remains a contentious subject. Some units insist that all measurements be taken with the cursor lined up with the direction of flow at a fixed angle of 60° whereas other departments use the smallest angle of insonation possible (see Ch. 6). The position of the angle correction cursor should be carefully lined up with the vessel wall, or the direction of blood flow, to minimize angle-related errors. There are three possible reasons why a Doppler signal may be displayed both above and below the baseline, and the sonographer should be able to identify these:

1. Aliasing (see Fig. 3.14A)
2. Mirroring due to the gain being set too high (see Fig. 6.4)
3. Flow reversal during the cardiac cycle (see Fig. 5.8).

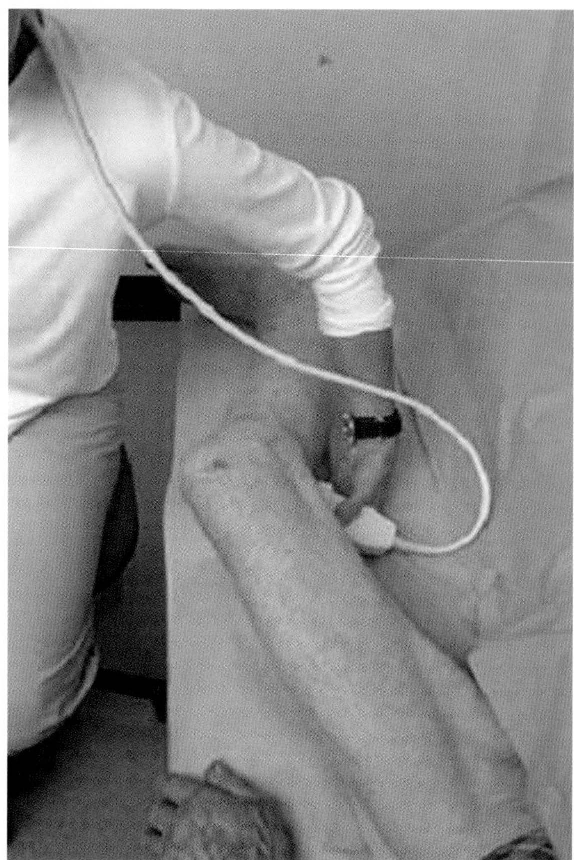

Figure 7.8 • An example of a very poor scanning posture, which is likely to result in repetitive strain injury to the shoulder, arm and wrist.

REPETITIVE STRAIN INJURY AND OCCUPATIONAL HAZARDS

Sonographers are at high risk of developing occupational injuries due to prolonged periods of bad posture during ultrasound examinations (Fig. 7.8). Back problems and repetitive strain injuries of the wrist and shoulder are increasingly common. To minimize the risk it is essential that vascular ultrasound units be equipped with variable-height examination tables that have adjustable upper and lower sections. Ideally, it should be possible to tilt the table, especially for venous examinations. The operator's chair should have a variable-height adjustment, adjustable back rest, and swivel capability. Sonographers should vary the workload and types of scans performed during the day and take regular breaks. The ability to scan with either hand also reduces strain on one side. The probe should not be gripped too hard, and excessive pressure should not be used to make contact between the patient and the probe. Most vascular examinations can be performed with relatively light probe contact. If the sonographer develops problems, these should be treated at an early stage as long-term chronic problems may be difficult to resolve.

SAFETY OF DIAGNOSTIC ULTRASOUND

During the scan, the patient is exposed to ultrasound energy, and it is therefore important that the sonographer be aware of the possible risks and how to minimize them. Over the years there has been a steady increase in the output power generated by ultrasound systems. The potential risks have been regularly assessed by various safety committees, including that of the World Federation of Ultrasound in Medicine and Biology (WFUMB 1998). Information on safety issues can be found on the website of the European Federation of Societies for Ultrasound in Medicine and Biology

(EFSUMB 2006). The British Medical Ultrasound Society has also produced a statement on the safe use and potential hazards of diagnostic ultrasound equipment (BMUS Safety Group 2000).

It is believed that the two main potential risks of tissue damage due to ultrasound exposure are tissue heating and cavitation. Cavitation refers to the formation, growth, oscillation, and violent collapse of small, gas-filled cavities within the ultrasound beam. Inertial cavitation – that is, large variation in size and possible violent collapse of bubbles – occurs above a threshold of negative acoustic pressure (Duck & Shaw 2003).

Ultrasound intensity

The intensity is the energy crossing a unit area (usually 1 cm^2) in unit time. The spatial peak temporal average intensity, I_{spta}, is the peak within the beam averaged over time. Another value of intensity that is used is the spatial peak pulse average intensity, I_{sppa}, which is the spatial peak intensity averaged over the duration of the pulse. These have been used by the US Food and Drug Administration (FDA) to define the upper limit of exposure produced by ultrasound systems for diagnostic use (Table 7.1). Manufacturers often supply data on the maximum I_{spta} and I_{sppa} in the operator's manual.

Mechanical and thermal indices

The output power produced by a system will vary with the modality used and the control settings. So that the ultrasound user can be aware of the potential risks of any given scanner set-up, two, potentially more meaningful indices have been developed. These are the thermal index (TI) and the mechanical index (MI). These indices are displayed on the screen of modern scanners in real time and will demonstrate any changes in the potential risk as the scanner modalities or controls are altered.

The TI has been developed to indicate the potential risk of producing thermal effects during the scan. It is the ratio of acoustic power emitted at the time to the power required to heat the tissue by 1 °C. A TI of 1 would therefore indicate the potential to heat the tissue in the beam by 1 °C. A TI of 2 indicates a potential rise of 2 °C, and so forth. An ultrasound exposure that does not produce a temperature rise of greater than 1.5 °C above normal body temperature of 37 °C is not thought to pose any risk of producing thermal damage. The power required to heat the tissue will depend greatly on what tissue is lying in the path of the ultrasound beam and is especially affected by the presence of bone, as bone is a strongly absorbing medium. For this reason, three models for the TI have been developed:

1. Soft tissue (TIS)
2. Tissue with bone present at the focus (TIB)
3. The cranial thermal index (TIC), used in transcranial Doppler.

The appropriate TI should be displayed depending on the scanner examination set-up selected. The development of these indices suffers from some limitations, as it is not straightforward to estimate the heat lost from the various regions of the body that are scanned.

MI indicates the likelihood of the onset of inertial cavitation. It is related to the peak negative pressure of the ultrasound pulses being used at the time. For an MI of 0.7, the physical conditions probably cannot exist for bubble growth and collapse to occur (Duck & Shaw 2003). However, if this threshold is exceeded, it does not mean that

APPLICATION	DERATED I_{SPTA} (mW/cm^2)	DERATED I_{SPPA} (W/cm^2)	MI	TI
All except ophthalmology	720	190	1.9	(6.0)*
Ophthalmology	50	NS	0.23	1.0

*The upper limit of 6.0 is advisory. At least one of the quantities MI and I_{sppa} must be less than the specified limit.

I_{spta}, spatial peak temporal average intensity; I_{sppa}, spatial peak intensity averaged over the duration of the pulse; MI, mechanical index; TI, thermal index; NS, not specified.

Table 7.1 The upper limits of exposure required by the United States Food and Drug Administration

bioeffects due to cavitation will occur. The higher the value of MI above this threshold, the greater the potential risk. There is currently no evidence that diagnostic ultrasound causes cavitation in soft tissue, except in the presence of gas, such as in the lung and intestines, and in the presence of contrast agents.

Another potential thermal hazard of which the sonographer should be aware is heating of the transducer itself, which may occur if the transducer has been damaged. Malfunction of the scanner may potentially lead to a higher than expected output power.

User's responsibility

Diagnostic ultrasound has been used for many years with no reported evidence of harmful effects. However, it is prudent to keep patient exposure to the minimum required to obtain an optimal diagnostic result. This can be done by keeping the time of the examination of a particular area to a minimum, especially when using color and spectral Doppler ultrasound, as these modes are more likely to cause heating. Controls such as the gain should be optimized before increasing the output power. Changes in the TI and MI with changes in scanner set-up should be monitored. It is important to keep up to date with current guidelines on the safe use of diagnostic ultrasound (BMUS Safety Group 2000; EFSUMB 2006).

Probably the biggest risk of ultrasound is misdiagnosis, and it is therefore important to obtain an adequate scan. The sonographer should be aware of new technologies and new developments in scanning techniques. If the sonographer is in any doubt of the result at the end of the scan, the limitations of the scan should be reported.

Infection control

Cross-infection of patients by the ultrasound transducer is a possible risk, therefore the transducer should be cleaned between each examination. The front face of transducers can be made of delicate material and the use of strong cleaning fluids is often not recommended. Consult the operating manual or manufacturer for advice on suitable cleaning procedures. The best method to overcome this problem, when there is a known risk, is to use a disposable probe cover. If the scan is to be performed near an open wound, a sterile probe cover and sterile gel should be used. Alternatively, a sterile transparent plastic dressing may be used to cover the wound, insuring no air bubbles are trapped under the dressing that would prevent imaging. Disposable gloves should always be worn if scanning infected or discharging regions.

References

BMUS Safety Group 2000 British Medical Ultrasound Society statement on the safe use, and potential hazards of diagnostic ultrasound. Available online at: www.bmus.org

Duck F A, Shaw A 2003 Safety of diagnostic ultrasound. In: Hoskins P R, Thrush A, Martin K et al. (eds) Diagnostic ultrasound: physics and instrumentation. Greenwich Medical Media, London, pp 179–203

EFSUMB 2006 Clinical safety statement for diagnostic ultrasound. Available online at: www.efsumb.org/ecmus/

WFUMB 1998 Conclusions and recommendations on the thermal and non-thermal mechanisms for biological effects. Ultrasound in Medicine and Biology 24 (Suppl. 1): xv–xvi

Further reading

European Committee for Medical Ultrasound Safety (ECMUS) Tutorials on behalf of the European Federation for Societies of Ultrasound in Medicine and Biology (EFSUMB). Available online at: www.efsumb.org/ecmus/

ter Haar G, Duck F A (eds) 2000 The safe use of ultrasound in medical diagnosis. BMUS/BIR, London

Ultrasound assessment of the extracranial cerebral circulation

8

CONTENTS

INTRODUCTION

Ultrasound can be used to evaluate the extracranial cerebral circulation in order to investigate patients who may be at risk of suffering a stroke (patients who have suffered a transient ischemic attack or TIA) or who have already suffered a stroke. Stroke is the third most common cause of death in the UK, with the stroke rate being approximately 2 in 1000 of the population per year. Approximately 80% of strokes are ischemic (i.e., thrombotic or embolic or both) as opposed to hemorrhagic. Up to 80% of ischemic strokes occur in the carotid territory, the area of the brain supplied by the carotid arteries. Trials have shown that patients with significant carotid artery disease and relevant symptoms benefit from surgery in order to prevent a stroke. The majority of carotid artery disease develops at the carotid bifurcation, and in the presence of a significant stenosis, carotid endarterectomy (CEA) can be performed. In this procedure, the diseased inner wall of the artery is removed, thus eliminating a potential source of emboli or flow-limiting stenosis. Carotid ultrasound examinations can be used to screen patients for carotid artery disease before further investigation. Alternatively, many centers now use ultrasound examination to select patients directly for surgery, without preoperative angiography, as angiography is known to carry its own small risk of transient and permanent neurological deficit. If the ultrasound scan is inconclusive and further imaging is required, magnetic resonance angiography (MRA) or computed tomography angiography (CTA) may make safer alternatives to X-ray angiography for confirming ultrasound findings prior to surgery or for further investigations, when ultrasound has provided only limited results. Some centers perform CEA for significant carotid disease prior to or combined with coronary artery bypass graft (CABG) surgery, with the aim of reducing the stroke rate associated with CABG surgery. In these centers the cardiologist or cardiac surgeons may require a carotid disease screening service to detect the presence of any significant disease.

ANATOMY

The brain is supplied by four vessels – the right and left internal carotid and vertebral arteries – and receives 15% of the cardiac output. The term extracranial cerebral arteries refers to all the arteries that carry blood from the heart up to the base of the skull. The left and right sides of the extracranial circulation are not symmetrical (Fig. 8.1). On the left side, the common carotid artery (CCA) and subclavian artery arise directly from the aortic arch, whereas on the right side the brachiocephalic artery, also known as the innominate artery, arises from the aorta and divides into the subclavian artery and CCA. The CCA, which has no branches, divides into the internal and external carotid arteries (ICA and ECA, respectively), but the level of the carotid bifurcation in the neck is highly variable. In approximately 90% of cases, the ICA lies posterolateral or lateral to the ECA and, unlike the ECA, has no branches below the skull. The proximal branches of the ECA are the superior thyroid, lingual, facial, and maxillary arteries. The carotid artery widens, at the level of the bifurcation, to form the carotid bulb. In some cases, the carotid bulb may only involve the proximal ICA, and not the distal CCA, and the degree of widening of the carotid bulb is quite variable. Within the skull, the distal segment of the ICA follows a U-shaped curved path, known as the carotid siphon. The most important branch of the ICA is the ophthalmic artery, which supplies the eye. The terminal branches of the ophthalmic artery, the supratrochlear and supraorbital arteries, unite with the terminal branches of the ECA. The ICA finally divides into the middle cerebral artery (MCA) and the anterior cerebral artery (ACA).

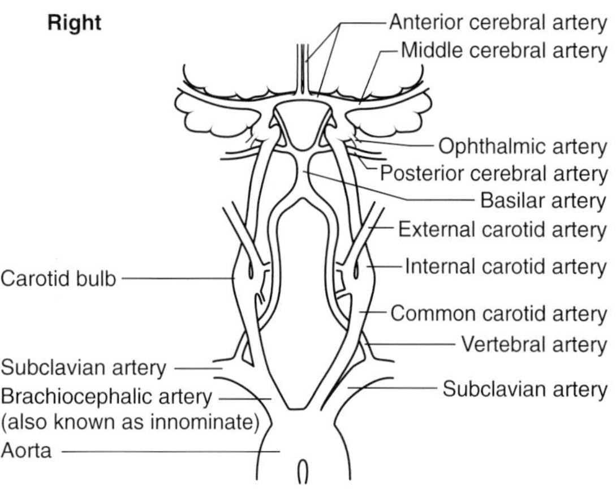

Figure 8.1 • Diagram of cerebrovascular anatomy.

The posterior circulation of the brain is mainly supplied by the left and right vertebral arteries, via the basilar artery. The vertebral artery is the first branch of the subclavian artery, arising from the highest point of the subclavian arch. At the sixth cervical vertebra, the vertebral artery runs posteriorly to travel upward through the transverse foramen of the cervical vertebrae. It is common for one vertebral artery to be larger than the other, with the left often being larger than the right. The two vertebral arteries join, at the base of the skull, to form the basilar artery, which then divides to form the posterior cerebral arteries. Figure 8.2A shows how the circle of Willis, situated at the base of the brain, joins the cerebral branches of the ICAs and basilar artery via the anterior and posterior communicating arteries. Blood flow to the brain is regulated by changes in cerebrovascular resistance, with carbon dioxide playing a major role in vasodilation.

Collateral pathways and anatomical variants

In the presence of severe vascular disease, the cerebral circulation has many possible collateral (alternative) pathways, both extracranially and intracranially. Not all of these can be assessed using ultrasound; however, two pathways that can be assessed are the following:

- The ophthalmic artery.

The ECAs do not normally supply blood to the brain, but in the presence of severe ICA disease, branches of the ECA can act as important collateral pathways. One such pathway is via the terminal branches of the ECA, communicating with the terminal branches of the ophthalmic artery. This collateral pathway can be observed using continuous-wave (CW) Doppler to detect reversal of flow in the supraorbital artery, a terminal branch of the

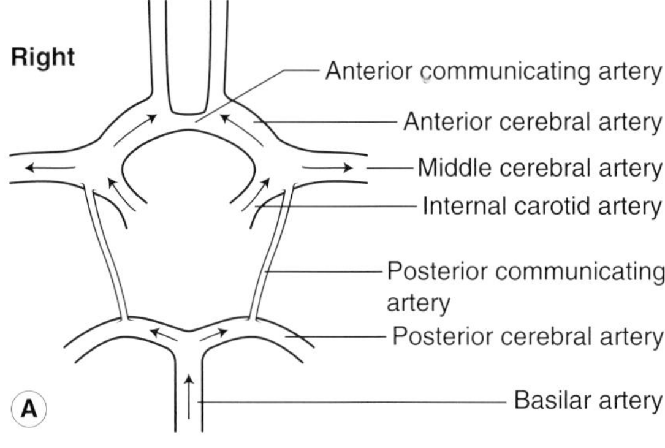

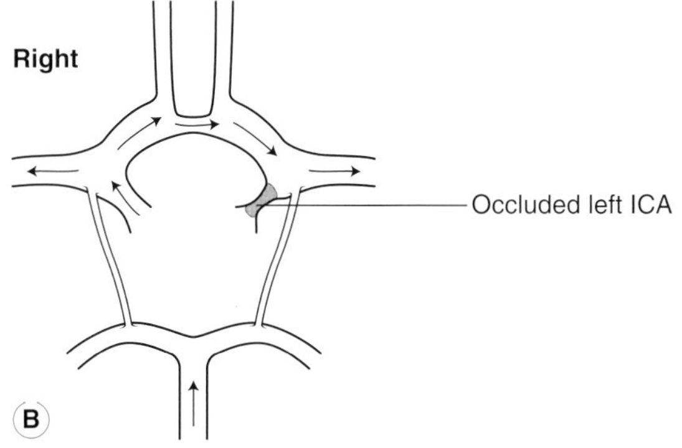

Figure 8.2 • Diagram of the circle of Willis. (A) Arrows indicate normal flow direction. (B) Arrows indicate cross-over flow from the right internal carotid artery (ICA) to the left middle cerebral artery (MCA) in the presence of a left ICA occlusion.

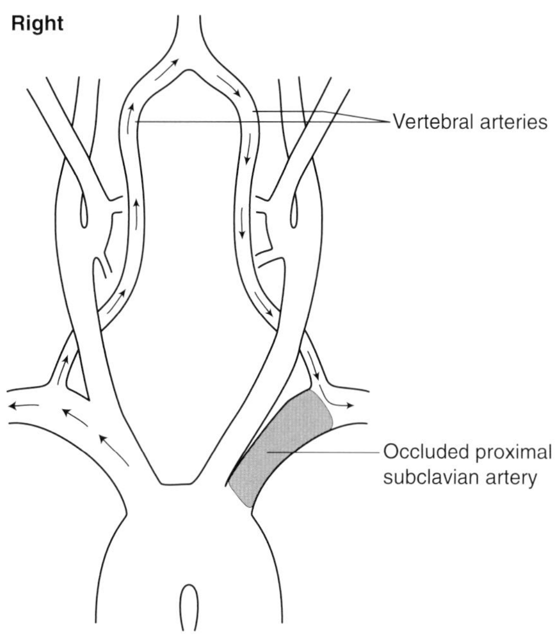

Figure 8.3 • Arrows indicate the direction of collateral flow in subclavian steal syndrome, via reverse flow in the vertebral artery to supply the arm, in the presence of a severe stenosis or occlusion of the proximal subclavian artery.

ophthalmic artery, as retrograde flow travels from the ECA branches toward the brain.

- The circle of Willis.

In the normal circulation, there is little blood flow through the communicating arteries in the circle of Willis, but in the presence of severe vascular disease they perform an important role in flow distribution. For example, in the presence of a left ICA occlusion, it is possible for the right ICA to supply blood flow to the left MCA via the right ACA, the anterior communicating artery and the left ACA, with flow reversal occurring in the left ACA (Fig. 8.2B).

The vertebral arteries may also supply flow to the MCA via the posterior communicating arteries of the circle of Willis. If the circle is well developed, it is possible for a single extracranial artery to provide adequate cerebral blood flow. However, in about 75% of the population, parts of the circle may be hypoplastic (very small) or absent, making the circle incomplete and therefore preventing the development of good collateral flow (von Reutern & von Büdingen 1993), but this may only become apparent in the presence of severe disease. Adequate collateral pathways have a better chance of developing in the presence of slowly developing disease.

An unusual collateral pathway can occur when the CCA is occluded and flow in the proximal ECA reverses, being supplied by retrograde flow in an ECA branch, to supply a patent ICA. Severe narrowing or occlusion of the proximal subclavian or brachiocephalic artery can result in a collateral pathway that 'steals' blood from the brain to supply the arm. In this case, blood will be seen to flow retrogradely down the ipsilateral vertebral artery to supply the distal subclavian artery beyond the diseased segment (Fig. 8.3). This is known as subclavian steal syndrome.

There are few variations in the extracranial circulation. In rare cases, the left CCA and subclavian artery may share a common origin or a single trunk. Other anomalies are the left vertebral artery arising directly from the aortic arch and, even more unusually, the right vertebral origin arising from the aortic arch.

SYMPTOMS OF CAROTID AND VERTEBRAL ARTERY DISEASE

Patients with carotid artery stenosis may suffer from TIA, stroke, or amaurosis fugax, a form of visual disturbance. Symptoms of TIA may only last a few minutes and the patient will make a full recovery within 24 h, whereas patients suffering from a stroke will have symptoms lasting more than 24 h and may not make a full recovery. Symptoms include single or multiple episodes of loss of power or sensation in an arm or leg (monoparesis), in both (hemiparesis), or in one side of the face; slurring or loss of speech (dysphasia); or visuospatial neglect.

As the right side of the brain controls the left-hand side of the body and the converse, the symptoms will relate to the contralateral carotid artery. Speech is usually controlled by the dominant side of the brain (i.e., a right-handed patient's speech will typically be controlled by the left side of the brain). Patients suffering from episodes of amaurosis fugax often complain of 'a curtain drawing across one eye' lasting for a few minutes, which is due to emboli within the retinal circulation. In this situation, the symptoms in the eye will relate to the ipsilateral carotid artery. Typical vertebrobasilar symptoms are shown in Box 8.1. Vague symptoms, such as dizziness and blackout, are not usually associated with carotid artery disease. Subclavian steal syndrome does not usually cause significant symptoms. Only about 15% of patients suffer symptoms of TIA before a stroke. Fifty percent of ischemic carotid territory strokes are due to thromboembolism of the ICA, whereas 25% are due to small-vessel disease and 15% are due to emboli originating from the heart. Only 1–2% of all strokes are hemodynamic strokes (i.e., due to flow-limiting stenoses) (Naylor et al. 1998).

Patients with symptoms of TIA or minor stroke are at a cumulative recurrent risk of a stroke due to large-vessel disease of 4% at 7 days following symptoms, 12.6% at 1 month, and 19.2% at 3 months (Naylor 2008). In other words, about 20% of people suffering a TIA will have a stroke within four weeks. Ultrasound can be used to help select those patients who would benefit from CEA to reduce the risk of stroke (method discussed later in the chapter). It has been shown that the benefit of CEA is greatest when the surgery is performed within 2 weeks of the patient's symptoms and that the benefit is reduced by almost a third if surgery is performed more than 4 weeks following the last symptom (Rothwell et al. 2004). In symptomatic patients with a 70–99% stenosis, the absolute risk reduction of CEA is 23% if surgery is performed within 2 weeks compared to 7.4% if performed at more than 12 weeks after symptoms. Guidelines from the American Heart Association/American Stroke Association (Sacco et al. 2006) suggest that patients suffering from TIA or minor stroke should be assessed and, if appropriate, have surgery within 2 weeks. This, therefore, requires patients suffering TIA or minor stroke to have rapid access to carotid duplex scanning to enable early diagnosis and treatment.

Symptoms similar to TIA can also be caused by other neurological problems, such as epilepsy, intracranial tumor, multiple sclerosis, or migraine. Asymptomatic carotid disease is usually discovered clinically by the presence of a carotid bruit, heard

BOX 8.1 Typical carotid territory and vertebrobasilar symptoms (after Naylor et al. 1998, With permission)

TYPICAL CAROTID TERRITORY SYMPTOMS

- Hemimotor/hemisensory signs
- Monocular visual loss (amaurosis fugax)
- Higher cortical dysfunction (dysphasia – incomplete language function, visuospatial neglect)

TYPICAL VERTEBROBASILAR SYMPTOMS

- Bilateral blindness
- Problems with gait and stance
- Hemi- or bilateral motor/sensory signs
- Dysarthria
- Homonymous hemianopia (loss of visual fields in both eyes)
- Diplopia, vertigo, and nystagmus (provided it is not the only symptom)

as a murmur when listening to the neck with a stethoscope. However, the presence of a carotid bruit may not be due to an ICA stenosis, but could instead relate to an ECA or aortic stenosis or to no stenosis at all. A large proportion of patients with a >70% stenosis will not have a carotid bruit, and therefore its presence or absence is not accurate enough to predict the presence of disease.

Trauma to the neck can lead to dissection of the carotid artery wall, possibly causing the vessel to occlude. This condition may be suspected in patients suffering a stroke following a neck injury. Ultrasound examination may also be requested in the presence of a pulsatile swelling in the neck to identify the presence of a carotid aneurysm or carotid body tumor, both of which are quite rare.

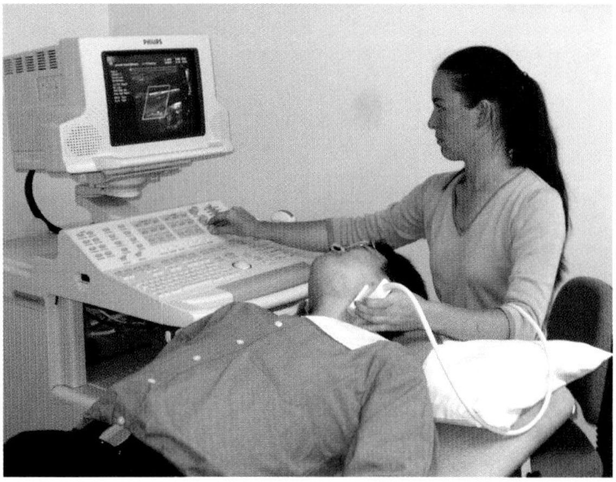

Figure 8.4 • The optimal position for scanning the carotid arteries.

SCANNING

Objectives and preparation

Purpose of scan

The purpose of the carotid scan is to identify the extent of any atheroma within the common carotid artery and extracranial internal and external carotid artery and to determine the degree of narrowing of the vessels. The examination should also demonstrate the presence and direction of flow in the vertebral arteries.

No specific preparation is required, but the patient must be capable of lying or sitting still during the examination. The optimal position for scanning the carotid arteries is with the sonographer sitting behind the patient's head. This allows easy access to the neck and enables the operator to rest the arm on the examination table while performing the scan (Fig. 8.4). Alternatively the sonographer can sit by the side of the patient while resting the arm on the patient's upper chest. The patient should lie supine on the couch with the head resting on a pillow. The neck should be extended and the head turned in the opposite direction to the side being examined. If the patient has difficulty in breathing or has back problems it may be necessary to sit the patient in a more upright position. If the patient is in a wheelchair (e.g., following a disabling stroke), it may be easier to do the scan in the wheelchair with the head resting on a pillow for support, preventing unnecessary movement of the patient. However, being in an upright position may affect the velocity values recorded and more care may be required in grading any significance disease (Pemble 2008).

The examination can be performed with a medium- to high-frequency flat linear array transducer, depending on the size of the patient's neck. The higher the frequency, the better the resolution of the vessel wall structure; however, in some cases the carotid bifurcation lies deep in the neck, requiring a lower-frequency transducer for visualization. Blood flow velocities detected in the majority of normal and diseased carotid arteries are reasonably high, so the scanner should be configured to visualize high-velocity pulsatile flow. Most ultrasound systems have examination presets available that are suitable for the majority of carotid examinations, but it may be necessary to alter these to enable the detection of low-velocity flow when differentiating carotid artery occlusion from a subtotal occlusion. A small spectral Doppler sample volume is usually used to interrogate the carotid arteries, as it allows for more selective investigation of areas of velocity increase or flow disturbance.

Technique

The carotid arteries are best visualized through the sternocleidomastoid muscle, which provides a good ultrasonic window, and this is done using a

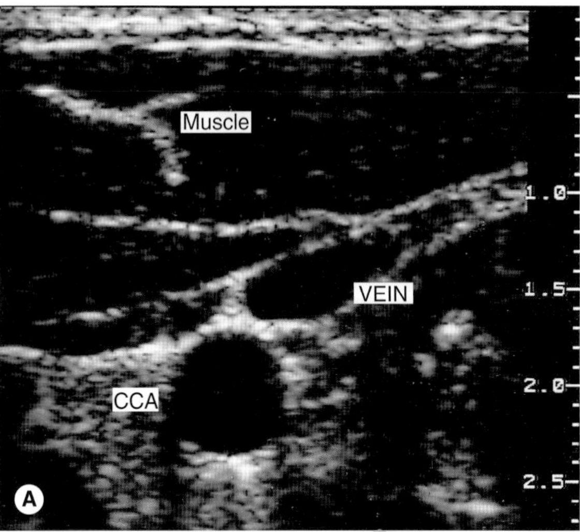

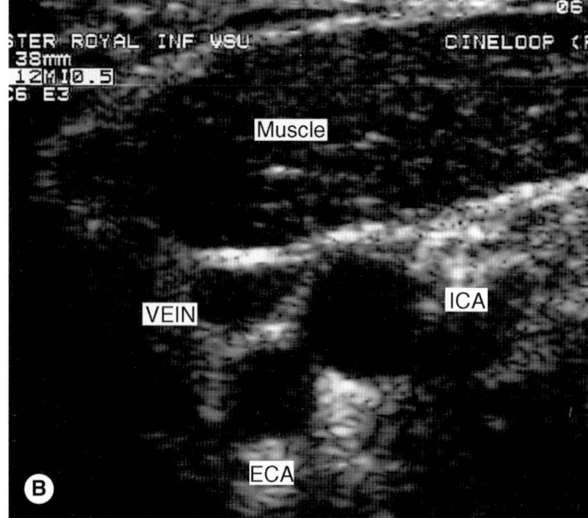

Figure 8.5 • Transverse B-mode images. (A) Common carotid artery (CCA) and jugular vein. (B) The internal (ICA) and external carotid arteries (ECA) just above the carotid bifurcation.

lateral rather than an anterior approach. The procedure is as follows:

1 Using B-mode imaging only, the CCA should be visualized in transverse section (Fig. 8.5A), starting at the base of the neck. On the right side, it is usually possible to visualize the distal brachiocephalic artery and the origin of the CCA and subclavian arteries. On the left side, the origin of the CCA cannot be visualized as it lies too deep in the chest. The CCA should be scanned along its length, in transverse section, up to the bifurcation, and along the ICA and ECA (Fig. 8.5B) as high up the neck as can be seen. This allows the sonographer to ascertain the level and orientation of the carotid bifurcation and also gives the first indications of the presence and location of any arterial disease. The jugular vein lies over the CCA (Fig. 8.5A) and is usually easily compressed. However, it is important not to apply too much transducer pressure when scanning the carotid arteries as there is a possibility of dislodging an embolus from the vessel wall.

2 The CCA is now visualized in longitudinal section using B-mode imaging, starting at the base of the neck. A longitudinal image of the CCA can be easily obtained by imaging the CCA in transverse section and then, keeping the CCA in the center of the image, rotating the probe so the CCA first appears as an ellipse and finally can be seen in longitudinal section. Prior knowledge of the orientation of the ICA and ECA gained from transverse imaging is helpful for locating the correct longitudinal imaging plane to view the bifurcation. It is necessary to use a range of longitudinal scan planes to visualize the carotid arteries, especially at the bifurcation (Fig. 8.6). Typically, the ICA lies posterolateral or lateral

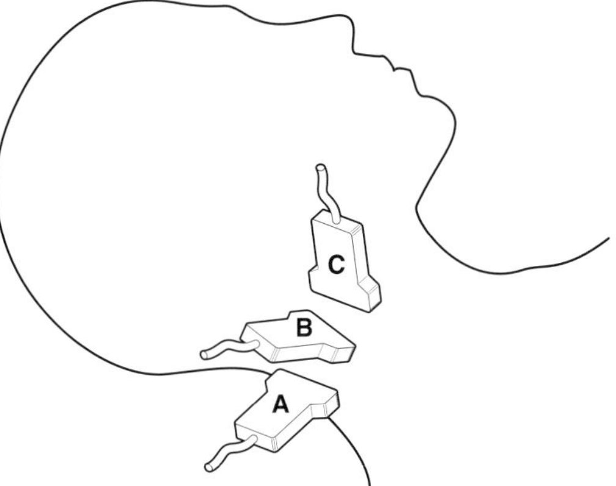

Figure 8.6 • Longitudinal scan planes used to visualize the carotid arteries. (A) Posterior. (B) Lateral. (C) Anterior.

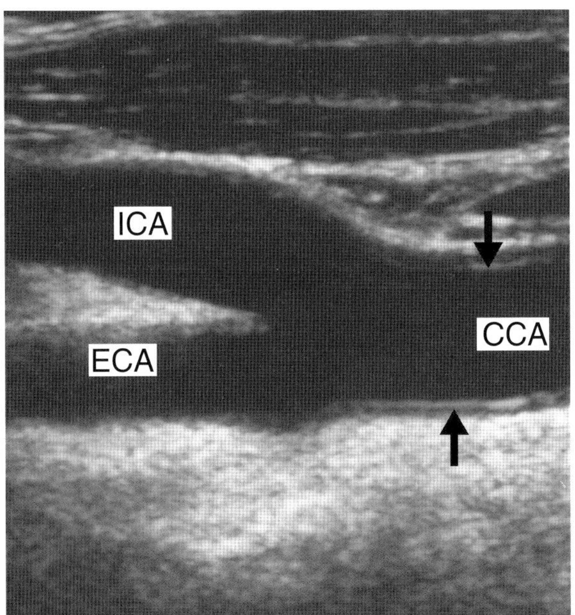

Figure 8.7 • Longitudinal B-mode image of the carotid bifurcation with the internal (ICA) and external carotid arteries (ECA) seen in the same plane. The arrows mark where the intima-media layer can be seen.

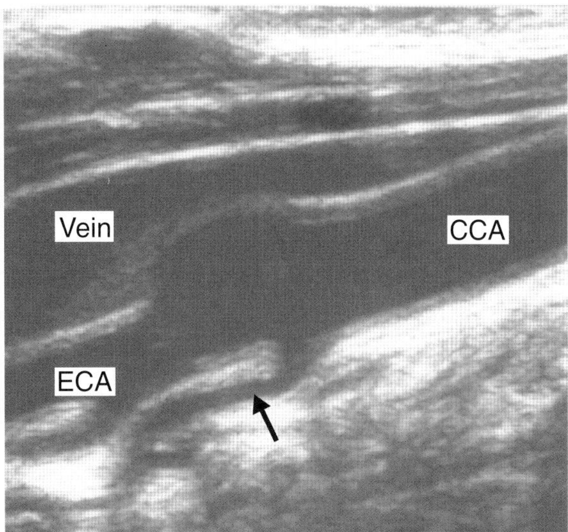

Figure 8.8 • B-mode image of the external carotid artery (ECA) showing the superior thyroid branch (arrow). CCA, common carotid artery.

to the ECA and is usually the larger of the two vessels. In a small percentage of cases, the bifurcation will appear as a tuning fork arrangement (Fig. 8.7), but in the majority of cases the ECA and ICA will not be seen in the same plane and will have to be imaged individually. This is achieved by keeping the lower portion of the probe face over the CCA and slowly rotating the upper portion through a small angle to image first the ICA and then the ECA, or vice versa. Only small probe movements are required when imaging the ICA and ECA, as the vessels usually lie close together.

3 Having located the three vessels and observed any evidence of disease in the B-mode image, color flow imaging can be used to investigate the flow from the proximal CCA up into the ICA and ECA. Identification of ECA branches (either on B-mode or color imaging) serves as a further indication as to which vessel is the ECA, as the ICA has no branches below the jaw (Fig. 8.8). Color flow imaging can provide evidence of disease, such as velocity changes due to stenosis, areas of filling defects due to the presence of atheroma, and the absence of flow due to occlusion. Diagnosis should not be made based on the color flow imaging alone, but it greatly aids the sonographer in selecting areas that require close investigation with the spectral Doppler.

4 The spectral Doppler is now used to observe the inflow to the carotid arteries by placing the sample volume in the proximal CCA at the base of the neck. The shape of the waveform may reveal the presence of proximal or distal disease, such as an ICA occlusion. In the absence of significant distal or proximal disease, the left and right CCA waveforms should appear symmetrical.

5 The examination so far has provided many clues as to which of the two vessels beyond the bifurcation is the ICA, such as the relative size and position of the two vessels and the presence of ECA branches. Spectral Doppler can now be used to confirm the identification of the ICA and ECA, as the ICA waveform shape is less pulsatile and has higher diastolic flow than the ECA (Fig. 8.9). Differentiation of the vessels may be further helped by tapping the temporal

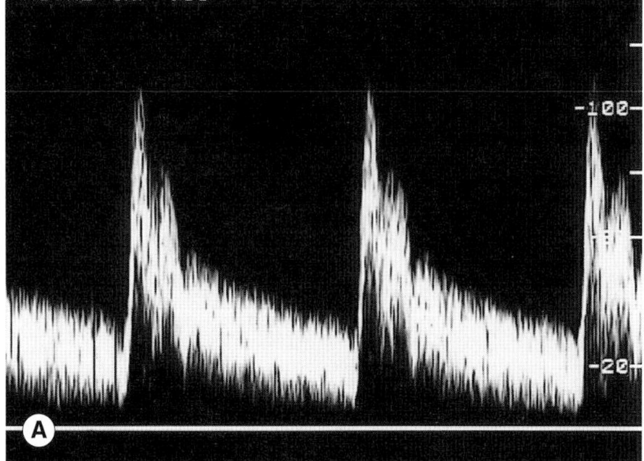

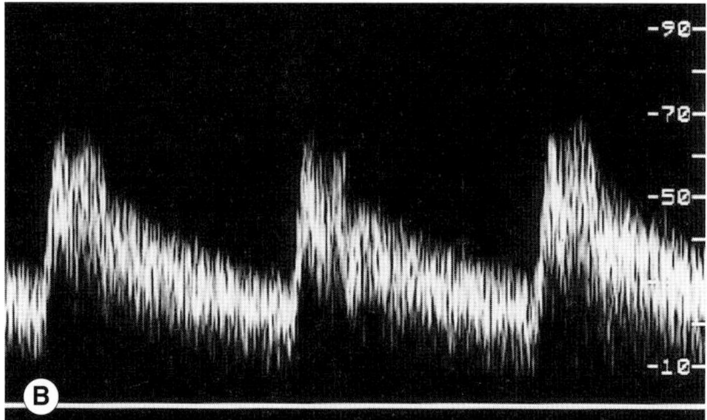

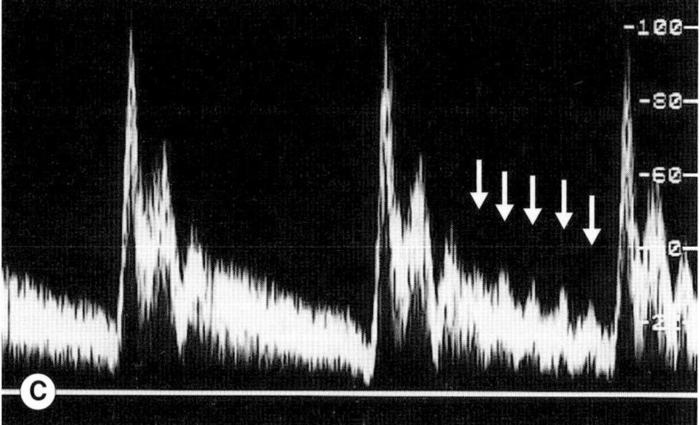

Figure 8.9 • Typical normal Doppler spectra obtained from the common carotid artery (A), the internal carotid artery (B), and the external carotid artery (ECA) (C). The effect of temporal tapping on ECA diastolic flow is marked with arrows.

artery, an ECA branch (which runs in front of the upper part of the ear), as this will cause changes in the ECA flow during diastole (Fig. 8.9C) but will have little effect on the ICA. It is imperative that the ICA and ECA should be correctly identified, as it is the presence of disease in the carotid bifurcation and ICA, not the ECA, that is the possible cause of carotid artery symptoms. If significant disease is present in the ICA, the upper limit of the disease in relation to the level of the jaw should be assessed. If no clear vessel can be seen beyond the stenosis, angiography may be required to confirm the endpoint of the disease.

6 Using spectral Doppler, peak systolic and end-diastolic velocity (EDV) measurements should be made in the CCA, ICA, and ECA and at the site of the maximum velocity increase within any stenoses to allow the degree of narrowing to be graded. Atypical waveform shapes should also be noted.

7 If no flow is detected in the ICA (Fig. 8.10) or CCA using the default carotid preset scanner settings, it is necessary to rule out the presence of low-volume flow due to a critical stenosis or subtotal occlusion (Fig. 8.11) before reporting the vessel to be occluded. This is achieved by optimizing the scanner controls to detect low-velocity flow (i.e., by lowering the pulse repetition frequency [PRF] and high-pass filter setting). If low-velocity flow is detected, the cause should be identified. For example, low-velocity flow may be detected in the CCA because of an ICA occlusion (Fig. 8.10B), or it may be detected in the ICA due to a severe stenosis of the ICA origin.

8 To conclude the first side of the examination, the vertebral artery should be located using B-mode or color imaging. The patient's head should be turned slightly to one side. First image the mid-CCA in longitudinal section and then slowly angle the transducer into a more anteroposterior plane. The vertebral processes, seen as bright echoes, should slowly be seen to stand out. Only short sections of the vertebral artery and vein can be seen at this level as they run through the transverse foramen of the vertebrae. The walls of the vertebral artery and vein can often be seen on the B-mode image, but color flow imaging can also help visualize the vessels (Fig. 8.12). Spectral Doppler is then used to confirm the direction and quality of flow in the vertebral artery.

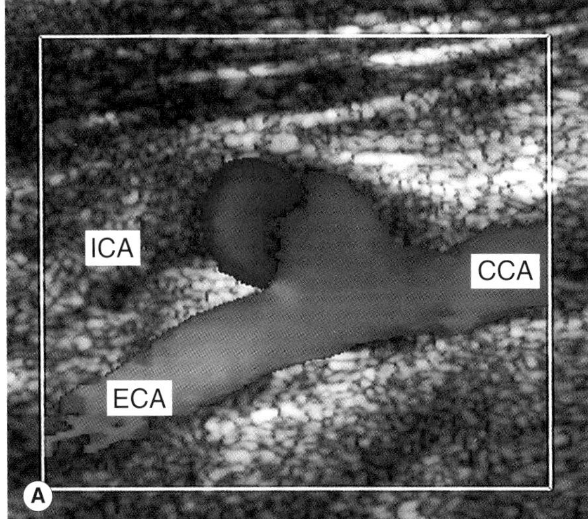

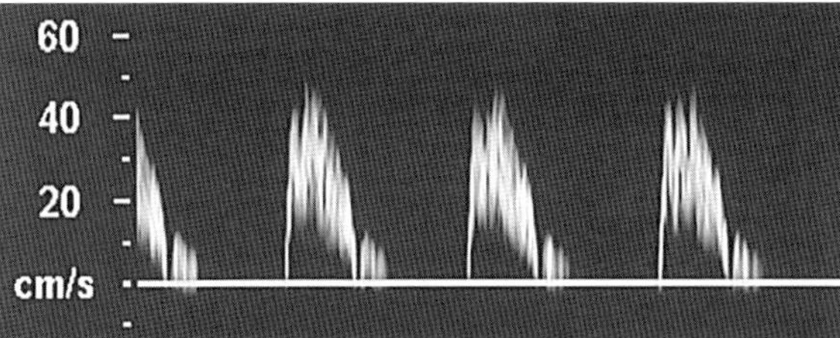

Figure 8.10 • (A) A color image of an occluded internal carotid artery (ICA) showing flow in the common carotid artery (CCA) with retrograde flow seen in the stump of the ICA occlusion and an absence of flow in the ICA beyond. (ECA, external carotid artery). (B) Doppler spectrum obtained from a CCA proximal to an ICA occlusion showing low-volume, high-resistance flow with a lack of diastolic flow.

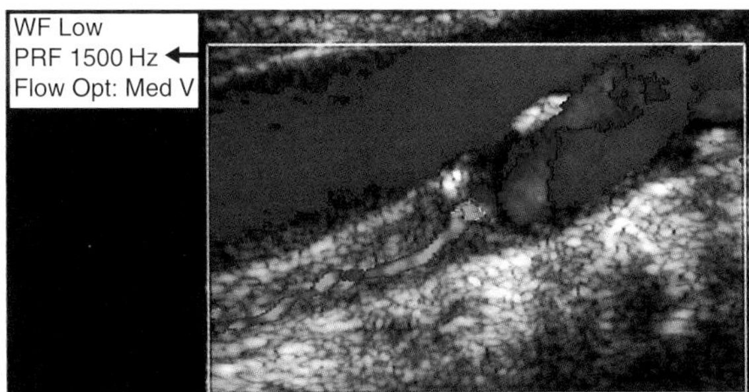

Figure 8.11 • Color image showing a narrow channel of low-velocity flow detected in a subtotal occlusion of the internal carotid artery. A low pulse repetition frequency (arrow) is required to detect the low-velocity flow.

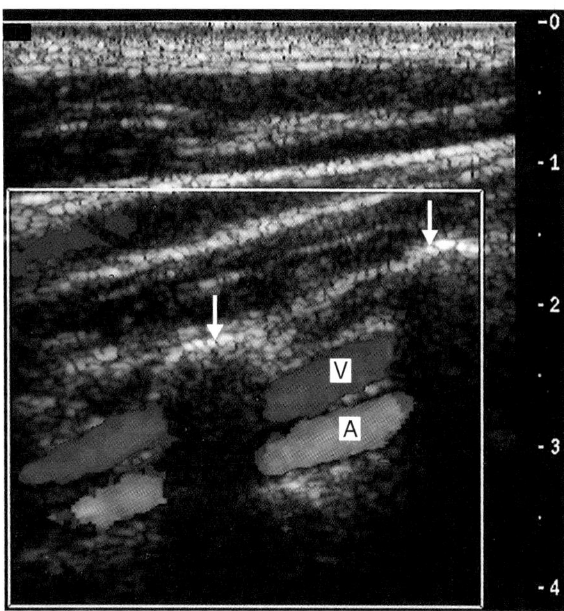

Figure 8.12 • Color flow image of the vertebral artery (A) and vein (V) seen between the vertebral processes of the spine (marked by the arrows).

9 Having completed the first side of the examination, the patient is asked to turn the head in the opposite direction, and the other side is examined in the same way. It is important to remember that the carotid and vertebral arteries on both sides are linked via several possible collateral pathways and that the presence of severe disease in one extracranial vessel may affect flow in another extracranial vessel if it is supplying a collateral pathway.

Recommendation

The peak systolic velocity (PSV) and end-diastolic velocity (EDV) should be measured in the common carotid artery 1–2 cm below the bifurcation and at the site of maximum velocity within any internal carotid artery (ICA) stenosis. If no narrowing is seen in the ICA, the PSV and EDV should be measured in the ICA just beyond the carotid bulb. These velocity measurements and ratios obtained from the measurements can be used to grade the degree of narrowing within the bifurcation.

B-MODE IMAGING

Normal appearance

The normal vessel walls will often appear as a double-layer structure when imaged in longitudinal section (Fig. 8.7), especially if a high-frequency transducer is used. This represents the intima-media layer and adventitia (Ch. 5) and is most clearly seen on the posterior wall in the CCA, when the vessel lies at right angles to the ultrasound beam. The normal thickness of the intima-media layer is of the order of 0.5–0.9 mm, when measured on ultrasound. A normal vessel lumen should appear hypoechoic; however it is possible for the sonographer to remove echoes from within the lumen by reducing the time gain compensation (Ch. 2), so careful use of the imaging controls is important. The B-mode imaging focal zone should be placed in the region of the vessel to insure optimal imaging of the vessel walls. Occasionally, it is difficult to obtain adequate B-mode images of the bifurcation. In this case, color flow imaging may help locate the vessels and enable spectral Doppler measurements to be made.

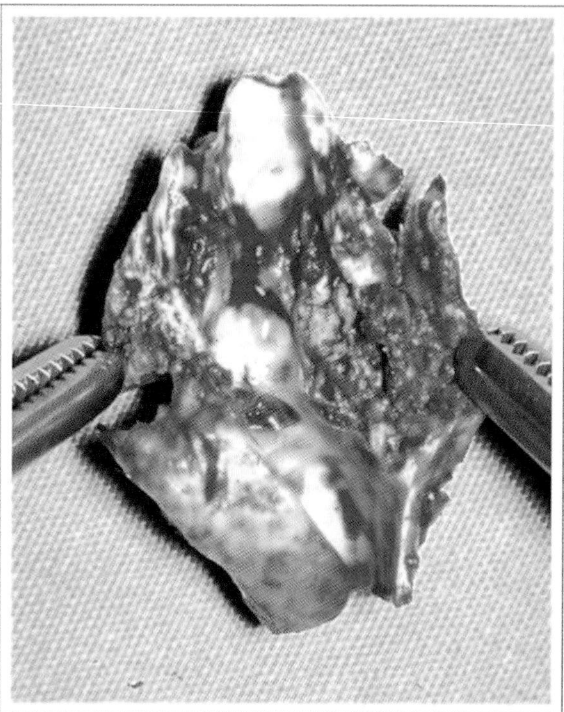

Figure 8.13 • Atheroma removed from the carotid bifurcation during carotid endarterectomy.

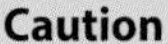

Caution

Reverberation artifacts can give the appearance of structures within the lumen. Reverberation artifacts can be generated from large boundaries within the imaging plane, such as muscle or vein wall, overlying the carotid artery. Changing the angle at which the carotid artery is viewed, either by heel-toeing the transducer or using a different scan plane, can minimize these artifacts. (see Fig. 7.2)

Abnormal appearance

The ultrasound appearance of the early stages of carotid artery disease is a thickening of the intima-media layer. As the disease progresses, more substantial areas of atheroma can be visualized, and this is most likely to occur at the carotid bifurcation. However, in a small proportion of patients, significant disease may be seen in the CCA and may even involve the CCA origin. It is important to remember the way ultrasound interacts with tissue and the effects of scanner set-up, such as gain control and compression curve selection (Ch. 2), before drawing conclusions about the appearance of plaque surface or composition. A high-frequency transducer should be used when investigating plaque composition. Many studies have been carried out comparing the ultrasound appearance of atheromatous plaque with histological investigation of specimens removed during CEA (Fig. 8.13) in an attempt to predict which plaques are more likely to be the source of emboli. Several of these studies show an association between the symptoms and the presence of intraplaque hemorrhage (i.e., bleeding into the plaque) (Merrit & Bluth 1992). If the surface of a plaque containing intraplaque hemorrhage or lipid pools ruptures, the contents of the plaque are discharged into the vessel lumen, causing distal embolization and leading to symptoms such as TIA or stroke. A multicenter European study (European Carotid Plaque Study Group 1995) showed that the echogenicity on the B-mode image was inversely related to the content of soft tissue (including hemorrhage or lipid) and directly related to the presence of calcification. In this study, they described the plaque using a scale of 1 to 3,

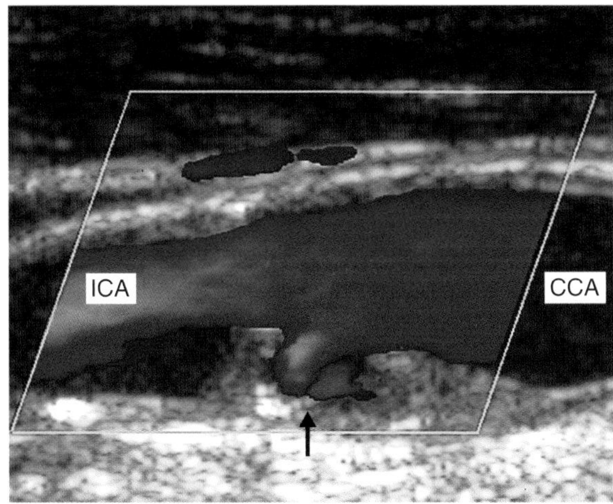

Figure 8.14 • An image of a heterogeneous plaque with a crater (arrow) suggesting an ulcer. ICA, internal carotid artery; CCA, common carotid artery.

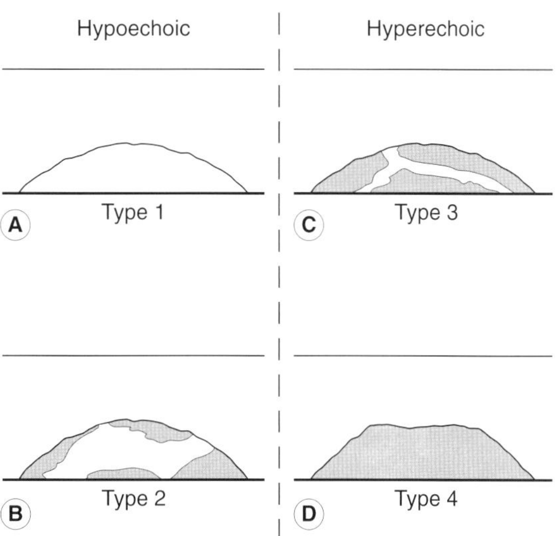

Figure 8.15 • Plaque categorization based on ultrasound imaging described by Bock & Lusby. (Bock and Lusby in Labs et al (eds), Diagnostic Vascular Ultrasound (Hodder Arnold, 1992). Reprinted by permission of Edward Arnold (Publishers) Ltd)

with 1 representing strong echoes (bright) and 3 representing low echogenicity or hypoechoic areas (dark). The plaques were also described as being homogeneous or heterogeneous. Irregularity of the plaque surface was not found to relate well to the presence of ulceration.

An international consensus meeting (de Bray et al. 1997) used a similar method of describing plaque features: echogenicity (from hypoechoic to hyperechoic), surface (from smooth to cavitated), and texture (from homogeneous to heterogeneous). It was suggested that echogenicity can be standardized against blood (hypoechoic), mastoid muscle (isoechogenic), or bone (hyperechogenic cervical vertebrae). Lumen surface was classified as regular, irregular (0.4–2 mm), and ulcerated (>2 mm depth and 2 mm in length with well-defined back wall at its base, with flow vortices seen on color imaging). Figure 8.14 shows a heterogeneous plaque with a crater, filled with blood flow, suggesting an ulcer.

A slightly different method of categorizing the plaque, imaged in longitudinal views, was reported by Bock & Lusby (1992) whereby the plaque was graded from 1 to 4, as shown in Figure 8.15. Type 1 appears as a hypoechoic area seen to have a thin cap (Fig. 8.16A). Hypoechoic areas were shown to relate to either lipid or intraplaque hemorrhage. Hyperechoic plaques were categorized as type 4 and were considered to be more benign. Figure 8.16D demonstrates a more hyperechoic plaque. Types 2 and 3 were heterogeneous plaques (Fig. 8.16B and C), with type 3 appearing more hyperechoic than type 2. Plaque types 1 and 2 were seen significantly more frequently in symptomatic patients, whereas types 3 and 4 were more commonly found in asymptomatic patients.

These and many other studies over recent years suggest that the most useful quality of the B-mode appearance of a plaque is the proportion of hypoechoic areas or areas of low echogenicity within the plaque. Clearly the appearance of a plaque is dependent on the scanner controls being set to give an optimal image.

Several research centers have used computer-assisted image analysis methods in an attempt to quantify features in images of plaques objectively (Gronholdt et al. 2001; Fosse et al. 2006). This involves using the digital ultrasound image and outlining areas that represent the plaque, the vessel lumen, and the brightest adventitia. The median gray-scale value within each of these areas is then calculated using image analysis software. The median gray-scale values obtained from the blood and the adventitia are used to standardize the gray-scale median value obtained from the plaque, with the lumen and adventitia values used as hypoechoic

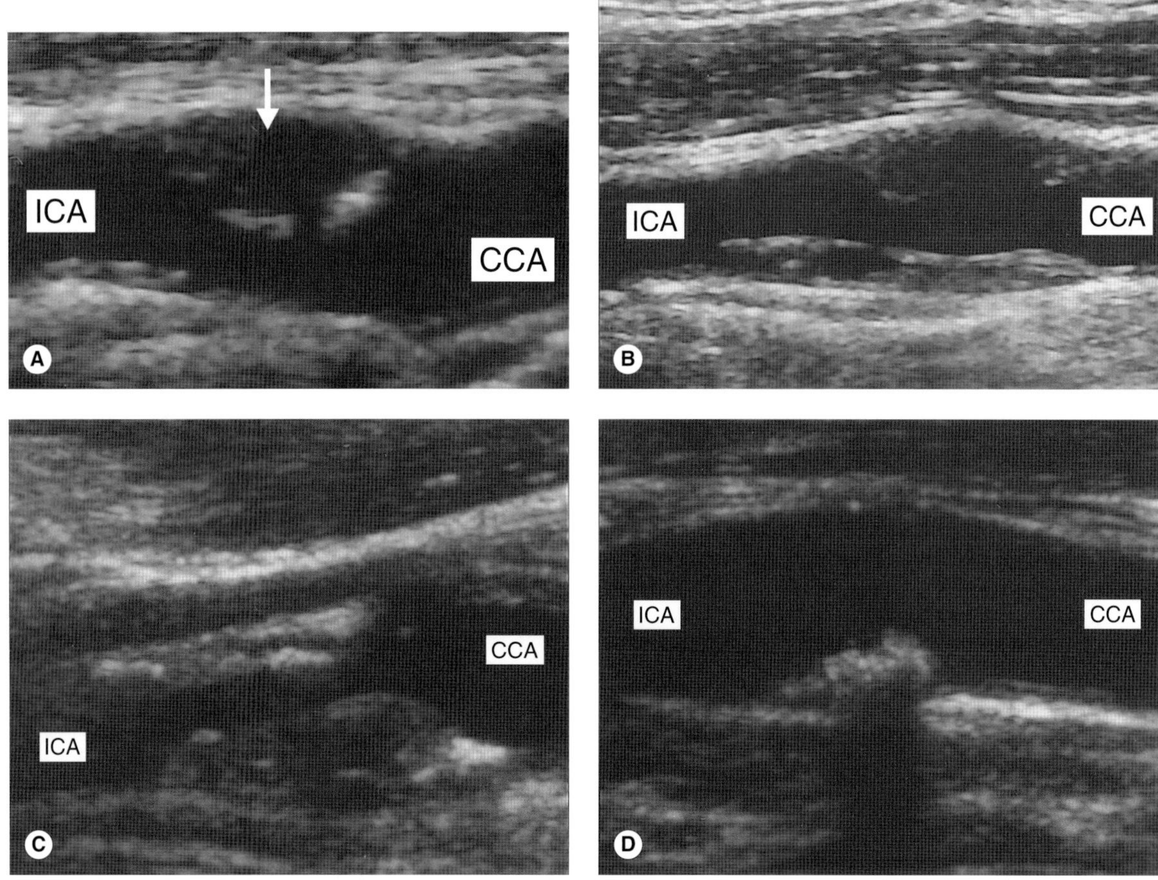

Figure 8.16 • (A) Hypoechoic plaque (arrow) with a thin cap, type 1. (B) Type 2 plaque. (C) Type 3 plaque. Types 2 and 3 are heterogeneous, with type 3 appearing more hyperechoic than type 2. (D) Homogeneous hyperechoic plaque, type 4. ICA, internal carotid artery; CCA, common carotid artery.

and hyperechoic reference structures respectively. This is done to reduce interscanner variability and gain level variability.

Fosse et al. (2006) found visual classification of the plaque echogenicity on ultrasound to be subjective and highly observer-dependent. They reported better reproducibility for computer-assisted offline classification of plaque; however, viability in selecting the region of interest can have an effect on the resulting gray-scale median value. Gronholdt et al (2001) found computer-assisted assessment of plaque echolucency in ≥ 50% stenosis to be associated with a risk of stroke in symptomatic but not asymptomatic individuals. . Studies have shown a correlation of histological appearance with an increased risk of ischemic cerebrovascular events (Mathiesen et al. 2001); however, the benefit of surgery over medical treatment in the management of asymptomatic patients based on the visual appearance of the plaque on ultrasound has not been proven. Further developments of computer-assisted classification may, in time, improve plaque characterization.

Comment

Large areas of atheroma will often be seen in the origin of an occluded internal carotid artery and, if the occlusion is long-standing, the occluded internal carotid artery may appear much smaller as its lumen contracts over time (Fig. 8.17).

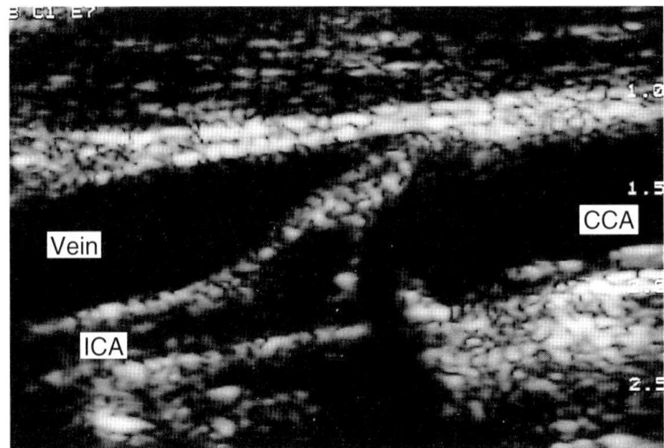

Figure 8.17 • A long-standing internal carotid artery (ICA) occlusion. CCA, common carotid artery.

COLOR IMAGING

Normal appearance

Flow in normal carotid arteries is pulsatile, with forward flow present throughout the cardiac cycle. With the appropriate PRF selected, color should continually fill the vessel lumen up to the walls and the peak systolic velocity (PSV) should be represented by a color near to the top of the color scale. For some patients it may be necessary to optimize the PRF from the pre-set value. The flow usually appears more pulsatile in the ECA than in the ICA and CCA. At the bifurcation, changes in the vessel geometry often lead to areas of flow reversal within the bifurcation, on the opposite side of the vessel to the ECA origin, giving the normal appearance seen in Chapter 5 (see Fig. 5.13A).

Abnormal appearance

The lack of color filling to the vessel wall may indicate the presence of atheroma. However, it is important to insure that filling defects are not due to a poor Doppler angle, inappropriately high PRF or high-pass filter setting, or to the presence of an image artifact preventing the color from being displayed. The presence of a filling defect at the vessel wall, where atheroma is not apparent on the B-mode image, may indicate an area of hypoechoic atheroma.

Increased velocity within a stenosis usually causes a change in the color displayed on the image, often associated with aliasing (Fig. 8.18A) and sometimes with flow recirculation (see Fig. 5.19). The color flow image can help to locate the area of greatest narrowing within a diseased segment of a vessel, which should then be investigated with the spectral Doppler (Fig. 8.18B). High-velocity jets may be seen within and just beyond a stenosis and the path of the flow may no longer be parallel to the vessel wall. In this case, the color image allows more accurate angle correction for velocity measurements. An area of flow reversal may be seen distal to a stenosis where the vessel lumen opens up again beyond the narrowing (see Fig. 5.19).Turbulent flow may also be seen beyond a stenosis (see Fig. 5.21) The complete absence of color Doppler filling within a vessel could indicate

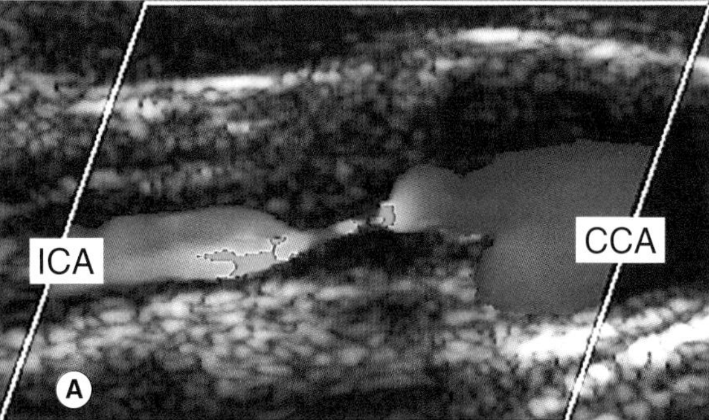

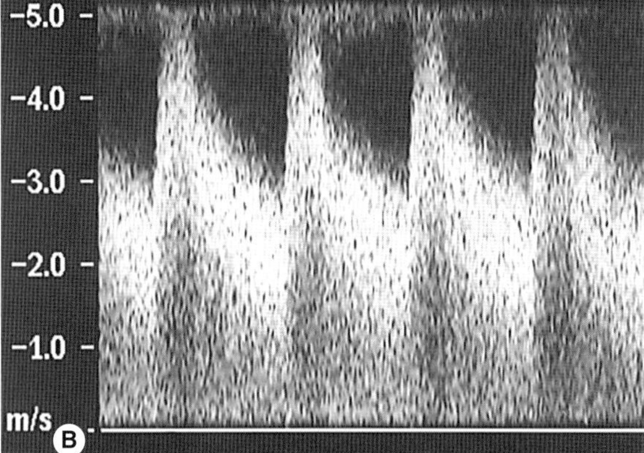

Figure 8.18 • (A) Color image showing a narrowed proximal internal carotid artery (ICA). (B) Doppler recording obtained from within the narrowing, demonstrating a significant velocity increase (peak systolic velocity 500 cm/s, end-diastolic velocity 300 cm/s) with increased spectral broadening, suggesting a significant stenosis (>80% diameter reduction). CCA, common carotid artery.

that the vessel is occluded, but this should be confirmed by optimizing the color controls for detection of low-velocity flow to rule out the presence of a very tight stenosis somewhere along the vessel. The apparent lack of color filling within the CCA or ICA during diastole may indicate high-resistance flow due to an occlusion or tight stenosis distal to that point. Spectral Doppler should be used to confirm the absence of diastolic flow, and both color and spectral Doppler should be used to investigate the distal vessels carefully.

SPECTRAL DOPPLER WAVEFORMS

Normal appearance

Spectral Doppler recordings obtained from the ECA show a higher-resistance flow pattern compared to the ICA with a pulsatile waveform shape and low diastolic flow (Fig. 8.9C) compared with the low-resistance waveform shape seen in the ICA (Fig. 8.9B). The normal CCA waveform (Fig. 8.9A) has a shape somewhere between that of the ICA and the ECA. The peak systolic velocities seen in the carotid arteries depend on the relative size of the vessel but are typically less than 110 cm/s in the normal ICA. The flow profiles in the normal bifurcation seen in color flow imaging (see Fig. 5.13) will affect the spectral Doppler waveform shapes detected in the ICA origin, which may appear disturbed or demonstrate areas of reverse flow. Distal to the bifurcation and carotid bulb, the waveform shapes should no longer appear disturbed.

Abnormal appearance

The presence of a narrowing within the carotid arteries will lead to an increase in the velocity of the blood across the stenosis, and this can be measured using spectral Doppler. Significant changes in the velocity within and just beyond a stenosis will be detected once the vessel is narrowed by a >50% reduction in diameter. The increase in velocity is related to the degree of narrowing (see Ch. 5). These velocity changes can be used to grade the degree of narrowing. The Doppler waveforms obtained within or just beyond a significant stenosis will also demonstrate an increase in spectral broadening (Fig. 8.18B).

Unusually low velocities can indicate the presence of disease proximal or distal to the site at which the Doppler recording is made. High-resistance waveforms, with an absence of flow during diastole, obtained from the CCA may indicate a severe ICA stenosis or occlusion (Fig. 8.10B). Figure 8.19 shows another example of a high-resistance waveform, obtained from a disease-free origin of the ICA proximal to an MCA occlusion. A reversal of flow during the whole of diastole in the carotid arteries (Fig. 8.20) may relate to a heart problem, such as aortic valve regurgitation (Malaterre et al. 2001). In this case this abnormal appearance will be seen in both the left and right carotid arteries and not be associated with only one side. The waveform detected distal to a very severe, flow-limiting stenosis will often demonstrate turbulent

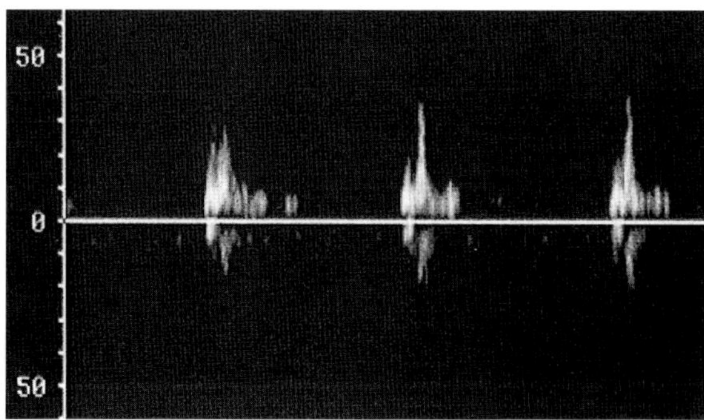

Figure 8.19 • High-resistance waveform detected in a nondiseased internal carotid artery origin proximal to a middle cerebral artery occlusion.

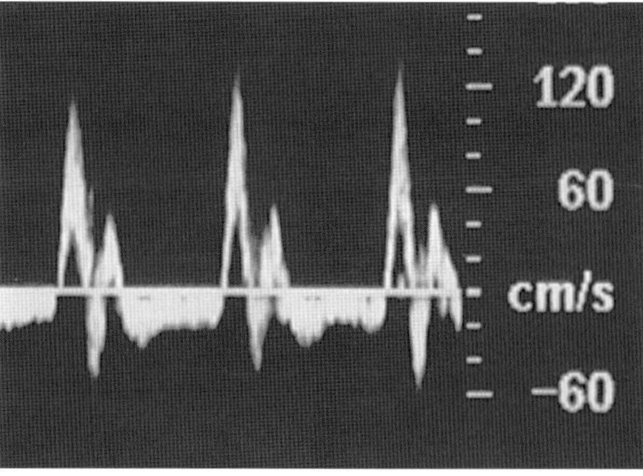

Figure 8.20 • Common carotid artery waveform showing reverse diastolic flow in the presence of aortic valve regurgitation.

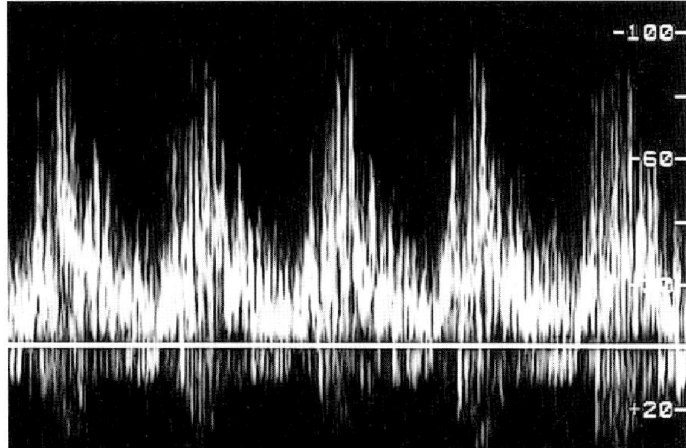

Figure 8.21 • Doppler recording demonstrating turbulent flow beyond a significant stenosis.

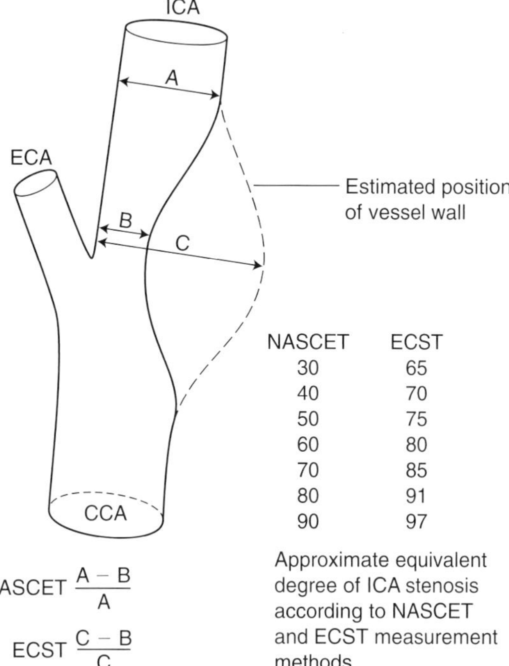

Figure 8.22 • The North American Symptomatic Carotid Endarterectomy Trial Collaborators (NASCET) and European Carotid Surgery Trialists' Collaborative Group (ECST) trials used different methods of reporting the degree of narrowing seen on carotid angiograms. ICA, internal carotid artery; ECA, external carotid artery; CCA, common carotid artery. (Reprinted with permission from Elsevier (The Lancet, 1998, 351: 1372–1373)

flow with an increased systolic rise time (Fig. 8.21). These abnormal waveform shapes can give the sonographer useful clues as to the presence of significant disease. The total absence of flow within a vessel, as demonstrated by color flow imaging, can be confirmed using spectral Doppler. However, it is sometimes possible to pick up low-velocity signals, due to wall thump, at a point just within the occluded vessel. The presence of small veins in the area of the bifurcation can also produce misleading Doppler signals, as venous flow in the neck can appear pulsatile.

Comment

It is possible for the carotid artery bifurcation to appear normal on B-mode and color imaging but for the spectral waveforms to appear abnormal due to disease proximal or distal to the bifurcation.

SELECTION OF TREATMENT FOR CAROTID ARTERY DISEASE

The results from two large multicenter trials have been published, the North American Symptomatic Carotid Endarterectomy Trial Collaborators (NASCET) (1991, 1998) and the European Carotid Surgery Trialists' Collaborative Group (ECST) (1998). These trials compared the benefits of carotid surgery, which carries some risk of mortality and morbidity, with the best medical treatment for patients with symptomatic carotid artery disease. The carotid disease was quantified using angiography. However, the method used to report the degree of narrowing from an angiogram differed between the European and North American trials. In the ECST trial, the degree of stenosis was measured by comparing the residual lumen diameter with the estimated diameter of the carotid bulb, whereas the NASCET trial compared the residual lumen diameter with the diameter of the normal distal ICA, as shown in Figure 8.22. Using these two different methods can lead to significant differences in grading the disease. For example, the narrowing in Figure 8.22 would be reported as a 70% diameter reduction by the European method but as only a 50% reduction by the North American method. Figure 8.22 also gives the approximate equivalent degree of stenosis, measured (from the same stenoses) using the different methods employed by the NASCET and ECST trials. Figure 8.23 shows an ultrasound B-mode image of a plaque with a

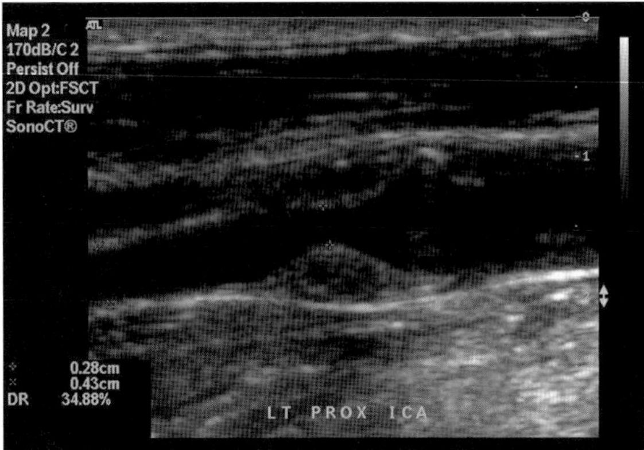

Figure 8.23 • B-mode image of a plaque in the carotid bifurcation showing a diameter reduction measurement made using the North American Symptomatic Carotid Endarterectomy Trial Collaborators (NASCET) method.

diameter measurement made using the NASCET method. It is possible, in a patient with large carotid bulbs, for the bulb to contain a large plaque without it causing a significant stenosis. In this situation it is important to describe this in the scan report as this may affect the choice of treatment, especially if the patient is symptomatic.

The difference in methods used to grade the degree of narrowing has made the comparison of the results from the two trials complicated. The ECST study showed that surgery reduced the risk of stroke in patients with ^{ECST}80–99% stenosis. However the NASCET reported similar results for patients with ^{NASCET}70–99%, which is equivalent to an ^{ECST}80–99% stenosis. Rothwell et al. (2003) remeasured the ESCT angiograms using the NASCET method and, analyzing the results of both trials together, concluded that CEA was of marginal benefit in symptomatic patients with a ^{NASCET}50–69% and was highly beneficial in those with a ^{NASCET} ≥70% stenosis but without near occlusion. Rothwell et al. indicate that it would be necessary to operate on about 6 patients to prevent one stroke. The trials suggest that surgery did not provide any significant benefit in patients with the string sign, near occlusion.

Another trial studying patients with significant (60–99%) asymptomatic stenosis, the Asymptomatic Carotid Atherosclerosis Study (ACAS) (1995), showed limited benefit of surgery in this group. Redgrave & Rothwell (2007) reviewed the evidence for medical and surgical intervention in these patients and concluded that the absolute benefit from endarterectony for aysmptomatic carotid stenosis is small, but can sometimes be justified in men. Future developments in patient selection may enable the group of patients at high risk of stroke to be more closely targeted. The fact that the symptoms are likely to relate to embolic rather than hemodynamic phenomena means that there is still some clinical debate as to whether plaque type and volume, along with the degree of vessel narrowing, are critical factors in the cause of stroke.

An alternative treatment for significant carotid disease is carotid angioplasty and stenting (CAS). Stents are expandable mesh tubes that can be used to keep a diseased vessel patent. Although stent placement does not involve a general anesthetic, sometimes used in CEA, there is a potential risk of stroke during the procedure. Carotid stents may be deployed with the use of some form of protection device such as a filter similar to a small umbrella positioned above the angioplasty site during stent placement to collect any emboli that may be dislodged in the process.

It is still controversial as to what role CAS has in the treatment of carotid artery disease. However it may be an appropriate treatment in a specific group of high-risk patients (Veith et al. 2001). In 2004 the US Food and Drug Administration approved a stent for use in carotid arteries in symptomatic patients with a ≥ 80% narrowing who are poor candidates for surgery. Randomized trials comparing CEA and CAS in recently symptomatic patients are still ongoing and the results of these may make the role of the two treatments clearer. Both CEA and CAS can be followed up using ultrasound and this is discussed later in the chapter.

Comment

It is important that the sonographer is up to date with the criteria for selection of treatment for patients with carotid artery stenosis as the ultrasound scan results will form an important part of the diagnostic process.

GRADING THE DISEASE

Imaging

Angiographic grading of carotid artery disease, as with other arterial disease, is described in terms of diameter reduction. Therefore as ultrasound criteria have been developed using angiography as the gold standard, ultrasound grading of stenoses is also typically described in terms of diameter reduction. However, the use of area reduction would seem more appropriate, especially in the presence of eccentric disease. Table 8.1 gives the percentage area reduction associated with a given percentage diameter reduction, assuming a symmetrical lumen reduction; however, these values are not correct in the presence of eccentric disease. B-mode imaging is the most appropriate method to evaluate the degree of narrowing, if the degree of lumen diameter reduction is less than 50%. However, if disease is eccentric, it is possible to overestimate the degree of narrowing if the atheroma lies on the anterior or posterior wall when imaged longitudinally. It is equally possible to underestimate the degree of narrowing on a longitudinal image if the plaque is situated on the lateral walls (Fig. 8.24). Therefore, the diseased vessel should be visualized in transverse section first, in order to select the optimal longitudinal imaging plane, although this is limited by the range of longitudinal scan planes available.

The percentage diameter reduction can be estimated from diameter measurements as follows:

$$\%\ \text{diameter reduction} = (1 - [\text{diameter of patent lumen}/\text{total diameter of vessel}]) \times 100$$

Color flow imaging can help in identifying any lumen reduction. It is possible to obtain a color flow image in longitudinal and transverse section and this may help in estimating the degree of narrowing, but there are potential pitfalls. Spurious flow voids can be created due to a poor angle of insonation or inappropriate PRF or filter settings, which may lead to an overestimate of the degree of narrowing. If the color gain is set too high, it is possible for the color to appear to 'bleed' out of the vessel lumen, and this can lead to an underestimate of the degree of narrowing (see Fig. 7.6).

DIAMETER REDUCTION (%)	CROSS-SECTIONAL AREA REDUCTION (%)
30	50
50	75
70	90

Table 8.1 Relationship between diameter reduction and cross-sectional area reduction assuming a concentric stenosis

Spectral Doppler

As the quantity of atheroma in the vessel increases, it becomes more difficult to estimate the degree of narrowing from the image, especially in the presence of calcified or hypoechoic atheroma. However, velocity criteria are used to grade the degree of stenosis once the vessel becomes narrowed by a >50% reduction in diameter. Over the years, several criteria have been produced for grading carotid artery disease, many of which have been published, and this has revealed many discrepancies.

The various criteria have been produced by comparing Doppler measurements with those of angiography, which has its own limitations, as the gold standard.

Most criteria for grading carotid stenoses are based on the PSV and EDV in the ICA, and the ratio of the PSV in the ICA to that in the CCA. Unlike the grading of stenosis in other parts of the arterial system, where there is often a proximal segment of normal vessel which can be used to calculate a velocity ratio, the geometry of the carotid bulb makes the situation less straightforward. The ratio of the PSV in the ICA to that in the CCA will partly depend on the relative dimensions of the CCA and ICA, and this is further complicated by the variable geometry of the carotid bulb. The presence of a large branch in the form of the ECA also complicates matters. Many criteria use absolute velocities in grading the narrowing. Using a combination of absolute velocity measurements and velocity ratios potentially reduces the pitfalls of using velocity criteria alone. For example, an increase in PSV can arise due to hypertension, age-related changes in vessel wall compliance, or increased flow to supply a collateral pathway. However, an increase would be seen in both the

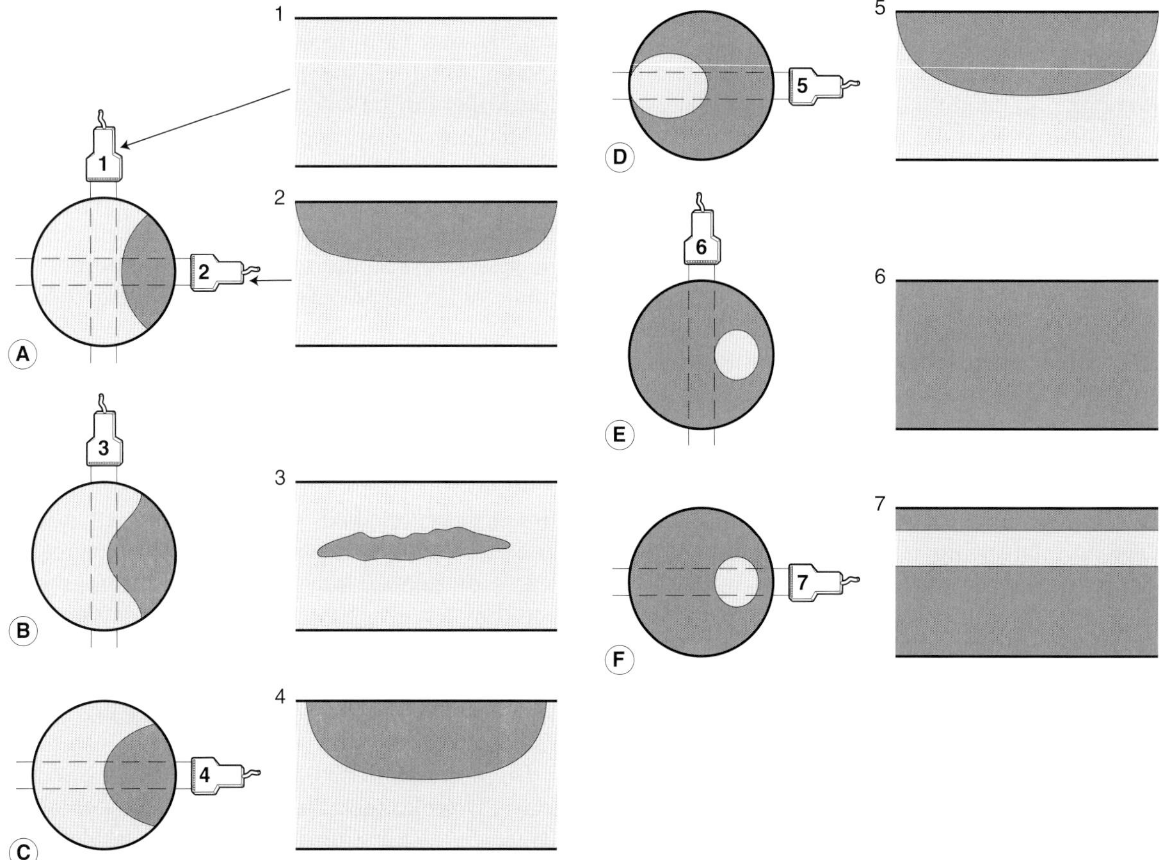

Figure 8.24 • It is possible to overestimate and underestimate eccentric disease when imaging in longitudinal section. The schematic diagrams show examples of disease imaged in transverse and longitudinal section from the numbered transducer positions. (A) An area of atheroma may not be seen in one longitudinal plane (1) and may appear more significant in another (2). (B) Atheroma on the lateral walls may protrude into the center of the vessel and give the appearance of atheroma floating in the vessel. (C, D) These longitudinal images give a similar appearance despite very different degrees of narrowing. (E, F): The longitudinal image may give the appearance of the vessel being occluded (E) or stenosed (F) depending on the imaging plane used.

CCA and ICA, and the absence of a significant velocity increase along the vesse would reassure the sonographer that there was no significant evidence of a stenosis. Conversely, an abnormal velocity ratio in the presence of low velocities, possibly due to low cardiac output, may help to identify a stenosis.

Table 8.2 gives some examples of criteria for grading carotid stenosis that have been developed by investigators at different centers over the years. These centers have divided the degree of narrowing into different bands. Following the ECST and NASCET trials, it is especially useful to distinguish between stenoses of <70% and ≥70% in order to select the group of patients who would benefit from surgery, given the appropriate symptoms. Bluth et al. (1988) produced their criteria using an early duplex scanner with a stand-off Doppler element, as opposed to a linear array transducer. These older systems were less prone to intrinsic spectral broadening and therefore produced different results from many modern linear array systems, which tend to overestimate peak velocities. Intrinsic spectral broadening (see Ch. 6) may lead to errors in velocity measurements that are dependent on the angle of insonation.

AUTHOR	PERCENTAGE STENOSIS DIAMETER REDUCTION	ICA PSV (cm/s)	ICA EDV (cm/s)	ICA PSV TO CCA PSV RATIO
Bluth et al. (1988)	40–59	<130	40*	<1.8
	60–79	>130	>40*	<1.8
	80–99	>250	>100*	>3.7
Robinson et al. (1988) (NASCET)	<50	<150	<50	<2
	>50	>150	>50	>2
	>70	>225	>75	>3
Hunink et al. (1993)	70–99	≥230		
Fraught et al. (1994) (NASCET)	50–69	<130	≤100	
	70–99	>130	>100	
Sidhu & Allan (1997)	50–59	>130	<40	<3.2
	60–69	>130	40–110	3.2–4
	70–79	>230	110–140	>4
	80–95	>230	140	>4
	96–99	"String flow"		
	100	"No flow"		
Filis et al. (2002) (NASCET)	<50	<150	<50	<1.8
	50–59	150–200	50–70	<2.2
	60–69	200–250	70–90	2.2–2.8
	70–79	250–330	90–130	2.8–3.8
	80–89	330–400	130–180	3.8–5
	90–99	>400	>180	>5
	Occlusion	"No flow detected at ICA by PW/CDI using sensitive scale settings. Unilateral blunted CCA flow"		
Stalkov et al. (2002)	70–99 (NASCET)	≥220	≥80	
	70–99 (ECST and CC[†])	≥190	≥65	
	80–99 (ECST)	≥215	≥90	
Grant et al. (2003) (NASCET)	<50	<125	<40	<2.0
	50–69	125–230	40–100	2.0–4.0
	≥70 but less than near occlusion	>230	>100	>4.0
	Near occlusion	High, low, or undetectable	Variable	Variable
	Total occlusion	Undetectable	Not applicable	Not applicable

*Peak diastolic velocity; [†]common carotid method.

ICA, internal carotid artery; PSV, peak systolic velocity; EDV, end-diastolic velocity; PW/CDI, pulsed-wave/color Doppler imaging; CCA, common carotid artery; NASCET, North American Symptomatic Carotid Endarterectomy Trial Collaborators; ECST, European Carotid Surgery Trialists' Collaborative Group.

Table 8.2 Summary of a selection of reported Doppler ultrasound criteria for diagnosing stenosis

Comment

Some centers choose to overcome angle-dependent variations in velocity recordings by using a fixed angle of 60°. In practice this may not always be possible. Aiming to take measurements with an angle between 45 and 60° may be a practical solution.

Most of the sets of criteria listed in Table 8.2 have been correlated against angiography using the NASCET method of reporting angiographic findings. Therefore a ≥70% stenosis as defined by these criteria would relate to a >80% diameter reduction as measured by the ECST method. Staikov et al. (2002) compared ultrasound criteria for detecting stenosis using both the NASCET and ECST methods of measuring angiograms and showed that the velocity criteria produced for a ≥70% stenosis by the NASCET method are similar to the criteria produced for a ≥80% stenosis using the ECST method. The criteria suggested by Sidhu & Allan (1997) are based on results reported by Moneta et al (1993, 1995). Table 8.2 includes criteria published following the Carotid Artery Stenosis Consensus conference (Grant et al. 2003). The consensus makes many recommendations, including the use of plaque estimate (percentage diameter reduction) with B-mode and color Doppler ultrasound, along with ICA PSV criteria as primary parameters. ICA/CCA PSV ratio and ICA EDV are recommended as additional parameters. Grant et al. (2003) reviewed many published ultrasound criteria for grading carotid disease in order to form the consensus criteria.

Table 8.3 shows the diagnostic criteria published in a paper presenting the recommendations for reporting carotid ultrasound investigations in the UK (Oates et al. 2008). These criteria are based on publications by Grant et al. (2003) and Filis et al. (2002) (shown in Table 8.2) and also includes the St Mary's ratio, the ICA PSV to CCA EDV ratio, published by Nicolaides et al. (1996). Oates et al. (2008) also provide advice on measurement technique and situations where caution is required in quantifying disease using these criteria. The St Mary's ratio (Nicolaides et al. 1996) should not be used in the absence of CCA diastolic flow or the presence of reversal of CCA diastolic flow, for example due to aortic valve disease (Fig. 8.20).

PERCENTAGE STENOSIS (NASCET)	INTERNAL CAROTID PEAK SYSTOLIC VELOCITY CM/S	PEAK SYSTOLIC VELOCITY RATIO ICA_{PSV}/CCA_{PSV}	ST MARY'S RATIO‡ ICA_{PSV}/CCA_{EDV}
<50	<125*	<2*	<8
50–59	>125*	2–4*	8–10
60–69			11–13
70–79	>230*	>4*	14–21
80–89			22–29
>90	>400†	>5†	>30
Near occlusion	High, low, or string flow	Variable	Variable
Occlusion	No flow	Not applicable	Not applicable

*Grant et al. (2003).
†Filis et al. (2002).
‡Nicolaides et al. (1996).
NASCET, North American Symptomatic Carotid Endarterectomy Trial Collaborators; ICA, internal carotid artery; PSV, peak systolic velocity; CCA, common carotid artery; EDV, end-diastolic velocity.

Table 8.3 Joint recommendations for reporting carotid ultrasound investigations in the UK: diagnostic criteria (Reprinted from European Journal of Vascular and Endovascular Surgery, 37/3, Oates, Naylor, Hartshorne, et al, 2008, with permission from Elsevier)

An important factor that may affect the criteria selected for grading stenoses is whether ultrasound is to be used as a screening test before angiography, MRA, or CTA, for which a high sensitivity is required (see Appendix B), or to select patients for surgery, without angiography, for which sensitivity and specificity should both be equally high, to keep the number of false-positive results as low as possible. The publications describing the criteria listed in Table 8.2 include details of the sensitivity and specificity obtained by these criteria. Each center should verify its criteria locally by comparing the ultrasound findings with alternative imaging such as MRA, CTA, or angiography. If a department has more than one scanner, it is necessary to check the criteria used on each machine as different models of scanner may give different results. It is important for sonographers to understand how the results of their scans are used by the surgical or medical teams that have requested them and that these teams are aware of the method the sonographers use to define the degree of disease.

COMBINING B-MODE, COLOR IMAGING, AND SPECTRAL DOPPLER INFORMATION

The information obtained from all three modalities should be used to estimate the degree of narrowing, as all modalities have their strengths and weaknesses. Figure 8.25 gives an example of how this can be done. Figure 8.25A shows a transverse image of a diseased ICA, with evidence of atheroma, part of which appears calcified (shown by the arrow). This image suggests a diameter reduction of 50–70%. Figure 8.25B shows a longitudinal image of the same vessel with an absence of flow seen in the proximal ICA. However, when the same vessel is imaged in a different longitudinal plane (Fig. 8.25C) the flow can now be seen within the vessel. Although the vessel lumen appears to be only slightly narrowed on this color image (Fig. 8.25C), the presence of a velocity increase, demonstrated by aliasing, should alert the sonographer to the possible presence of a more significant narrowing. Spectral Doppler velocity measurement (Fig. 8.25D) gives a PSV of 200 cm/s and an EDV of 75 cm/s in the ICA. Using the velocity criteria of Grant et al. (2003) (Table 8.2) these velocity measurements would indicate a narrowing of 50–69% (NASCET) diameter reduction. An ICA PSV to CCA PSV ratio should be measured to support this conclusion.

By using the appearance of both B-mode and color images in transverse and a variety of longitudinal imaging planes, along with velocity measurements and velocity ratios, the sonographer is able to estimate the degree of narrowing. There will, however, be situations in which imaging and velocity measurement are limited and the sonographer is unable to make a judgment on the severity of the disease, and this should be made clear in the scan report.

NORMAL AND ABNORMAL APPEARANCES OF VERTEBRAL ARTERY FLOW

The vertebral artery and vein can be seen between the vertebral processes. The vein normally lies above the artery, and flow in the artery is normally seen traveling toward the head (cephalad flow) (Figs 8.12 and 8.26A). It is not uncommon to see a larger vertebral artery or higher velocities on one side, usually the left, compared with the other. Occasionally, it may only be possible to visualize one of the vertebral arteries. The Doppler spectrum obtained from the vertebral artery demonstrates a low-resistance waveform shape with high diastolic flow (Fig. 8.26A).

Reverse flow (i.e., flow away from the head) in one of the vertebral arteries would suggest subclavian steal syndrome (Figs 8.3 and 8.26B). Doppler recordings obtained from the ipsilateral distal subclavian artery will appear damped (see Ch. 10), and sometimes it is possible to detect a stenotic jet in the proximal subclavian artery due to a stenosis. In some cases the appearance of the vertebral artery flow can be confusing, showing flow away from the head during systole and toward the head during diastole, as shown in Figure 8.26C. Here, the pressure drop across the diseased subclavian artery is not sufficient to cause flow reversal in the vertebral artery throughout the whole cardiac cycle. To confirm that this abnormal flow is due to subclavian steal, the patient should be asked to exercise the arm ipsilateral to the abnormal vertebral flow, by bending the forearm toward the shoulder once per second for 1 min. Alternatively, a sphygmomanometer cuff can be used to induce hyperemia by inflating the cuff around the upper

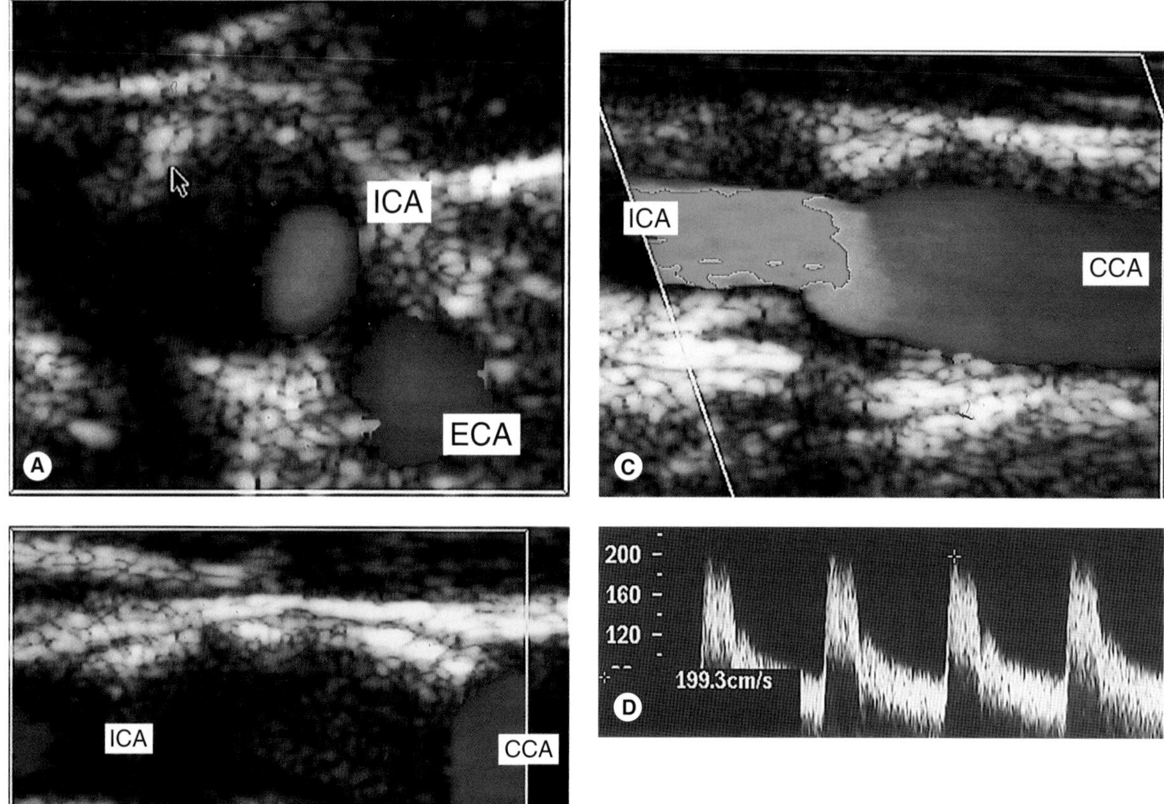

Figure 8.25 • A combination of B-mode, color flow imaging, and spectral Doppler can be used to assess carotid disease. (A) A transverse image of a diseased internal carotid artery (ICA), with atheroma, part of which appears calcified (arrow), suggesting a 50–70% diameter reduction (ECA, external carotid artery). (B) A longitudinal image of the vessel with an absence of flow seen in the proximal ICA. (C) When the vessel is imaged in a different plane, flow can be seen within the vessel. Although the vessel lumen appears to be only slightly narrowed in this plane, a velocity increase, demonstrated by aliasing, is seen. (D) Spectral Doppler velocity measurement gives a peak systolic velocity of 200 cm/s and an end-diastolic velocity of 75 cm/s in the ICA, indicating a 60–69% (North American Symptomatic Carotid Endarterectomy Trial Collaborators: NASCET) diameter reduction.

arm to a pressure above systolic pressure for 2–3 min and then deflating. The exercise or hyperemia will increase the blood flow to the arm and cause the flow in the vertebral artery to reverse throughout the whole cardiac cycle. It is not possible to scan the entire length of the vertebral artery because sections of it are obscured by the vertebral processes; however, if indicated, it is sometimes possible to image the vertebral artery origins in the base of the neck, although this can be quite difficult.

PROBLEMS ENCOUNTERED IN IMAGING CAROTID ARTERY FLOW

Calcified atheroma

Extensive calcified plaque within the carotid bifurcation leading to significant shadowing on the image can cause problems with grading the disease. Calcification may prevent any B-mode, color, or spectral Doppler information from being obtained from within the vessel. The initial appearance of the absence of flow detected by the color

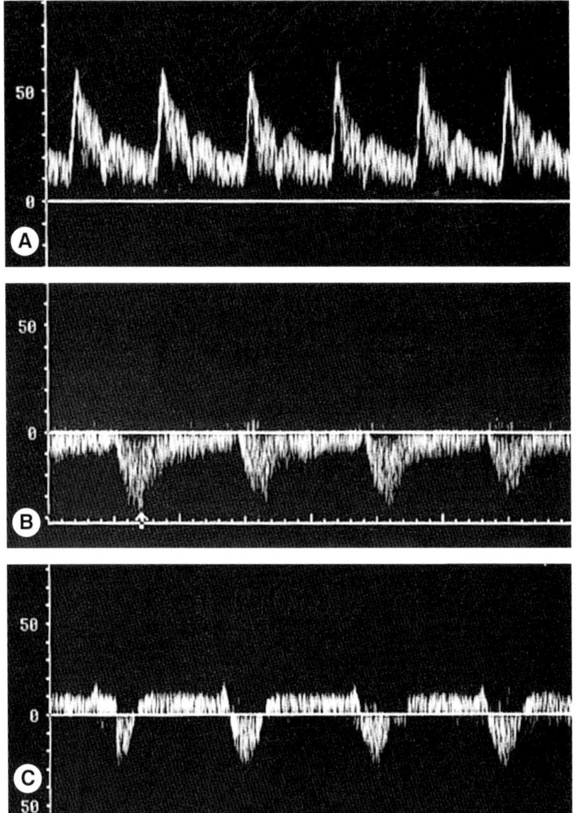

Figure 8.26 • (A) Flow seen in a normal vertebral artery. (B) Complete flow reversal. (C) Partial flow reversal seen in the vertebral artery due to subclavian steal syndrome.

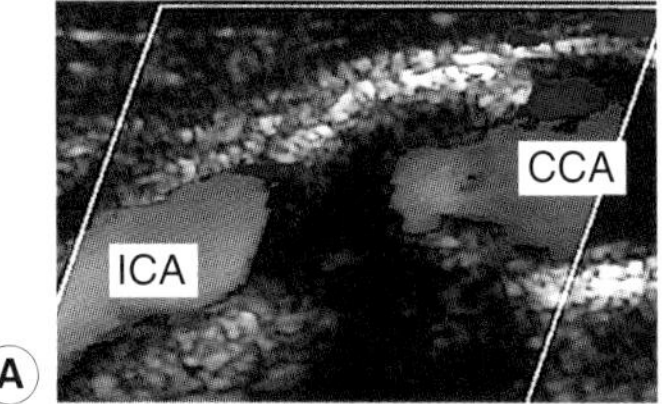

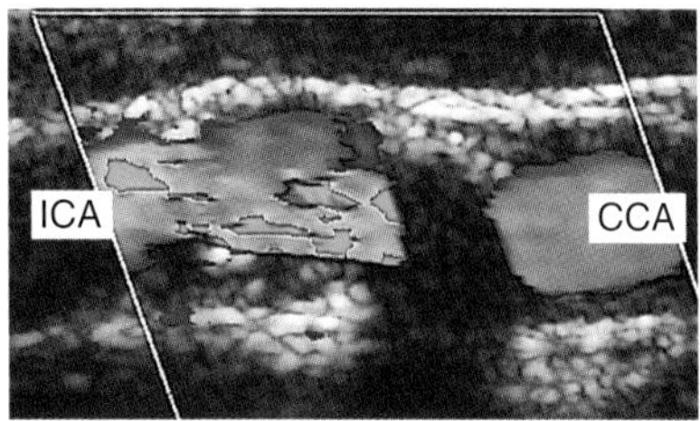

Figure 8.27 • Calcification of the anterior arterial wall may prevent B-mode imaging, color flow imaging, and spectral Doppler recordings within the calcified segment of vessel. (A) Color flow imaging does not suggest a significant change in velocity across the calcified segment. (B) Marked flow disturbance (increased velocity and flow recirculation) is seen beyond the area of calcification.

flow imaging may mislead the sonographer into thinking that the vessel is occluded. However, the presence of bright echoes on the anterior wall and an absence of echoes below this should suggest calcification (Fig. 8.27). Images of the vessel distal to the calcification should be obtained and the presence of flow established. If the distal vessel can be seen clearly, with no evidence of further calcification, but no flow is detected even when the scanner is optimized to detect low-velocity flow, the vessel is probably occluded. If flow is detected distal to a calcified area, the spectral Doppler waveform may assist in grading the degree of stenosis present within the calcified area.

The presence of extensive calcified atheroma may not necessarily relate to a significant narrowing. If the calcified atheroma only extends a short way along the vessel wall, the presence of a normal Doppler waveform beyond it would suggest that it was not causing a severe stenosis. If, however, the calcification extends for more than 1 cm, a normal waveform beyond it cannot be used to indicate the absence of any significant narrowing as normal flow can be established within a short distance distal to a stenosis. If an abnormal waveform is detected beyond the calcification, the presence of a significant stenosis can be more confidently predicted. High PSV and EDV (Fig. 8.18B) produced by a jet extending beyond a stenosis, poststenotic flow turbulence (Fig. 8.21), or low-velocity, damped flow would all suggest the presence of a significant stenosis. If any doubt about the presence or absence of significant disease remains at the end of the examination, the sonographer should make this clear in the report, as alternative imaging may be required to clarify the degree of narrowing. In cases of less severe calcification, the sonographer may be able to overcome poor imaging by viewing the vessels in a different plane (Fig. 8.25).

Vessel tortuosity

Imaging tortuous vessels can be a problem as the vessel may not appear in a single plane. Its path may run parallel to the ultrasound beam, thus producing poor images of the vessel walls. Color Doppler imaging can be used to assist in following tortuous arteries (Fig. 8.28), but the changing direction of the vessel may require regular changes in the steering angle of the color box to allow the flow to be visualized. Poor Doppler angles may limit the color flow imaging and, in this situation, power Doppler may help to image the vessel and assist in ruling out filling defects in the vessel due to the presence of atheroma.

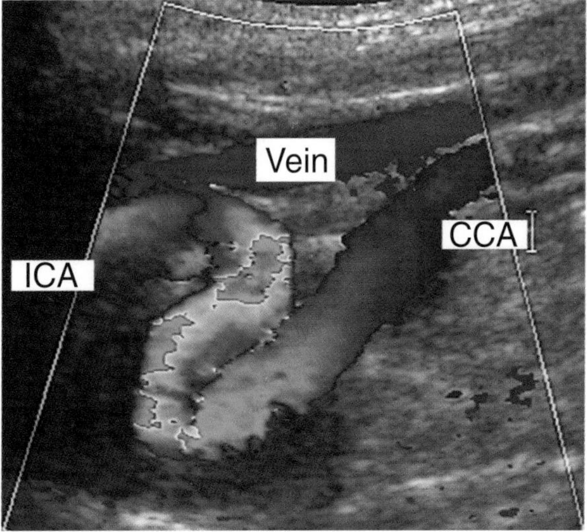

Figure 8.28 • Color flow image of a tortuous internal carotid artery (ICA). CCA, common carotid artery.

POSTOPERATIVE CAROTID ARTERY APPEARANCE ON ULTRASOUND

Only a small percentage of patients develop severe recurrent stenosis or occlusion following surgery and, of these, only a few suffer from any symptoms. It has been shown that routine postoperative ultrasound surveillance does not significantly affect patient management, and patients are often rescanned only if symptoms recur. The scan procedure is the same as that already described, but the postoperative appearance differs slightly from the appearance of a normal carotid bifurcation. First, the vessel wall no longer has the double-layer appearance where the plaque has been removed. It is often possible to see a step in the posterior CCA wall at the beginning of the site of the endarterectomy (Fig. 8.29). A vein or prosthetic patch may be used to close the site of the endarterectomy, as it is thought that this may reduce the risk of early postoperative thrombosis or late restenosis. If a patch has been used to widen the vessel, it will often produce a slightly dilated bifurcation compared to normal. A prosthetic patch produces a brighter echo than a vein patch or adjacent arterial wall, and it can therefore usually be easily seen on the image. Vein patches can be susceptible to rupture whereas prosthetic

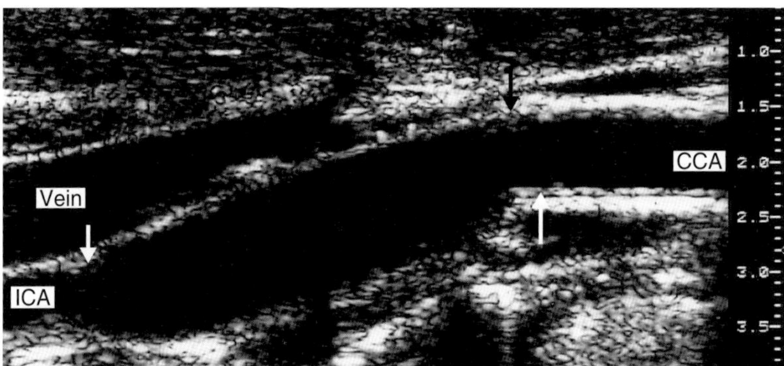

Figure 8.29 • A montage image of a postoperative carotid endarterectomy site. The small arrows demonstrate the length of the endarterectomy site. The large arrow demonstrates the intima-media layer proximal to the endarterectomy site. ICA, internal carotid artery; CCA, common carotid artery.

patches can be susceptible to infection, which can produce a rucked appearance to the patch. Ultrasound can be used to measure the dimensions of the endarterectomy site and investigate any recurrent disease.

POST CAROTID ARTERY ANGIOPLASTY AND STENTING APPEARANCE ON ULTRASOUND

Ultrasound can also be used to follow up patients who have had a carotid stenosis treated by angioplasty and stenting. Figure 8.30A shows how with B-mode imaging the stent can be clearly seen within the carotid artery with evidence of the plaque seen between the stent and the carotid artery wall. Color flow imaging and spectral Doppler (Figure 8.30B) can be used to assess the residual lumen poststenting and to monitor any restenosis within the stent. One issue that has arisen with ultrasound assessment of stented carotid arteries is that the velocities detected in the stented vessels without significant narrowings are on average higher than the velocities seen in normal carotid arteries. Lal et al. (2008) found that velocity criteria developed for native arteries overestimate the degree of in-stent restenosis It has been suggested that this may be due to the difference in the mechanical properties, that is the wall compliance, of the stent compared to the native vessel. New velocity criteria, specifically for assessing stented carotid arteries, have been developed and two of these (Lal et al. 2008, Zhou et al. 2008) are shown in Table 8.4. Significant restenosis of the stent, especially in the presence of further symptoms, will probably require further treatment.

NONATHEROMATOUS CAROTID ARTERY DISEASES

Nonatheromatous extracranial carotid diseases include aneurysms, carotid body tumors, and dissection, but all are relatively rare. Patients may have a pulsatile swelling in the neck that can be investigated with ultrasound to rule out an aneurysm. The carotid arteries should be scanned along their length, especially in the area of the suspected swelling, and the cross-sectional diameter measured. Any unusual appearances relating to the arteries should be reported. In many cases, the 'pulsatile swelling' is due to a superficial brachiocephalic bifurcation or carotid bifurcation, often associated with tortuous vessels, leading to the vessel being easily palpated. Another possible cause of a pulsatile swelling is the presence of a

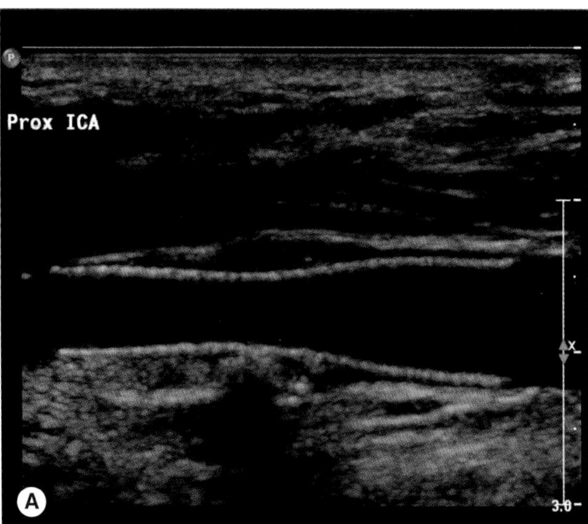

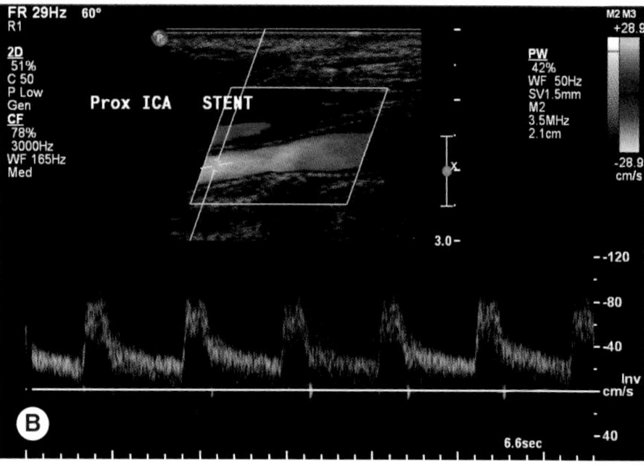

Figure 8.30 • (A) B-mode image showing a carotid artery that has been treated with angioplasty and stenting. (B) Color flow imaging and spectral Doppler can be used to assess the residual lumen post angioplasty and stenting. ICA, internal carotid artery.

AUTHOR	PERCENTAGE STENOSIS DIAMETER REDUCTION	ICA PSV (cm/s)	ICA EDV (cm/s)	ICA PSV TO CCA PSV RATIO
Lal et al. (2008)	0–19%	<150*		<2.15*
	20–49%	150–219		
	50–79%	220–339		≥2.7
	80–99%	≥340		≥4.15
Zhou et al. (2008)	>70%	>300	>90	>4

*PSV and EDV measurements for stented carotid arteries are performed within the stented segments.
ICA, internal carotid artery; PSV, peak systolic velocity; EDV, end-diastolic velocity; CCA, common carotid artery.

Table 8.4 Two new criteria developed for the assessing stenosis in stented carotid arteries (ICA PSV measured from within stented segment)

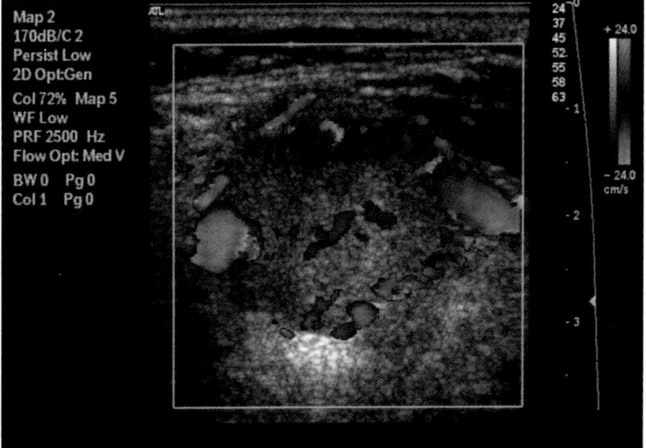

Figure 8.31 • Transverse image of a carotid body tumor lying between the internal carotid artery (ICA: right) and external carotid artery (ECA: left).

carotid body tumor. The carotid body is a small structure within the vessel wall, situated at the carotid bifurcation, and is responsible for detecting blood gases and pH. As a carotid body tumor grows, it causes the ICA and ECA to be splayed apart, and the tumor usually appears highly vascular on color flow imaging (Fig. 8.31). However, further investigation is required to confirm any ultrasound findings.

Carotid artery wall dissection, which can be due to trauma such as whiplash, can create a false lumen within the carotid arteries (Fig. 8.32). This may remain patent and be seen as a second flow lumen on color flow imaging. Alternatively, the false lumen may occlude, causing a reduction in the residual vessel lumen or possibly a complete occlusion of the vessel. An intimal flap may be seen on the image as a fine line within the lumen that may move due to the pulsatile blood flow; however, it can be difficult to image.

TRANSCRANIAL DOPPLER ULTRASOUND

Generally, ultrasound is not easily transmitted through bone, making imaging within the skull difficult. However, the temporal bone is thinner than the rest of the skull and, by using low-frequency ultrasound (e.g., 2 MHz), it is possible to obtain both color flow images and spectral Doppler recordings from segments of some of the intracranial vessels. Nonimaging transcranial Doppler has been used to monitor flow in the MCA during carotid surgery for many years. CEA involves exposing the carotid bifurcation and clamping the CCA, ICA, and ECA. This can lead to compromised cerebral circulation, and, where appropriate, a temporary plastic shunt can be used to maintain flow between the CCA and ICA while the plaque is surgically removed. Transcranial Doppler enables MCA blood velocity to be measured, allowing failure of the shunts to be detected. Air and particulate emboli generated at the site of the endarterectomy can be detected, using Doppler ultrasound, as they travel through the MCA. Emboli give a characteristic 'chirp' on the audible Doppler signal and may appear as a brighter line on the spectral Doppler waveform.

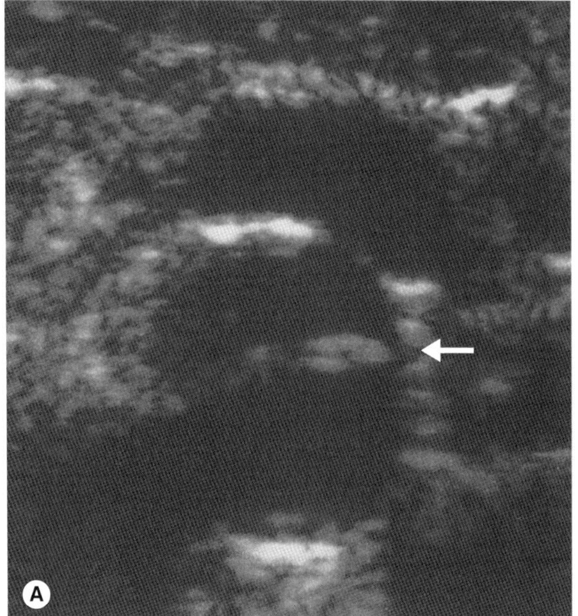

Figure 8.32 • B-mode image of a carotid artery wall dissection (arrow) showing a false lumen imaged in transverse section (A) and in longitudinal section (B). ICA, internal carotid artery; CCA, common carotid artery.

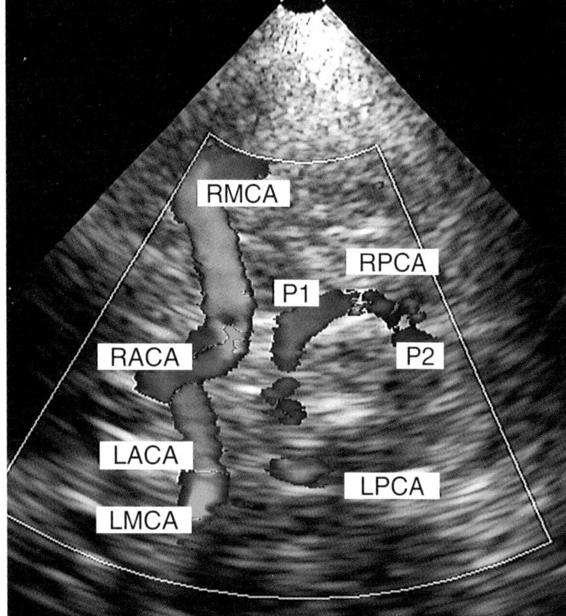

Figure 8.33 • Transcranial color flow imaging can be used to investigate the intracerebral circulation (see Fig. 8.2A). RMCA, right middle cerebral artery; RPCA, right posterior cerebral artery; RACA, right anterior cerebral artery; LACA, left anterior cerebral artery; LMCA, left middle cerebral artery; LPCA, left posterior cerebral artery.

Transcranial color flow imaging is performed using low-frequency phased array transducers and can provide a color map of part or all of the MCA, ACA, posterior cerebral artery, and circle of Willis (Fig. 8.33). However, views can sometimes be limited by attenuation caused by the temporal bone. Transcranial color flow imaging requires an indepth understanding of possible collateral pathways and, as yet, does not have a clear role in routine ultrasound assessment of the cerebral circulation. The techniques used in transcranial Doppler assessment are beyond the remit of this book, and the reader is referred to the further reading section at the end of this chapter.

REPORTING

The ultrasound report should describe the presence, location, and appearance of any atheroma seen within the CCA and ICA. In the presence of extensive disease (Fig. 8.34) the lower and upper extent of the disease should be clearly stated in the report. Any significant velocity increases along the carotid arteries should be reported and interpreted to estimate the degree of narrowing present. Abnormal waveforms seen within the CCA, ICA, or ECA should also be described, along with a suggestion as to what they may indicate. The presence and direction of vertebral artery flow should be noted. The report should make it very clear if there was

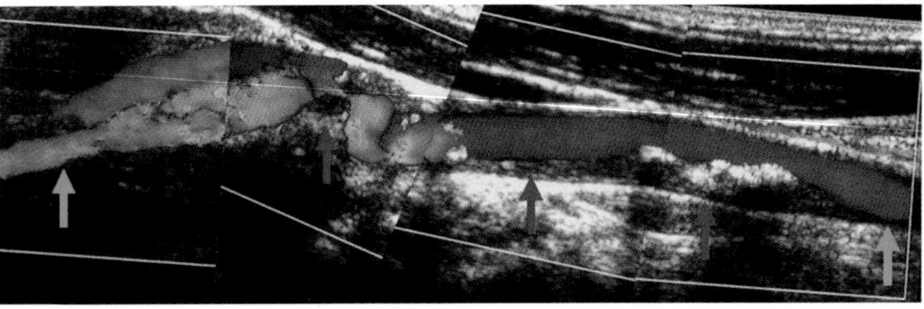

Figure 8.34 • Color image of extensive disease in the common carotid artery (right) and internal carotid artery (left). The green arrows represent the lower and upper limit of the carotid artery disease. The red arrows mark areas of plaque, with the plaque in the bulb (left red arrow) causing a tight stenosis. The ultrasound report should clearly state the extent of the disease.

BOX 8.2 Information to include in a carotid scan report, especially when surgery is performed on the basis of ultrasound alone

- Locations and appearance of any atheroma seen within the common carotid artery (CCA), bifurcation, and internal carotid artery (ICA)
- Significant velocity increases seen in the carotid arteries and an estimation of the degree of narrowing present
- Abnormal waveforms seen within the CCA, ICA, and external carotid artery
- Endpoint of ICA disease
- Presence and direction of vertebral artery flow
- Level of the carotid bifurcation in relation to the angle of the jaw
- Evidence of subocclusion
- Small ICA distal to disease that may preclude the use of a shunt
- Limitations of the examination

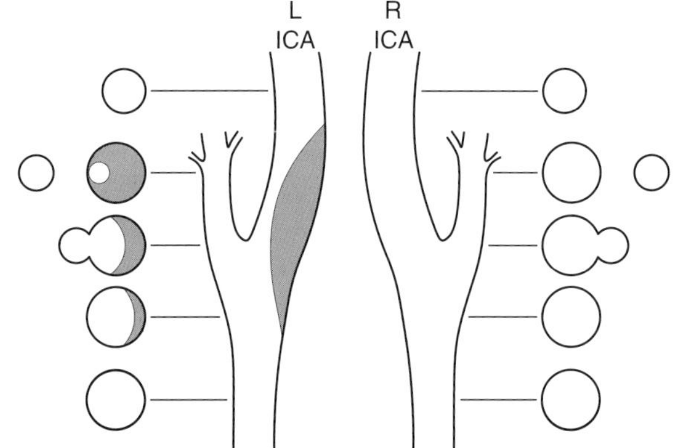

Figure 8.35 • Example of a diagrammatic method of reporting a carotid ultrasound scan result. ICA, internal carotid artery.

any limitation of the carotid examination, such as the following:

- Inconclusive identification of an occlusion or subocclusion
- Calcification obscuring the vessel for more than 1 cm
- No visible endpoint to ICA disease
- Whether the scan was otherwise suboptimal
- Whether waveforms obtained suggest possible significant vascular disease proximal or distal to the bifurcation which may require further investigation.

When ultrasound is to be used to select patients for surgery, without the use of any other alternative imaging, it is essential that the examination and report should cover the points listed in Box 8.2. The report can consist of a written report alone or may include images of atheroma and waveforms seen. Alternatively, a diagrammatic representation of the disease seen can be produced. Figure 8.35 is an example of a diagrammatic method of producing a report. It is important that the department has a written protocol, including the criteria used to interpret the Doppler findings and the method of reporting to be used.

References

Asymptomatic Carotid Atherosclerosis Study Group 1995 Carotid endarterectomy for patients with asymptomatic internal carotid artery stenosis. Journal of the American Medical Association 273: 1421–1428

Bluth E I, Stavros A T, Marich K W et al. 1988 Carotid duplex sonography: a multicenter recommendation for standardized imaging and Doppler criteria. Radiographics 8: 487–506

Bock R W, Lusby R J 1992 Carotid plaque morphology and interpretation of the echolucent lesions. In: Labs K H, Jager K A, Fitzgerald D E (eds) Diagnostic vascular ultrasound. Edward Arnold, London, pp 225–236

de Bray J M, Baud J M, Dauzat M 1997 Consensus concerning the morphology and the risk of carotid plaques. Cerebrovascular Disease 7: 289–296

Donnan G A, Davis S M, Chambers B R et al. 1998 Surgery for prevention of stroke. Lancet 351: 1372–1373

European Carotid Plaque Study Group 1995 Carotid artery plaque composition – relationship to clinical presentation and ultrasound B-mode imaging. European Journal of Endovascular Surgery 10: 23–30

European Carotid Surgery Trialists' Collaborative Group 1998 Randomised trial of endarterectomy for recently symptomatic carotid stenosis: final results of the MRC European Carotid Surgery Trial (ECST). Lancet 351: 1379–1387

Filis K A, Arko F R, Johnson B L et al. 2002 Duplex ultrasound criteria for defining the severity of carotid stenosis. Annals of Vascular Surgery 16: 413–421

Fosse E, Johnsen SH, Stensland-Bugge E et al. 2006 Repeated visual and computer-assisted carotid plaque characterization in a longitudinal population-based ultrasound study: the Tromso study. Ultrasound in Medicine and Biology 32: 3–11

Fraught W E, Mattos M A, van Bemmelen P S et al. 1994 Color-flow duplex scanning of carotid arteries: new velocity criteria based on receiver operator characteristic analysis for threshold stenosis used in the symptomatic and asymptomatic carotid trials. Journal of Vascular Surgery 19: 818–828

Grant E G, Benson C B, Moneta G L et al. 2003 Carotid artery stenosis: gray-scale and Doppler US diagnosis. Society of Radiologists in Ultrasound Consensus Conference. Radiology 229: 340–346

Gronholdt M L, Nordestgaard B G, Schroeder T V et al. 2001 Ultrasound echolucent carotid plaques predict future strokes. Circulation 104: 68–73

Hunink M G M, Polak J F, Barlan M M et al. 1993 Detection and quantification of carotid artery stenosis: efficacy of various Doppler velocity parameters. American Journal of Roentgenology 160: 619–625

Lal B K, Hobson II,R W, Tofighi B et al. 2008 Duplex ultrasound velocity criteria for the stented carotid artery. Journal of Vascular Surgery 47: 63–73

Malaterre H R, Kallee K, Giusiano B et al. 2001 Holodiastolic reversal flow in the common carotid: another indicator of the severity of aortic regurgitation. International Journal of Cardiovascular Imaging 17: 333–337

Mathiesen E B, Bonaa K H, Joakimsen O 2001 Echolucent plaques are associated with high risk of ischemic cerebrovascular events in carotid stenosis. Circulation 103: 2171

Merrit C R B, Bluth E I 1992 Ultrasound identification of plaque composition. In: Labs K H, Jager K A, Fitzgerald D E (eds) Diagnostic vascular ultrasound. Edward Arnold, London, pp 213–224

Moneta G L, Edwards J M, Chitwood R W et al. 1993 Correlation of North American Symptomatic Carotid Endarterectomy Trial (NASCET) angiographic definition of 70% to 99% internal carotid stenosis with duplex scanning. Journal of Vascular Surgery 17: 152–159

Moneta G L, Edwards J M, Papanicolaou G et al. 1995 Screening for asymptomatic internal carotid artery stenosis: duplex criteria for discriminating 60% to 99% stenosis. Journal of Vascular Surgery 21: 989–994

Naylor A R 2008 Delay may reduce procedural risk, but at what price to the patient? European Journal of Vascular and Endovascular Surgery 35: 383–391

Naylor A R, Beard J D, Gaines P A 1998 Extracranial carotid disease. In: Beard J D, Gaines P A (eds) Vascular and endovascular surgery. WB Saunders, London, pp 317–350

Nicolaides A N, Shifrin E G, Bradbury A et al. 1996 Angiographic and duplex grading of internal carotid stenosis: can we overcome confusion? Journal of Endovascular Surgery 3: 158–165

North American Symptomatic Carotid Endarterectomy Trial Collaborators (NASCET) 1991 Beneficial effect of carotid endarterectomy in symptomatic patients with high-grade carotid stenosis. New England Journal of Medicine 325: 445–453

North American Symptomatic Carotid Endarterectomy Trial Collaborators 1998 The final results of the NASCET trial. New England Journal of Medicine 339: 1415–1425

Oates C P, Naylor A R, Hartshorne T et al. (2008) Joint recommendations for reporting carotid ultrasound investigations in the United Kingdom. European Journal of Vascular and Endorascular Surgery (in press)

Pemble L 2008 A study of the validity of performing carotid duplex ultrasound with the patient in a seated position. Ultrasound 16: 80–82

Redgrave J, Rothwell P 2007 Asymptomatic carotid stenosis: what to do. Current Opinion in Neurology 20: 58–64

Robinson M L, Sacks D, Perlmutter G S et al. 1988 Diagnostic criteria for carotid duplex sonography. American Journal of Roentgenology 151: 1045–1049

Rothwell P M, Eliasziw M, Gutnikov S A et al. 2003 Analysis of pooled data from the randomised controlled trials of endarterectomy for symptomatic carotid stenosis. Lancet 361: 107–116

Rothwell P M, Eliasziw M, Gutnikov S A 2004 Endarterectomy for symptomatic carotid stenosis in relation to clinical subgroups and timing of surgery. Lancet 363: 915–924

Sacco R L, Adams R, Albers G et al. 2006 Guidelines for the prevention of stroke in patients with ischaemic stroke or transient ischaemic attack: a statement for healthcare professionals from the American Heart Association/American Stroke Council on Stroke. Stroke 37: 577–617

Sidhu P S, Allan P L 1997 Ultrasound assessment of internal carotid artery stenosis. Clinical Radiology 52: 654–658

Staikov I N, Nedeltchev K, Arnold M et al. 2002 Duplex sonographic criteria for measuring carotid stenoses. Journal of Clinical Ultrasound 30: 275–281

Veith F J, Amor M, Ohki T et al. 2001 Current status of carotid bifurcation angioplasty and stenting based on a consensus of opinion leaders. Journal of Vascular Surgery 33: S111–S116

von Reutern G M, von Büdingen H J 1993 Ultrasound diagnosis of cerebrovascular disease. Thieme Verlag, Stuttgart

Zhou W, Felkai D D, Evans M et al. 2008 Ultrasound criteria for severe in-stent restenosis following carotid artery stenting. Journal of Vascular Surgery 47: 74–80

Further reading

Allan P L, Dubbins P A, Pozniak M A et al. 2006 Clinical Doppler ultrasound. Churchill Livingstone, London

Babikan V, Wechsler L 1999 Transcranial Doppler ultrasonography. Butterworth Heinemann, Woburn

Newell D W, Aaslid R 1992 Transcranial Doppler. Raven Press, New York

Zwiebel WJ, Pellerito JS 2005 Introduction to vascular ultrasound, 5th edn. Elsevier Saunders, Philadelphia

Duplex assessment of lower-limb arterial disease

CONTENTS

INTRODUCTION

The symptoms of lower-limb arterial disease can range from mild muscle pain on exercise (claudication) to severe ischemia resulting in potential amputation. The prevalence of lower-limb arterial disease has been estimated to be in the region of 3–10%, increasing to 15–20% in persons over the age of 70 years. The disease mainly affects persons >50 years old. It was with the introduction of color flow imaging in the 1980s that duplex scanning became a practical method of assessing the lower-limb arteries. A number of studies comparing the accuracy of duplex scanning with angiography have been undertaken and published and these indicated that duplex ultrasound scanning provided comparable results to angiography (Legemate et al. 1989; Pemberton & London 1997). Although little has changed in scanning techniques over the last decade, duplex scanning continues to play a central role in the patient management pathway by allowing clinicians to formulate treatment plans without the need for diagnostic arteriograms, which, like all invasive tests, carry a small risk of complications (Egglin et al. 1995). Figure 9.1 summarizes the current role of ultrasound. It can be seen that vascular radiologists can spend less time performing diagnostic arteriograms and instead concentrate their skills on therapeutic treatment by balloon angioplasty. In some instances, the decision may be taken to treat the patent conservatively due to the location or extent of the disease, avoiding the risk of intervention. Ultrasound also has an important role to play in the acute surgical admissions unit, where acute arterial occlusions can be rapidly located and identified or other pathologies, such as false aneurysms, diagnosed. This chapter provides an overview of lower-limb arterial disorders and offers practical advice on color duplex scanning of peripheral arteries.

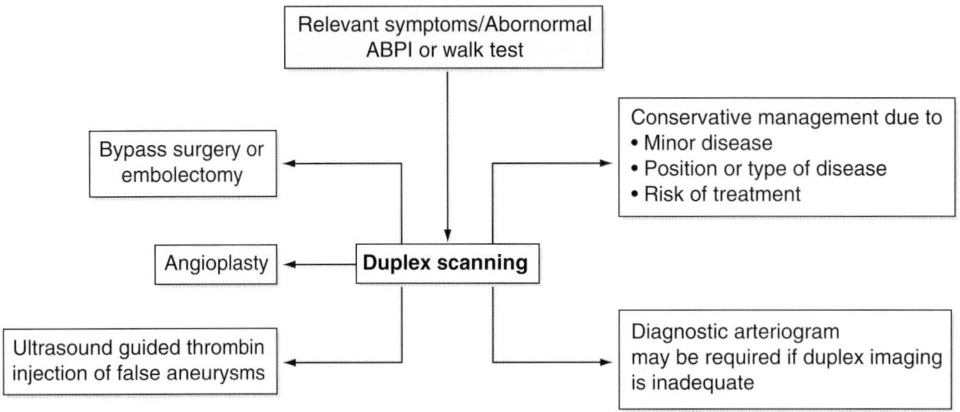

Figure 9.1 • The current role of ultrasound.

ANATOMY OF THE LOWER-LIMB ARTERIAL SYSTEM

The anatomy of the lower-limb arterial system is demonstrated in Figure 9.2. The abdominal aorta has been included in this section, as it can be a source of lower-limb symptoms.

The aorta lies slightly to the left of the midline in the abdomen, and its bifurcation is located at the level of the fourth lumbar vertebra in the region of the umbilicus. The aorta divides into the left and right common iliac arteries (CIA) at the aortic bifurcation. The CIA is variable in length (3.5–12 cm) and in some cases it is very short, with the iliac bifurcation occurring close to the aorta. The CIA divides into the external and internal iliac arteries at the iliac bifurcation, which lies deep in the pelvis. The internal iliac artery supplies blood to the pelvis and pelvic viscera. The external iliac artery varies in length (6–12 cm) and is normally superficial to the iliac vein. It gives off the deep circumflex iliac artery and inferior epigastric artery, before becoming the common femoral artery (CFA) at the level of the inguinal ligament. The aorta and iliac arteries lie behind the peritoneum, containing the bowel, which can make imaging of these vessels difficult due to overlying bowel gas. One branch of the CFA that can often be identified with ultrasound is the superficial epigastric artery.

The CFA divides into the deep femoral artery, also known as the profunda femoris artery, and the superficial femoral artery (SFA) at the level of the groin. The profunda femoris artery usually runs posterolateral to the SFA and supplies blood to the thigh tissue and muscles. It also acts as an important collateral pathway in the presence of an SFA occlusion. The profunda femoris artery usually gives off the medial and lateral circumflex arteries just beyond its origin. The SFA follows a medial course down the thigh, becoming the popliteal artery at the level of the adductor canal above the knee. The SFA gives off relatively few major branches, although the descending genicular artery can act as an important collateral pathway. The popliteal artery then runs behind the knee, or popliteal fossa, and bifurcates below the knee into the anterior tibial (AT) artery and tibioperoneal trunk. The popliteal artery has a number of genicular and sural branches supplying blood to the knee joint and gastrocnemius and soleus muscles. The proximal AT artery runs in an anterolateral direction through the interosseous membrane to the anterolateral aspect of the upper calf. It then continues to run to the lower calf, becoming the dorsalis pedis artery over the dorsum of the foot. The tibioperoneal trunk can vary in length and bifurcates into the posterior tibial (PT) and peroneal arteries (Fig. 9.2B). The PT artery follows a medial course along the calf and runs behind the medial malleolus (or ankle bone) in its distal segment. The peroneal artery lies deeper than the PT artery against the border of the fibula and runs toward the lateral malleolus (outer aspect of the ankle) in its distal segment, dividing into lateral malleolar, calcaneal, and perforating branches. It is important to note that the peroneal artery is often spared in the presence of tibial artery disease. This is why its identification can be useful if a distal bypass procedure is being considered.

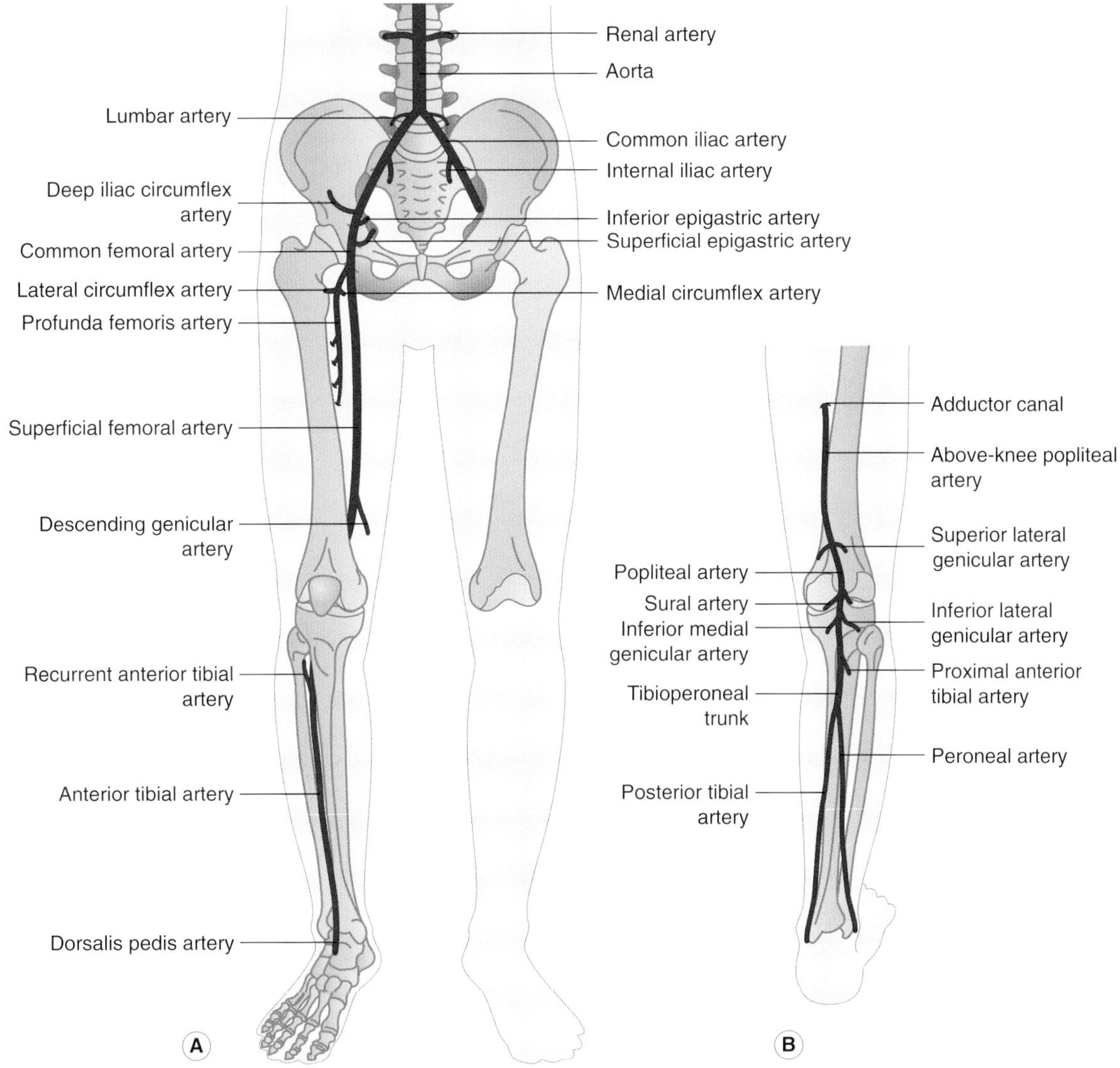

Figure 9.2 • (A) Arterial anatomy of the aortoiliac and lower-limb arteries from an anterior view. (B) Arterial anatomy of the lower limb from a posterior view.

The forefoot is mainly supplied by the dorsalis pedis artery and the medial and lateral plantar arteries, which are terminal branches of the PT artery. The dorsalis pedis and plantar arteries anastomose to form the plantar arch, which supplies the arteries to the toes.

There are a number of anatomical variations in the lower-limb arterial system that may occasionally be encountered during routine examinations. The most common variations are listed in Table 9.1.

Collateral circulation and pathways

Although symptoms are generally proportional to the extent of disease, it is sometimes surprising to find patients with arterial occlusions but relatively minor symptoms. Conversely, some patients with one or two stenoses can experience significant impairment to their lifestyle. This variability is mainly due to the quality of the collateral circulation. If an arterial segment is severely diseased or occluded, there are often alternative pathways that are able to carry blood flow around the diseased

ARTERY	VARIATION
Common femoral artery bifurcation	The bifurcation can sometimes be very high; the proximal course of the profunda femoris artery can sometimes be variable and lies posterior and medial to the superficial femoral artery in a small number of cases
Anterior tibial artery	High origin across the knee joint
Anterior tibial artery	May be small or hypoplastic
Peroneal artery	Origin from anterior tibial artery rather than the tibioperoneal trunk

Table 9.1 Anatomical variations of the lower-limb arterial system

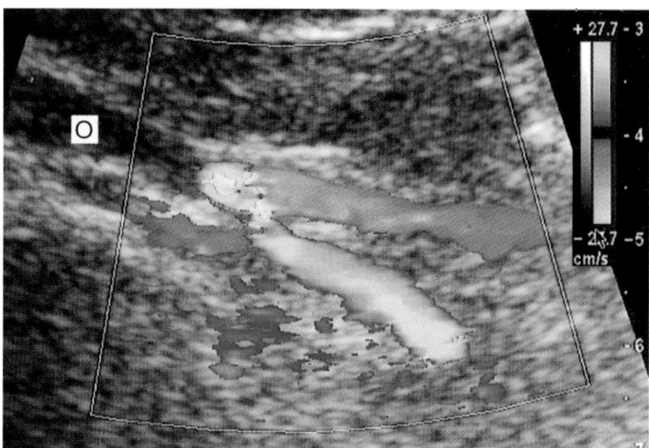

Figure 9.3 • An example of collateral flow. The common iliac artery is occluded (O) and reverse flow (blue) is demonstrated in the internal iliac artery, as it supplies flow to the external iliac artery (red).

segment, referred to as collateral vessels. In this situation, reverse flow is observed in major branches of arteries just distal to an area of severe disease, where they help to resupply blood flow to the main vessel. One such example is flow reversal observed in the internal iliac artery, supplying blood to the external iliac artery in the presence of a CIA occlusion (Fig. 9.3). It should be noted that it is very difficult to follow collateral vessels for any length using the duplex scanner, especially in the pelvis. This is not really a problem, as it is the length and severity of the disease in the main vessels that the sonographer is attempting to document. However, the quality of the collateral circulation is very important, and this can be determined by assessing the patient clinically and measuring the ankle–brachial pressure index (ABPI). Common collateral pathways are summarized in Table 9.2.

SYMPTOMS OF LOWER-LIMB ARTERIAL DISEASE

Classification of peripheral arterial disease: Fontaine's stages and Rutherford's categories (Rutherford et al. 1997; Reprinted from Journal of Vascular Surgery, 26/3, Rutherford et al. 1997, with permission from Elsevier)

FONTAINE		RUTHERFORD		
Stage	Clinical	Grade	Category	Clinical
I	Asymptomatic	0	0	Asymptomatic
IIa	Mild claudication	0	1	Mild claudication
IIb	Moderate to severe claudication	I	2	Moderate claudication
		I	3	Severe claudication
III	Ischemic rest pain	II	4	Ischemic rest pain
IV	Ulceration or gangrene	III	5	Minor tissue loss
		III	6	Major tissue loss

DISEASED ARTERY	DISTAL NORMAL ARTERY	COMMON COLLATERAL PATHWAY
Common iliac artery	External iliac artery	Lumbar arteries communicating with the iliolumbar arteries of the ipsilateral internal iliac artery, which supply the external iliac artery via retrograde flow; there can also be communication between the contralateral internal iliac artery and ipsilateral internal iliac artery
External iliac artery	Common femoral artery	Ipsilateral internal iliac artery via pelvic connections to the deep iliac circumflex artery or inferior epigastric artery
Common femoral artery	Femoral bifurcation	Ipsilateral pelvic arteries filling the profunda femoris artery via the femoral circumflex arteries, which supply the superficial femoral artery via retrograde flow
Superficial femoral artery	Above-knee popliteal artery	Flow via profunda femoris artery (or branches of the proximal superficial femoral artery if patent) to the descending or superior genicular arteries, depending on the length of the superficial femoral artery occlusion
Superficial femoral artery	Below-knee popliteal artery	Profunda femoris artery branches to inferior genicular branches of the popliteal artery
Popliteal artery	Distal popliteal artery	Flow via the superior genicular arteries to inferior genicular arteries, depending on the level of the occlusion
Proximal tibial arteries	Distal tibial arteries	There are numerous arterial collateral connections in the calf, but they may not be large enough to carry sufficient flow to the foot

Table 9.2 Common collateral pathways of the lower-limb arteries

Intermittent claudication

Atherosclerosis is a major health problem in developed countries where lifestyle factors, such as smoking and diet, can accelerate the progression of the disease. It is estimated that intermittent claudication affects approximately 4.5% of the population aged between 55 and 74 years, and there is evidence that persons with claudication have a significantly higher mortality rate from cardiac disease than nonclaudicants (Fowkes et al. 1991). Intermittent claudication is caused by arterial narrowing in the lower-limb arteries, and symptoms develop over a number of months or years. Claudication is typified by pain and cramping in the muscles of the leg while walking, which usually forces the patient to stop and rest for a few minutes in order to ease the symptoms. The severity of pain experienced and the distance a patient is able to walk can vary from day to day but, generally, walking briskly or on an incline will produce rapid onset of symptoms. The location of pain (i.e., calf, buttock, or thigh) is often associated with the distribution of disease. For instance, aortoiliac disease often produces thigh, buttock and calf claudication whereas femoropopliteal disease is associated with calf pain. There are sometimes physical signs of deteriorating blood flow in the lower limb, such as hair loss from the calf and an absence of nail growth. Claudication only occurs during exercise because, at rest, the muscle groups distal to a stenosis or occlusion remain adequately perfused with blood. However, during exercise the metabolic demand of the muscles increases rapidly, and the stenosis or occlusion will limit the amount of additional blood flow that can reach the muscles, so causing claudication.

Many patients with intermittent claudication are treated by conservative methods. This includes reduction or elimination of risk factors associated with atherosclerosis, such as smoking. Patients are also advised to undertake a controlled exercise program to build up the collateral circulation around the diseased vessel, which may ease symptoms over time. If necessary, serial ABPI measurements or exercise tests can be performed to monitor the patient's progress. Interventional treatment is mainly by angioplasty which involves the dilation of stenoses or occlusions with percutaneous balloon catheters (see Ch. 1). Arterial stents are sometimes used to prevent restenosis, although in-stent stenosis is known to occur in a proportion of cases due to the development of intimal hyperplasia (see Fig. 9.20). Surgical bypass is usually avoided, unless the patient is suffering from severe claudication, as there is a small potential risk of complications occurring during or after surgery, which in extreme cases could lead to amputation or even death.

Chronic critical lower-limb ischemia

Critical lower-limb ischemia occurs when blood flow beyond an arterial stenosis or occlusion is so low that the patient experiences pain in the leg at rest because the metabolic requirements of the distal tissues cannot be maintained (Fig. 9.4). This is frequently typified by severe rest pain at night, forcing the patient to sleep in a chair or to hang the leg in a dependent position over the side of the bed. This improves blood flow due to increased hydrostatic pressure. The Trans-Atlantic Inter-Society Consensus for the management of peripheral arterial disease (TASC II) (Norgren et al. 2007) makes the following recommendation for defining critical lower-limb ischemia:

> *The term critical limb ischemia (CLI) should be used for all patients with chronic ischemic rest pain, ulcers or gangrene attributable to objectively proven arterial occlusive disease. The term CLI implies chronicity and is to be distinguished from acute limb ischemia.*

In addition the documents also states:

> *The diagnosis of CLI should be confirmed by the ankle–brachial index (ABI), toe systolic pressure or transcutaneous oxygen tension. Ischemic rest pain most commonly occurs below an ankle pressure of 50 mmHg or a toe pressure less than 30 mmHg. Other causes of pain at rest should, therefore, be considered in a patient with an ankle pressure above 50 mmHg, although CLI could be the cause. For patients with ulcers or gangrene, the presence of CLI is suggested by an ankle pressure less than 70 mmHg or a toe systolic pressure less than 50 mmHg. (It is important to understand that there is not complete consensus regarding the vascular hemodynamic parameters required to make the diagnosis of CLI.)*

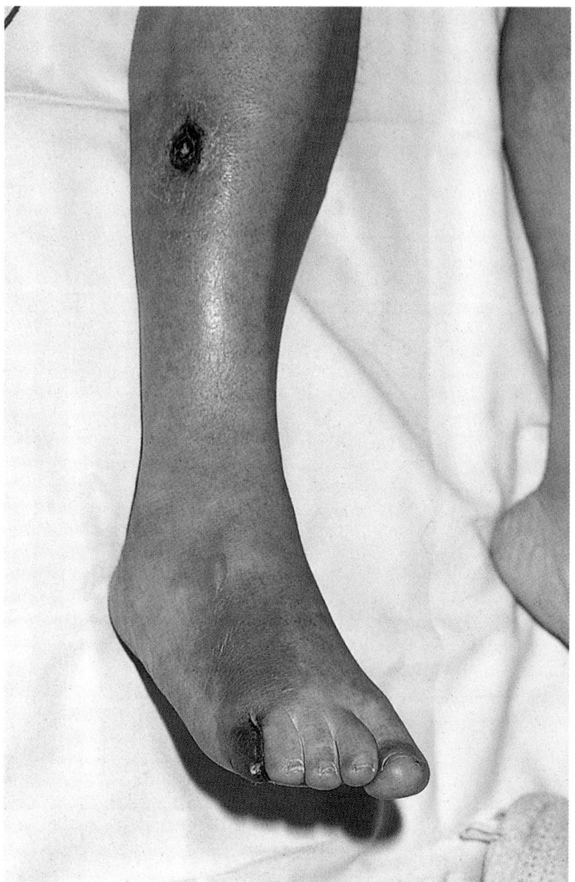

Figure 9.4 • The appearance of critical lower-limb ischemia with gangrene of the small toe.

The treatment of lower-limb ischemia includes angioplasty or arterial bypass grafting. Unfortunately, some patients are not suitable candidates for any form of limb salvage, and amputation is the inevitable outcome.

Acute limb ischemia

Acute limb ischemia, as the name suggests, is due to sudden arterial obstruction in the lower-limb arteries that may threaten limb viability. The position of the obstruction can be variable. Main causes of acute ischemia are listed in Box 9.1. Acute thrombosis of an existing arterial lesion, a so-called acute-on-chronic occlusion, can occur when the blood flow across a diseased segment of an artery

BOX 9.1 Cause of acute lower-limb ischemia

- Thrombosis of an atherosclerotic artery
- Embolism from heart, aneurysm, plaque, or critical stenosis upstream (including cholesterol or atherothrombotic emboli secondary to endovascular procedures)
- Thrombosed aneurysm with or without embolization
- Aortic/arterial dissection
- Arterial trauma
- Thrombosis of an arterial bypass graft
- Spontaneous thrombosis associated with a hypercoagulable state
- Popliteal entrapment with thrombosis
- Popliteal adventitial cyst with thrombosis

is so slow that it spontaneously thromboses. Long segments of an artery may occlude in this situation. Acute ischemia is more likely to occur if the collateral circulation around the disease is poorly developed. An embolus may be released from other areas of the body, such as the heart or from an aneurysm, and then travels distally down the leg, eventually obstructing the artery when the arterial diameter is less than that of the embolus. An embolus frequently obstructs bifurcations such as the common femoral bifurcation or distal popliteal artery and tibioperoneal trunk. Another example is obstruction of the aortic bifurcation by an embolus projecting down both CIA origins, referred to as a saddle embolus. The body has very little time to develop collateral circulation around embolic occlusions, and the limb may be very ischemic.

The classic symptoms of acute ischemia are shown in Box 9.2. In this situation, emergency intervention by surgical embolectomy, bypass surgery, or thrombolysis should be performed, provided that the patient is fit enough for treatment. Left untreated, acute ischemia can lead to muscle death or necrosis. This can cause swelling of the calf muscle, and eventually the sac, or fascia, surrounding the muscles will restrict any further swelling, leading to a pressure increase within the muscle compartments. This is known as compartment syndrome, and the acute increase in intramuscular pressure can further exacerbate the

BOX 9.2 The findings of acute limb ischemia may include the '5 ps'

1. Pain
2. Pulselessness: check with Doppler measurements
3. Pallor: change in color and temperature is a common finding in acute limb ischemia. Venous filling may be slow or absent
4. Paresthesia: numbness occurs in more than half of patients
5. Paralysis is a sign of poor prognosis

muscle ischemia. If limb salvage is possible, surgical splitting of the fascia, called a fasciotomy, may be required to release the excess pressure.

Severe muscle ischemia can produce toxins causing systemic symptoms that can lead to organ failure and death. An urgent amputation is usually performed if there is no viable option to restore blood flow to the limb.

Microembolization into the foot is often called 'trash foot' or 'blue-toe syndrome.' Localized tissue infarction occurs, leading to necrosis. It is not unusual for the patient to have a palpable ankle pulse. The outcome is often poor when a large area of tissue is affected and results in local amputation of toes, forefoot, or leg.

DISEASE PATTERNS AND LOWER-LIMB WAVEFORM SHAPES

Caution

Remember, if the patient has just walked briskly from the waiting room to the examination table the shape of observed waveforms in normal arteries may demonstrate continuous forward flow, due to changes in peripheral resistance. The patient should be allowed to relax for several minutes before starting the examination (see Fig. 5.11B).

It is important to have an understanding of the different patterns of disease that may be encountered during the examination as long segments of arteries are being interrogated. Common findings include isolated or multiple stenoses, occlusions, diffuse calcified wall disease, aneurysms, and, rarely, dissections. In addition, the ability to distinguish both visually and audibly between normal and abnormal Doppler waveforms is essential (Fig. 9.5). At rest, the normal spectral Doppler display recorded from a lower-limb extremity artery, excluding the aorta, is a triphasic flow pattern with a clear spectral window (Fig. 9.5A). This characteristic pulsatile waveform shape is due to a combination of compliant distensible arterial walls and pulse wave reflections from the periphery. It may even be possible to see four phases in young healthy adults. The triphasic pattern is easily distinguished from the audio output. In elderly patients or patients with poor cardiac output, the waveform may be biphasic or even monophasic.

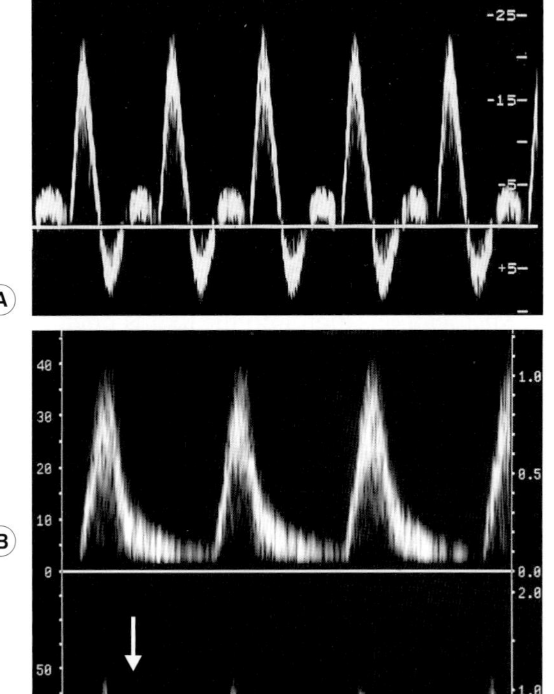

Figure 9.5 • Waveform shapes can reveal useful information about the condition of proximal and distal arteries. (A) A normal triphasic waveform recorded from the superficial femoral artery (SFA). (B) Damping of the common femoral artery (CFA) waveform with an increased systolic acceleration time and loss of pulsatility indicates significant proximal disease. (C) A waveform recorded from the SFA just proximal to an occlusion. Note the high-resistance, low-volume waveform shape and characteristic shoulder on the systolic downstroke (arrow), due to pulse wave reflection from distal disease.

Waveforms with an increased systolic rise time are characteristic of disease proximal to the point of measurement (Fig. 9.5B). For example, a study by Sensier et al. (1998) demonstrated that qualitative assessment of the CFA Doppler waveform has a sensitivity of 95%, a specificity of 80%, and an accuracy of 87% for the prediction of significant aortoiliac artery disease. This study therefore suggests that observation of the CFA waveform shape is a useful technique for the investigation of inflow disease. The presence of triphasic flow with a short systolic rise time is an indicator of normal inflow. However, care should be exercised when investigating younger patients who may have a very short proximal iliac stenosis, as the arterial waveform shape may have recovered at the level of the CFA, appearing normal. Conversely, high-resistance, low-volume flow waveforms are indicative of severe disease distal to the point of measurement. One such example is the characteristic shoulder seen on the systolic downstroke of an SFA waveform recorded proximal to severe disease in the SFA (Fig. 9.5C). This is due to a reflected wave from the disease or occlusion. Severe calcification of the arterial wall may also affect the shape of the recorded Doppler waveform due to changes in vessel compliance as the vessels become very rigid. This is commonly observed in the tibial vessels of diabetic patients, where the waveform shape may become monophasic with continuous forward flow throughout the cardiac cycle. A montage of different levels of disease and spectral waveforms is shown in Figure 9.6.

Advice

There are situations in which flow in nondiseased lower-limb arteries at rest may have reduced pulsatility or even be continuous. Examples include increased flow (hyperemia) due to limb infected ulcers, cellulitis, or the presence of arteriovenous fistulas. Hyperemic flow will be demonstrated as continuous flow in one direction.

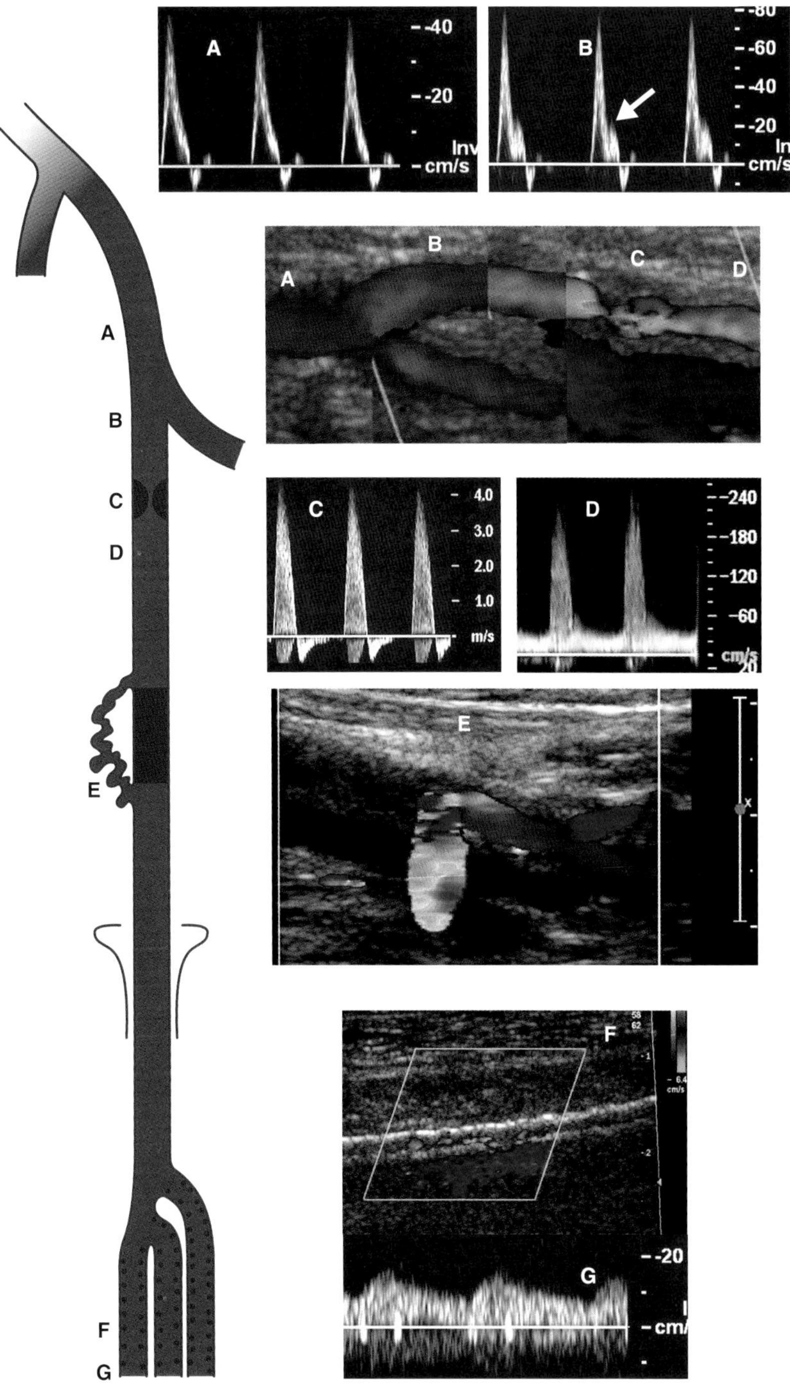

Figure 9.6 • A montage showing different levels of disease and corresponding Doppler recordings and images in the lower limb. A normal pulsatile waveform is recorded in the common femoral artery at point A. At point B just within the superficial femoral artery (SFA), a shoulder is seen on the systolic downstroke (arrow) of the Doppler waveform, indicating increased resistance due to the distal disease. A severe stenosis is demonstrated at point C. At point D poststenotic turbulence is recorded. A short SFA occlusion is present in the leg with refilling of the artery via collateral vessels at point E. There is significant calcification in the runoff vessels, as demonstrated by the bright echogenic walls of the posterior tibial artery at point F and a beaded appearance to the color display (coded red) in the artery. Doppler recordings from point G in the posterior tibial artery demonstrate abnormal damped low-velocity waveforms.

ANKLE BRACHIAL PRESSURE MEASUREMENTS AND EXERCISE TESTING

Sources of error

- Incompressibility of the calf vessels can be a problem, especially in patients with diabetes or significant renal disease, as medial calcification in the walls of the calf arteries can make them rigid and incompressible (Fig. 9.6F), leading to falsely elevated recordings. An example of such a measurement would be an ankle pressure of 280 mmHg and a brachial pressure of 120 mmHg (ankle–brachial pressure index (ABPI) = 2.3). An ABPI of >1.4 should be regarded as abnormal and further investigation may be required
- Accidental probe movement during cuff inflation can give an impression that the signal has disappeared. Make sure that the probe is kept stationary and motionless and hold it towards its base with a finger resting on the skin for greater control

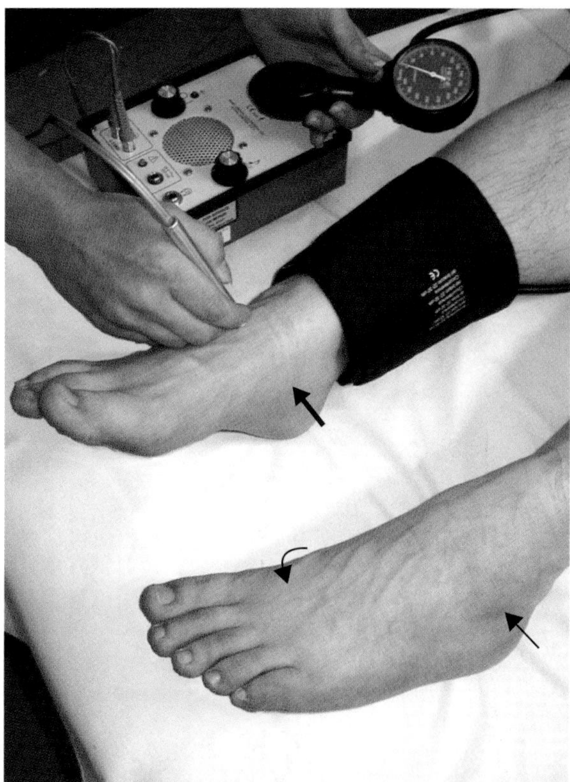

Figure 9.7 • Measurement of the ankle–brachial pressure index. Probe positions are shown to detect flow in the dorsalis pedis artery (probe) and the posterior tibial artery (large arrow). The peroneal artery is located on the outer aspect of the ankle (small arrow). The probe position has also been shown to detect flow from the plantar arch (curved arrow).

Before discussing the practical aspects of lower-limb scanning in detail it is useful to discuss the role of simple hand-held continuous-wave Doppler devices. The audio output of these devices can give a subjective impression of the quality of blood flow at specific sites, such as the ankle. However, for qualitative assessment, the measurement of the ABPI is a simple method of detecting and grading arterial disease. This is especially useful if the patient is presenting with leg ulceration and there is uncertainty whether this is primarily venous or arterial, as a normal ABPI would indicate a venous cause. The test normally takes 10–15 min and is performed as follows. Prior to the test the patient should be fully rested for at least 5–10 min and lying supine to remove the effect of hydrostatic pressure. A blood pressure cuff is then placed around the ankle. A high-frequency (8–10 MHz) continuous-wave Doppler probe is used to listen to the Doppler signals in the dorsalis pedis and Posterior tibial arteries at the ankle, as shown in Figure 9.7.

It is sometimes necessary to examine the peroneal artery, as it may be the only vessel supplying the foot in patients with severe arterial disease. The systolic blood pressure is measured at each of these points by briskly inflating the cuff to above the patient's systolic blood pressure, at which point the arterial flow signal disappears. The cuff should be inflated to at least 20–30 mmHg above the pressure that is required to occlude the artery. The cuff is then deflated, and the pressure at which the arterial signal reappears, corresponding to the systolic pressure at the position of the cuff, is recorded. The systolic brachial pressure is then measured in a similar way from both arms, in case there is upper-extremity disease. The highest recorded ankle pressure is then divided by the highest brachial pressure to calculate the ABPI. This index is independent of the patient's systemic blood pressure and can be used to grade the severity of arterial disease, as shown in Table 9.3 (adapted from AbuRahma 2000). The index ranges between 1 and 1.4 in

ABPI	COMMENT
1–1.4	Normal
0.99–0.9	Mild disease 'Considered normal'
0.89–0.5	Claudication
0.49–0.3	Severe occlusive disease
<0.3	Ischemia and possible rest pain

Table 9.3 Grading arterial disease using the ankle–brachial pressure index (ABPI)

normal subjects due to amplification of the arterial pulse wave along the limb and reflected waves from the periphery. However, it is worth noting that many scientific publications consider an index >0.9 to indicate a normal circulation.

Abnormal ABPI measurements can confirm the presence of arterial disease but do not give any indication of the position of the disease in the leg. Segmental pressures can help to isolate the diseased segment with the use of multiple pressure cuffs placed at the ankle, below the knee, above the knee, and at the top of the thigh. Significant pressure differences between cuffs would indicate disease between those segments.

Problems

There is no dorsalis pedis pulse:

- Make sure that the probe is not being pressed too hard on to the foot as this can occlude the artery underneath
- Ensure that the foot is relaxed and not excessively planter flexed (toes pointing down), as in some case the artery can be stretched and temporally occluded in this position
- As a normal variation, the artery can be small or hypoplastic. Check the posterior tibial artery instead

Resting ABPI measurements may be normal in patients with mild to moderate claudication. However, ABPI measurements can be carried out before and after exercise on a treadmill to measure the patient's walking distance until the patient claudicates and the degree of pressure reduction following exercise. This is because exercising muscles require increased blood flow. However, as flow increases, the pressure gradient across the stenosis increases and therefore a lower pressure will be recorded distal to the stenosis. Eventually a point will be reached at which the stenosis limits any further increase in flow and the patient experiences the onset of claudication in the muscle groups distal to the disease. Another alternative is to use commercially available foot flexion devices to exercise the calf muscles while the patient sits on the examination table. This reduces cardiac stress. Exercise testing is also a particularly useful screening test, as some patients exhibiting symptoms of claudication may have other disorders producing their symptoms, such as spinal stenosis, sciatica, or musculoskeletal problems. In these cases, the postexercise pressures will be normal. Unfortunately, there is a wide range of exercise protocols used by vascular laboratories (e.g., speed 2–4 km/h, exercise duration 2–5 min, and treadmill incline 10–12%). This can make comparisons of results among units difficult. However, individual patients' performance can be measured on sequential visits to monitor their treatment or progress.

Key point

It is important to monitor patients closely during exercise testing as many with claudication have associated coronary artery disease. It is essential to have an emergency call system close at hand. In the absence of a treadmill it is possible to exercise the patient along the known length of a corridor.

Problems

If the leg is too swollen or too painful to measure a blood pressure, a subjective audio assessment of the arterial waveform can be useful as a triphasic waveform generally indicates normal arterial flow, whereas a damped monophasic waveform indicates the likelihood of significant disease.

PRACTICAL CONSIDERATIONS FOR LOWER-EXTREMITY DUPLEX SCANNING

The scanning objectives are shown in Box 9.3. The time allocated for the examination depends on the number of segments that need assessing. The femoropopliteal segment can normally be examined in both legs in half an hour. However, a bilateral aortoiliac to ankle scan may take up to an hour, depending on sonographer experience. There is usually no special preparation required before a lower-limb duplex scan. Nevertheless, some vascular units request patients to fast overnight before an examination of the aortoiliac arteries to improve imaging of this region. In our experience this is of little help, especially if patients require scans at short notice. Bowel preparations have proved useful, although in practice they can be difficult to administer to elderly or diabetic patients and are impractical in a single-visit clinic.

The patient should have an empty bladder before an aortoiliac scan as this improves the visualization of these segments and also causes less patient discomfort if transducer pressure has to be applied. The examination room should be at a comfortable ambient temperature (>20°C) to avoid peripheral vasoconstriction.

Scanner setup

A peripheral arterial scanning option should be selected before starting the examination, but adjustment of the control settings will often be required in the presence of significant disease (see Ch. 7). The color pulse repetition frequency (PRF) is usually set in the 2.5–3 kHz range for demonstrating moderately high-velocity flow. By using the correct settings normal arterial segments can be interrogated rapidly using color flow imaging. There should be color filling to the vessel walls. The color image normally demonstrates a pulsatile flow pattern with the color alternating between red and blue due to flow reversal during the diastolic phase (see Ch. 5).

> **BOX 9.3 Scanning objectives**
>
> The sonographer should be able to:
>
> - locate the site or sites of disease
> - detect lesions at multiple levels and, where possible, identify the most hemodynamically significant
> - differentiate stenoses from occlusions
> - grade the severity of stenoses
> - measure the length of occlusions
> - identify the presence and location of aneurysms
>
> In addition, textural features of the disease such as excessive calcification (echogenic) or nonorganized thrombus (anechoic) can be described.

STARTING THE SCAN

It is useful to start the assessment by examining the CFA at the groin, as the observed blood flow patterns at this level can reveal information about the condition of the aortoiliac arteries and also provide some clues to the condition of the SFA, as described earlier in the chapter (Fig. 9.5). It is important to have a good understanding of the anatomy of the arteries and veins at the level of the groin and to be able to identify the major branches and junctions and their relationship to each other (Fig. 9.8). A mid-frequency linear array transducer is the most suitable probe for scanning the femoral, popliteal, and calf arteries. A low-frequency, curvilinear array abdominal transducer is used for the aortoiliac segment. The segmental guidelines can be used in any order. A combination of B-mode imaging, color flow imaging, and spectral Doppler recordings should be used throughout the examination. Color flow imaging is essential for identifying the aortoiliac and calf arteries. Spectral Doppler velocity measurements should be made at an angle of insonation of 60° or less.

Assessment of the aortoiliac artery and CFA

The patient should be relaxed and lying in a supine position with the head supported by a pillow. The patient should be asked to relax the abdominal muscles and to rest the arms by the sides. Sometimes, rolling patients on to their side can improve visualization of the iliac arteries if obscuring bowel gas is present. The scanning positions for assessing the inflow arteries are shown in Figure 9.9, and a color image of the arteries is shown in Figure 9.10. The procedure for assessment is as follows:

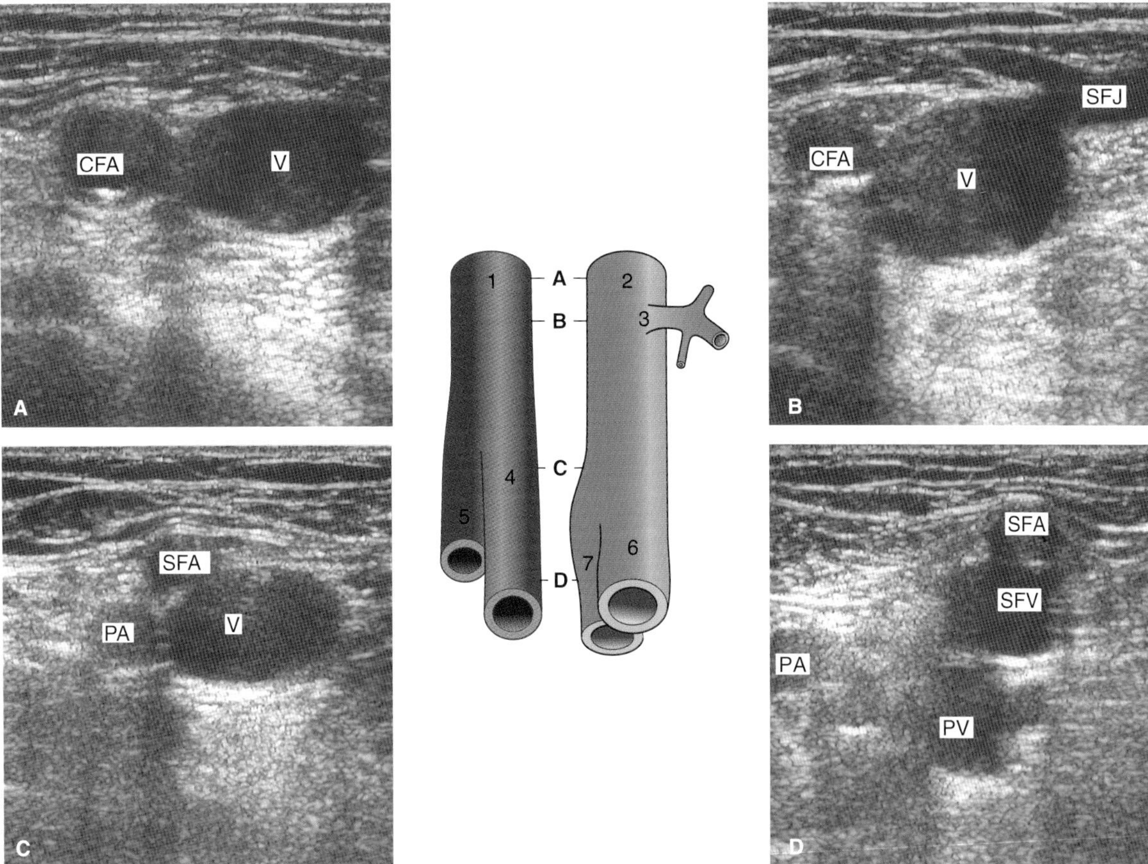

Figure 9.8 • The anatomy of the right femoral artery and vein at the groin, with corresponding transverse B-mode images at four different levels (A, B, C, D). Vessels shown on the diagram are: 1 common femoral artery, 2 common femoral vein, 3 saphenofemoral junction, 4 superficial femoral artery, 5 profunda femoris artery, 6 femoral vein, 7 profunda vein. Vessels demonstrated on the images are the common femoral vein (V), common femoral artery (CFA), saphenofemoral junction (SFJ), superficial femoral artery (SFA), profunda femoris artery (PA), femoral vein (SFV), and profunda vein (PV). Note that the femoral artery bifurcation is sometimes found above the level of the saphenofemoral junction. In addition, the superficial femoral artery tends to roll on top of the femoral vein, as shown in the B-mode image.

1 Using a mid-frequency linear array transducer, the CFA is identified at the level of the groin in transverse section, where it lies lateral to the common femoral vein (Figs 9.8 and 9.9A). The CFA is then followed proximally in longitudinal section until it runs deep under the inguinal ligament and can no longer be assessed with this probe. A low-frequency curvilinear transducer should then be selected. Using the probe to push any gas upwards and driving the color box toward the edge of the sector (field of view) can help in visualizing the aortoiliac region and in maintaining adequate spectral Doppler angles (Fig. 9.9D).

2 The external iliac artery is then identified in longitudinal section and followed proximally toward its origin using color flow imaging. The artery is normally seen to lie above the iliac vein. Sometimes, tilting or rolling of the transducer and the use of oblique and coronal probe positions along the abdominal wall are useful in imaging around areas of bowel gas.

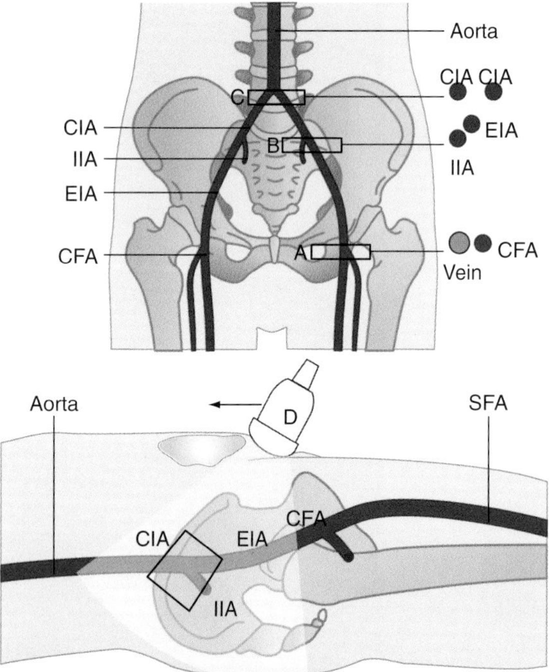

Figure 9.9 • Probe positions for imaging the common femoral artery (CFA) and aortoiliac arteries. (A) CFA transverse. (B) Origin of external and internal iliac arteries transverse. (C) Aortic bifurcation transverse. (D) Arteries in the longitudinal plane. Starting at the groin and pushing bowel gas upward with the transducer (arrow) can help visualization. Positioning the color box to the edge of the scan sector can improve the angle of insonation with spectral Doppler. CIA, common iliac artery; IIA, internal iliac artery; EIA, external iliac artery; SFA, superficial femoral artery.

3. The common iliac bifurcation should be identified by locating the origin of the external iliac and internal iliac arteries. This can be achieved in the longitudinal plane, but transverse imaging is also helpful for confirmation if the image is adequate, as the internal iliac artery usually divides in a posteromedial direction (Fig. 9.9B). This area serves as an important anatomical landmark for localizing areas of disease in the aortoiliac system. Sometimes it is not possible to identify the internal iliac artery, and the position of the common iliac bifurcation has to be inferred, as it usually lies in the deepest part of the pelvis, as seen on the scan image, although the CIA is sometime fairly short and this is not always a reliable feature.
4. The CIA is then followed back to the aortic bifurcation in longitudinal section (Fig. 9.9D). At this point, it is useful to confirm the level of the aortic bifurcation in transverse plane (Fig. 9.9C). The origins of the CIA are assessed in the longitudinal plane. The aorta should also be examined in transverse and longitudinal planes to exclude an aortic aneurysm or stenosis (see Ch. 11).

Assessment of the femoral and popliteal arteries

To start the examination, the patient should be lying reasonably flat with the leg rotated outward and the knee gently flexed and supported. A color image of the femoropopliteal and calf arteries is shown in Figure 9.11. The scanning positions for imaging the femoropopliteal arteries are shown in Figure 9.12. The procedure for assessment is as follows:

1. The CFA is identified in transverse section with a mid-range linear array transducer at the groin and followed distally to demonstrate the femoral bifurcation (Figs 9.8 and 9.12A). The CFA lies lateral to the common femoral vein (Fig. 9.8).
2. Turning to a longitudinal plane, the femoral bifurcation is examined (Fig. 9.12B). The profunda femoris artery usually lies posterolateral to the SFA, requiring a slight outward turn of the transducer. The profunda femoris artery can often be followed for a considerable distance, particularly if the SFA is occluded and it is supplying a collateral pathway to the lower thigh. The origin of the SFA is usually located anteromedial to the profunda femoris artery, requiring a slight inward turn of the transducer.
3. The SFA is then followed distally along the medial aspect of the thigh in a longitudinal plane, where it will lie above the superficial femoral vein (Fig. 9.12C). If the image of the SFA is lost it is easier to relocate in transverse section (Fig. 9.12D). In its distal segment the SFA runs deep and enters the

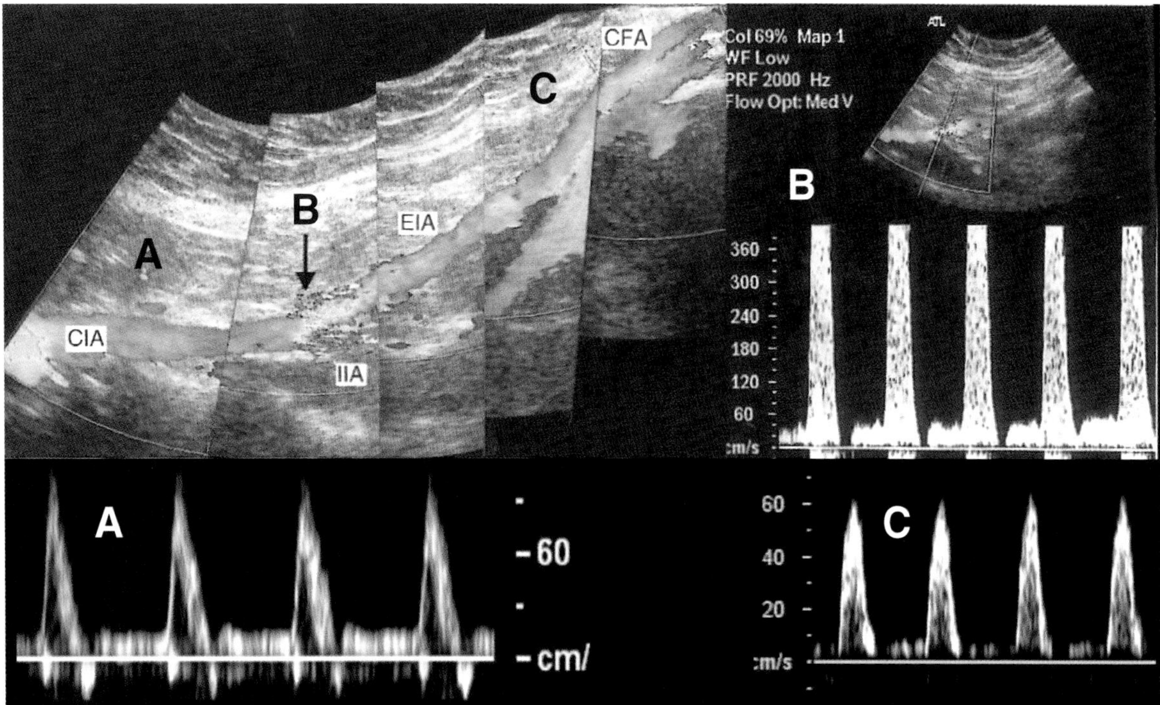

Figure 9.10 • A color montage of the inflow arteries showing the common iliac artery (CIA), external iliac (EIA) and internal iliac arteries (IIA), and the common femoral artery (CFA). Note the stenosis at the iliac artery bifurcation (arrow), demonstrated by aliasing. Spectral Doppler recordings are taken proximal to the stenosis (A), across the stenosis (B), and distal to the stenosis (C).High systolic velocity, aliasing, and spectral broadening at point B indicate a severe stenosis. There is an abnormal waveform distally at point C with increased systolic rise time and a loss of reverse flow.

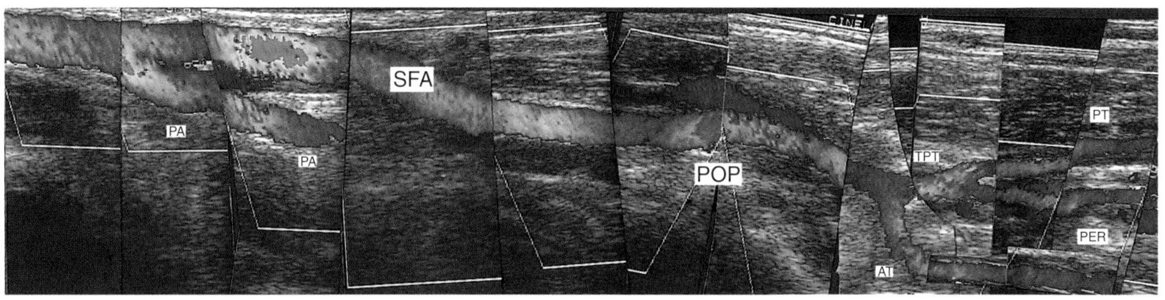

Figure 9.11 • A color montage of the femoropopliteal and calf arteries. The image shows the profunda femoris artery (PA), superficial femoral artery (SFA), popliteal artery (POP), tibial peroneal trunk (TPT), posterior tibial (PT), anterior tibial (AT), and peroneal artery (PER).

adductor canal, becoming the popliteal artery. It is usually possible to image the proximal popliteal artery to just above the knee level from this position (Fig. 9.12E). A low-frequency transducer can help to image the artery in a large thigh. Using an anterior position at point (Fig. 9.12I) can also improve visualization in some cases.

4 The popliteal artery can be examined by rolling the patient on to the side. Alterna-

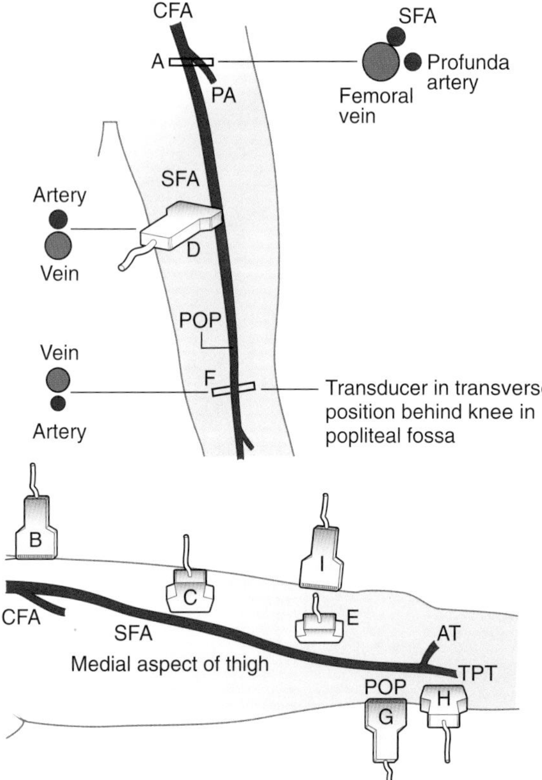

Figure 9.12 • Probe positions for imaging the femoropopliteal arteries. (A) Femoral artery bifurcation transverse. (B) Femoral bifurcation longitudinal. (C) Superficial femoral artery (SFA) longitudinal. (D) SFA transverse. (E) Proximal popliteal artery above-knee longitudinal. (F) Popliteal artery transverse. (G) Popliteal artery longitudinal, from the popliteal fossa. (H) Origin of the anterior tibial. Note that the distal SFA and proximal popliteal artery are sometimes easier to image by using a more anterior approach at point I. CFA, common femoral artery; PA, profunda femoris artery; POP, popliteal artery; TPT, tibial peroneal trunk.

tively, the patient can lie in a prone position, resting the foot on a pillow, although a lot of elderly patients are not able to tolerate this position. It is also possible to image the popliteal artery with the legs hanging over the edge of the examination table and the feet resting on a stool. Whichever method is used, it is important not to overextend the knee joint as this can make imaging difficult. Conversely, if the knee is too flexed, access to the popliteal fossa is difficult.

5. Starting in the middle of the popliteal fossa, the popliteal artery is located in transverse section and is seen posterior to the popliteal vein (Fig. 9.12F). Turning into a longitudinal plane, the popliteal artery is then followed proximally, above the popliteal fossa, to overlap the area previously examined from the lower medial thigh (Fig. 9.12G).
6. The popliteal artery is then examined longitudinally across and below the popliteal fossa, where it is possible to continue directly into the tibioperoneal trunk. The tibioperoneal trunk can be imaged from a number of positions.

Assessment of the tibial arteries

Practical tip

Patients with critical leg ischemia often hang the leg in a dependent position and cannot tolerate lying flat for long periods of time. In this situation it is easier to scan the popliteal arteries and calf vessels with the leg dependent as this will also improve the detection of flow and make the procedure more comfortable for the patient. The femoral vessels can be scanned with the end of the examination tilted down.

The tibial arteries can be imaged from several different transducer positions, as demonstrated in Figure 9.13. It is often easier to locate the tibial arteries in the distal calf and follow them proximally to the top of the calf. However, for the purposes of this section, the description of the examination starts just below the knee. It should be noted that imaging of the distal tibial arteries at the ankle is often easier with a high-frequency linear array transducer.

Anterior tibial artery

1. With the leg rolled outward and the knee slightly flexed, the origin of the AT artery is imaged from a posteromedial position just below the knee, where it will be seen to drop immediately away from the popliteal artery (Fig. 9.12H). Often it is only possible to see the first 1–2 cm of the AT from this position. The tibioperoneal trunk is

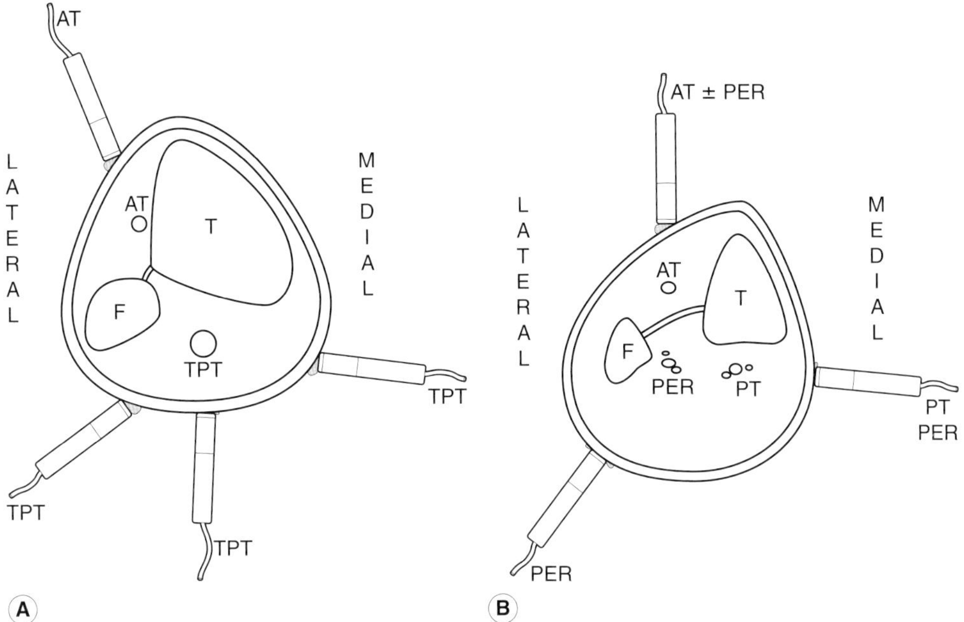

Figure 9.13 • Cross-sections of the calf to show longitudinal transducer positions for imaging the tibial arteries and veins in the calf. (A) Several positions can be used to image the vessels in the upper calf proximal to the bifurcation of the tibioperoneal trunk (TPT). (B) Probe positions to image the posterior tibial (PT), anterior tibial (AT), and peroneal artery (PER) in the mid and lower calf. Note that it is possible to image two vessels from a similar position, as shown. T, tibia; F, fibia.

usually seen as a direct continuation of the popliteal artery distal to the AT artery origin.

2 The proximal AT artery is then imaged from the anterolateral aspect of the upper calf, just below the knee, where it will be seen to rise toward the transducer in a curve, through the interosseous membrane. The membrane can be identified as a bright echogenic line running between the tibia and fibula in cross-section. The artery will lie on top of the membrane. The AT artery is then followed distally, along the anterolateral border of the calf, until it becomes the dorsalis pedis artery, over the top of the foot.

Posterior tibial artery

1 With the leg rolled outward and the knee flexed, the origin of the PT artery is imaged from a medial position, below the knee, where the tibioperoneal trunk divides into the PT artery and the peroneal artery. The proximal PT artery will gently rise toward the transducer, and the associated paired veins act as useful landmarks. The origin of the peroneal artery is often visible from this plane and will lie posterior to the PT artery origin.

2 The PT artery is then followed along the medial aspect of the calf toward the inner ankle or medial malleolus. The PT artery lies superficial to the peroneal artery when imaged from the medial aspect of the calf.

3 The origin and a short segment of the PT artery can often be visualized from a posterolateral position below the knee, where it will be seen to run deep as it divides from the tibioperoneal trunk.

Peroneal artery

Imaging of the peroneal artery may have to be performed from a number of different positions (Fig. 9.13B). The optimum position varies from patient to patient.

- View 1 The peroneal artery can be followed from its origin along the calf using the same medial calf position as that described to image the PT artery. From this position, the peroneal artery will be seen lying deeper than the PT artery against the border of the fibula, surrounded by the larger peroneal veins. Slight anterior or posterior longitudinal tilting of the probe may be needed to follow the artery distally.
- View 2 The peroneal artery can usually be followed distally from its origin using a posterolateral position, below the knee and along the calf.
- View 3 The peroneal artery can sometimes be imaged from the anterolateral aspect of the calf, where it will be seen lying deep to the AT artery. This is the most difficult position from which to obtain images of the peroneal artery.

Commonly encountered problems

There are a number of problems and pitfalls associated with lower-limb duplex scanning. Table 9.4 lists some of the more frequently encountered problems.

SCAN APPEARANCES

B-mode images

Normal appearance

Like the carotid arteries, the lumen of a normal peripheral artery should appear clear, and the walls should be uniform along each arterial segment, although noise may cause speckle within the image of the vessel. The intima-media layer of the arterial wall is sometimes seen in normal femoral and popliteal arteries. In practice, it is frequently difficult to image the vessels clearly in the aortoiliac segment, abductor canal region, and calf without the help of color flow imaging.

Abnormal appearance

Areas of atheroma, particularly if they are calcified, may be seen within the vessel lumen. The atheroma may be extensive and diffusely distributed, especially in the SFA (Fig. 9.14). Large plaques at the common femoral bifurcation are relatively easy

SEGMENT	PROBLEM	SOLUTIONS
Aortoiliac arteries	Bowel gas obscuring part or all of the image	Try different probe positions (medial, lateral or coronal positions); leave the segment and try again in a few minutes
Aortoiliac arteries	Tortuous arteries	Use the color display to follow the artery; considerable adjustment of the probe position is often needed
Femoropopliteal arteries	Severe calcification of the artery producing color image dropout	Try different transducer positions to work around the calcification
Femoropopliteal arteries	Obese patient with large thigh	When using a broad-band transducer, lower the color and spectral Doppler transmit frequencies for better penetration; consider switching to a 3.5 MHz curved linear array transducer in very difficult situations
Tibial arteries	Large calf with gross edema	Start the scan at the ankle and work proximally; a 3.5 MHz linear array probe can be used to image these vessels proximally
Tibial arteries	Very low flow due to proximal occlusions	Lower the pulse repetition frequency and wall filters; place the leg in a dependent position to increase distal blood flow

Table 9.4 Common problems encountered during duplex evaluation of the lower-limb arteries

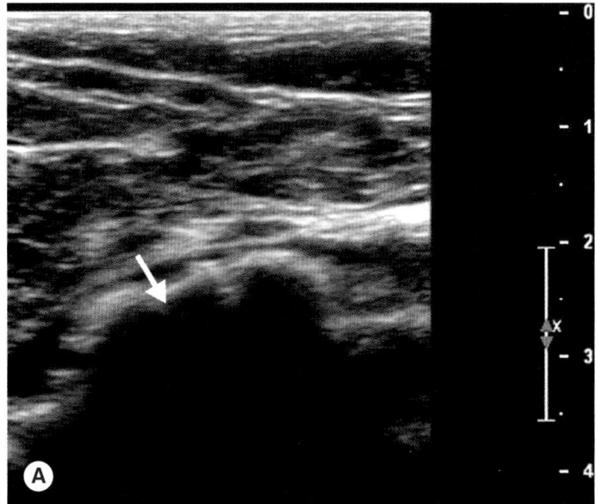

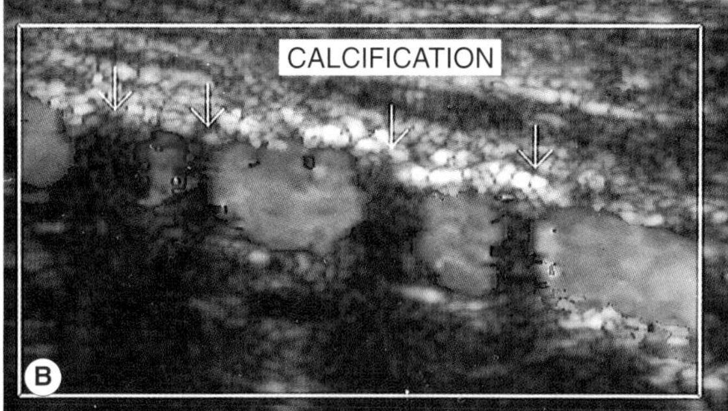

Figure 9.14 • (A) Calcified atheroma (arrow) is present in the common femoral artery, leading to drop-out of the B-mode signal. A large acoustic shadow is present. (B) Calcified atheroma in the superficial femoral artery is leading to drop-out of the color flow signal in parts of the lumen (arrows).

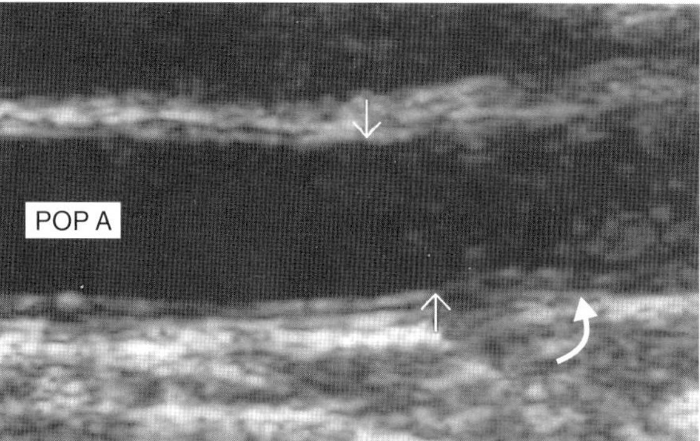

Figure 9.15 • An acute occlusion of the popliteal artery (POP A). The vessel is patent to the level of the two arrows. The occlusion is demonstrated by the relatively low-level echoes in the lumen distally. Note some intimal detail is still visible in the occluded section (curved arrow).

to image, and these may extend into the proximal profunda artery or SFA. Localized plaques of the CFA often produce a 'cauliflower' appearance and are normally located on the posterior wall. Calcification of the arterial wall, especially in diabetic patients, produces strong ultrasound reflections, and the walls of the calf arteries can appear particularly prominent (Fig. 9.6F). When an arterial segment has been occluded for some time, the vessel may contract and appear as a small cord adjacent to the corresponding vein. This appearance is most frequently seen in the SFA and popliteal artery. B-mode imaging in combination with color flow imaging is also very useful for identifying acute occlusions of the SFA or popliteal artery, where there may be fresh thrombus present in the vessel lumen. The lumen will appear clear or demonstrate minimal echoes on the image, because thrombus has a similar echogenicity to blood (Fig. 9.15). However, color flow imaging reveals an absence of flow in the occluded segment of the vessel. The start of the occlusion can often be very abrupt, with little disease seen proximally.

Abnormal dilatations or arterial aneurysms should be measured using the B-mode image, as described in Chapter 11.

Color flow images

Abnormal appearance

Utilizing the color controls as described in Chapter 7, arterial stenoses will be demonstrated as areas of color flow disturbance or aliasing. Severe stenoses frequently produce a disturbed color flow pattern extending 3–4 vessel diameters beyond the lesion (Figs 9.10 and 9.16). Any areas of color flow disturbance should be investigated with angle-corrected spectral Doppler to estimate the degree of narrowing. In addition, the color flow image of flow in a nondiseased artery distal to severe proximal disease may demonstrate damped low-velocity flow, which will be seen as continuous flow in one direction.

Occlusions of lower-limb arteries most frequently occur in the SFA and popliteal artery. An

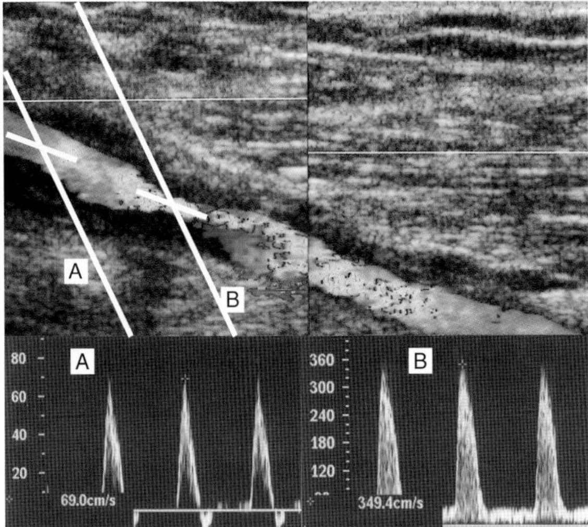

Figure 9.16 • Superficial femoral artery disease is demonstrated by color flow aliasing and marked flow disturbance just distal to the lesion. Flow is assessed using spectral Doppler. (A) Measurement of the peak systolic velocity just proximal to the stenosis. (B) Measurement of the peak systolic velocity across the stenosis. The peak systolic velocity ratio is calculated by dividing B by A, producing a velocity ratio of 5. This would confirm a severe stenosis.

occlusion is demonstrated by a total absence of color flow in the vessel. Occlusions can occur at the origins of arteries or in mid-segment. If an artery is occluded from its origin, at the level of a major bifurcation, flow will normally still be seen in the sister branch. For example, the profunda femoris artery is usually found to be patent when the SFA is occluded (Fig. 9.17). When an artery occludes in mid-segment, collateral vessels are normally seen dividing from the main trunk at the beginning of the occlusion. Similarly, collateral vessels resupply flow to the artery at the distal end of the occlusion (Fig. 9.18). Collateral vessels can follow tortuous routes as they divide from the main trunk, and they are sometimes only seen when the main artery is imaged in cross-section. It is therefore helpful to interrogate any suspected occlusion in both longitudinal and transverse imaging planes. The PRF often needs to be lowered (typically to 1 kHz) distal to an occlusion in order to increase the sensitivity of the scanner to lower flow velocities. The color flow image distal to an occlusion often demonstrates a continuous forward flow pattern with reduced pulsatility due to damping of the normal blood flow pattern.

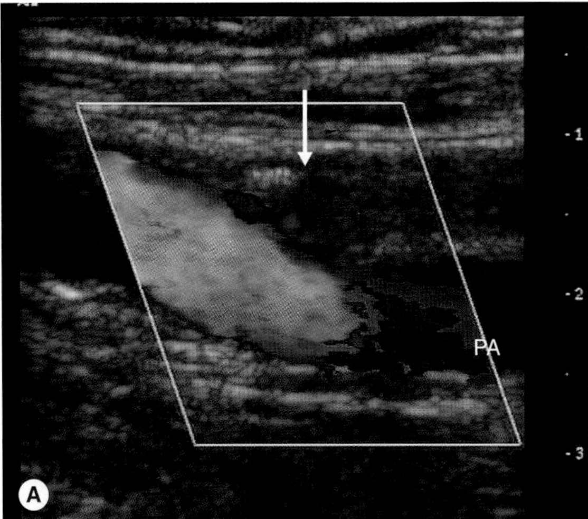

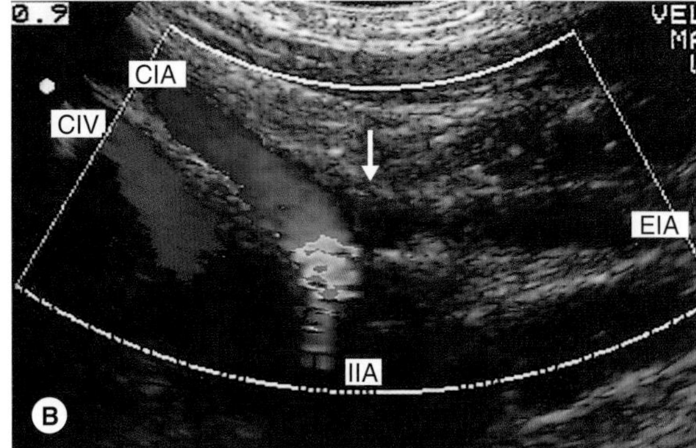

Figure 9.17 • (A) Color flow image of the femoral bifurcation demonstrating a superficial femoral artery origin occlusion (arrow). The profunda femoris artery (PA) is patent. (B) Color flow image of an external iliac artery (EIA) occlusion (arrow). The common iliac artery (CIA) and internal iliac artery (IIA) are patent. The common iliac vein (CIV) is visible in this image.

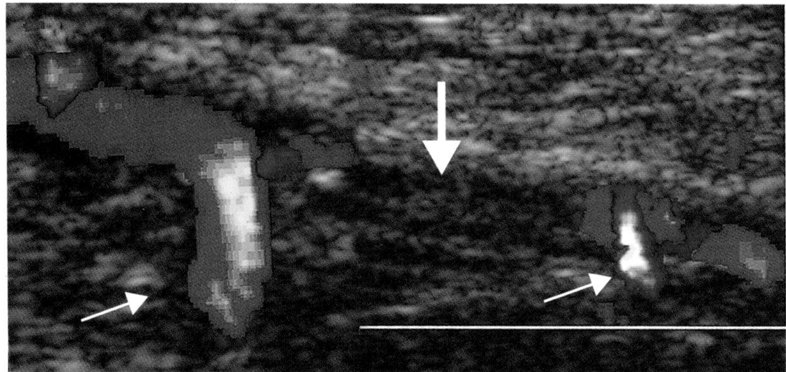

Figure 9.18 • A short mid-superficial femoral artery occlusion is demonstrated by an absence of color flow in the vessel (large arrow). Large collateral vessels are seen at both ends of the occlusion (small arrows).

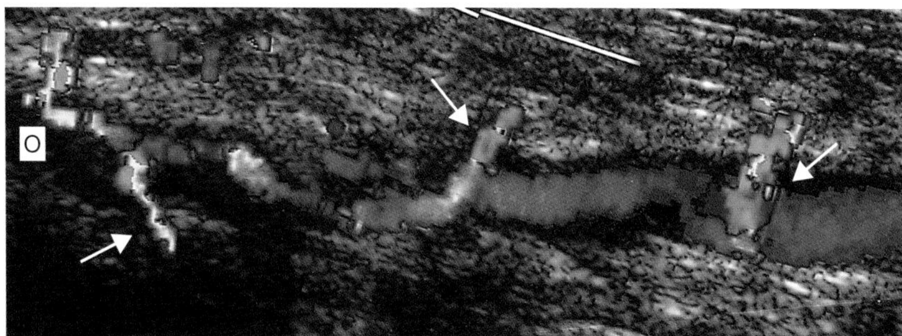

Figure 9.19 • A color montage demonstrates flow in the popliteal artery distal to an occlusion (O). The flow becomes progressively higher distal to the occlusion, as more collateral vessels join the main artery (arrows). Marked areas of flow disturbance can occur at points where collateral vessels feed the main artery, and these can be mistaken for stenoses.

Blood flow in the main artery may also improve progressively over the first few centimeters distal to the occlusion as more collateral vessels join the main trunk. This effect can be observed on the color flow image (Fig. 9.19). High-velocity flow in a collateral vessel can produce an area of marked color flow disturbance in the main artery at the point where the collateral joins. This can be misinterpreted as a stenosis. Spectral Doppler should be used to interrogate this area carefully. It is possible to misdiagnose a long stricture as an occlusion because of very slow flow through the stricture due to the development of good collateral flow around the diseased site. The PRF should be lowered to examine low-velocity flow across these lesions.

Spectral Doppler

Abnormal recordings and grading of stenosis

Reference velocities

Data have been published for the average peak systolic velocity found in normal external iliac, superficial femoral, and popliteal arteries which are 119, 90, and 68 cm/s, respectively (Jager et al. 1985).

Spectral Doppler should always be used to interrogate areas of color flow disturbance. The spectral Doppler sample can be increased in size to cover the lumen if there is difficulty in obtaining adequate signals. Measurements should be taken just proximal to, across, and just beyond the lesion. In the presence of a significant stenosis, there will be an increase in flow velocity across the lesion associated with spectral broadening and turbulence just distal to the lesion. As demonstrated previously (see Table 8.1), a concentric 50% diameter reduction of the arterial lumen will produce a 75% reduction in cross-sectional area, leading to significant flow changes. The main criterion used to grade the degree of narrowing in a lower-limb artery is the measurement of the peak systolic velocity ratio. The peak systolic velocity ratio is calculated by dividing the maximum peak systolic velocity recorded across the stenosis (V_s) by the peak systolic velocity recorded in a normal area of the artery just proximal to the stenosis (V_p), as demonstrated in Figures 9.10 and 9.16. Different protocols have been published for defining a 50%, or greater, diameter reduction in the lower-limb arteries. Many vascular units use a peak systolic velocity ratio of equal to or greater than 2 (Cossman et al. 1989; Sensier et al. 1996), although a ratio of 2.5 is used by other centers (Legemate et al. 1991). It is important to audit and evaluate the criteria used by your unit against other imaging techniques such as angiography or computed tomographic angiography (CTA) Table 9.5 shows how the velocity ratio can be used to grade the severity of lower-limb disease (Hennerici & Neuerburg-Heusler 1998). Velocity ratios can still be used to grade stenoses in the presence of multisegment disease. Grading lesions at bifurcations can be technically challenging, especially if there is a natural diameter change between the proximal artery and the daughter artery and in the absence of any published data, the calculated ratio should be interpreted cautiously. This situation is encountered at the common femoral bifurcation. Another potentially confusing situation occurs when the aortoiliac and CFAs are clear but the SFA is occluded and the profunda femoris artery is severely stenosed. This can give rise to a monophonic waveform pattern in the CFA with a high end-diastolic velocity, although the systolic acceleration time remains short. A great deal of care should be used in interpreting flow patterns in this situation.

Finally, areas of aneurysmal dilation typically demonstrate a reduction in peak systolic velocity, frequently associated with disturbed flow patterns.

Other methods of measurement have been used to grade lower-limb arterial disease, including pulsatility index, but these have tended to be used with continuous-wave Doppler and are probably less useful for duplex scanning where velocity changes can be measured directly.

DIAMETER REDUCTION	VELOCITY RATIO (V_S/V_P)	COMMENTS
0–49%	<2	Waveform is triphasic but mild spectral broadening and an increase in end-diastolic velocities are recorded as the degree of narrowing approaches 49%
50–74%	⩾2	Waveforms tend to become biphasic or monophasic; there is an increase in end-diastolic velocity; spectral broadening is present; flow disturbance and some damping are recorded distal to the stenosis
75–99%	⩾4	Waveform is usually monophasic with significant increase in end-diastolic velocity; marked turbulence and spectral broadening are demonstrated; flow is damped distal to the stenosis. If the stenosis is very short and in the absence of proximal disease, it is possible for biphasic flow to be recorded within the stenosis
Occluded	No flow detected	Doppler waveforms proximal to an occlusion often demonstrate a high-resistance flow pattern

Table 9.5 Suggested criteria for grading lower-limb arterial disease using velocity ratios, based on several references

SPECIALIZED APPLICATIONS

Assessment of tibial arteries and the plantar arch prior to bypass surgery

Duplex scanning in combination with continuous-wave Doppler recordings can be a useful method of determining which calf artery is supplying most blood to the distal region of the foot prior to distal bypass surgery (McCarthy et al. 1999). In this way, it is possible to select a target vessel to position the distal anastomosis. This is important as there needs to be a low-resistance arterial pathway to the foot, distal to a graft, to ensure that the graft remains patent and the foot perfused. The three tibial arteries of the calf have connections to the plantar arch, which is located toward the end of the foot. The PT and dorsalis pedis arteries usually contribute most flow to the arch via plantar arteries. The plantar arch supplies blood to the plantar metatarsal arteries and digital arteries of the toes. The patient should be assessed with the leg in a dependent position to maximize blood flow distal to the diseased part of the vessel. Using the duplex scanner, it is possible to assess the patency and quality of each of the tibial arteries to ankle level. A continuous-wave Doppler probe is then used to assess the Doppler signals from the plantar arch. The probe position for recording flow at the plantar arch is demonstrated in Figure 9.7. Selective digital pressure is then applied over the most suitable tibial artery, as previously demonstrated by duplex scanning of the target vessel, to occlude it at the ankle. A substantial reduction or cessation of flow at the plantar arch during compression would suggest that the arch is in continuation with the selected tibial artery. This type of assessment can be complex, as there may be more than one patent tibial artery supplying the plantar arch. The peroneal artery can also supply the distal AT artery or dorsalis pedis artery via branches, which in turn may supply the plantar arch.

ASSESSMENT OF ARTERIAL STENTS

Arterial stents are used to prevent restenosis, although some authorities suggest they are no more effective than standard angioplasty at maintaining long-term vessel patency. Stents are mainly deployed in the aortoiliac arteries and proximal CFA, although they are also used in the SFA and popliteal artery. Stents are available in different lengths and sizes, and multiple stents can be deployed if the disease is very extensive. They are usually visible on the B-mode image, producing a stronger reflection compared to the arterial wall. The cross-hatched, or lattice, metal structure can often be identified. It is sometimes possible to see nipping of the stent if the atheroma in the artery is very calcified or fibrous and has not been completely compressed to the vessel wall. Color flow imaging and spectral Doppler can be used to assess the flow across the stent (Fig. 9.20). It is not uncommon to find some localized flow disturbance in the region of the stent due to the step between the arterial wall and proximal and distal ends of the stent. Spectral Doppler should be used to grade the degree of any in-stent stenosis. Stents placed in arteries close to joints, such as the CFA or popliteal artery, can be stressed by joint movement and may kink or bend. Localized aneurysms can be excluded by inserting a covered stent across the aneurysm; this is discussed in Chapter 11.

OTHER ABNORMALITIES AND SYNDROMES

Lower-limb symptoms in younger patients are sometimes due to inflammatory or small-vessel disorders, such as Buerger's disease. Flow recordings are normal in the larger arteries proximally, but the distal vessels in the calf may demonstrate low-flow, high-resistance waveforms.

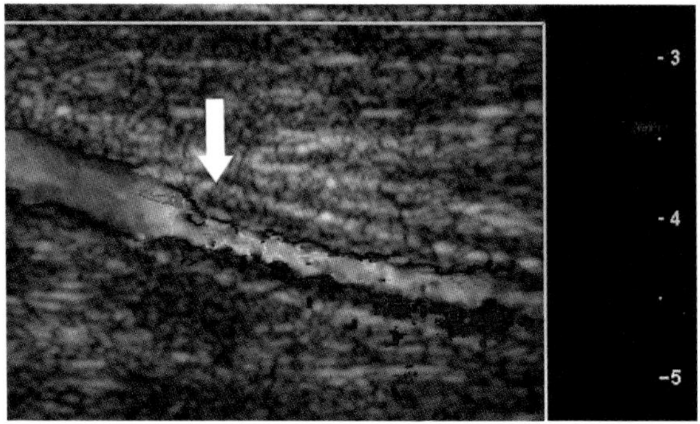

Figure 9.20 • Color flow imaging demonstrates a stenosis (arrow) at the proximal end of a superficial femoral artery stent.

Popliteal entrapment syndrome

Popliteal entrapment syndrome is also a rare but potential cause of claudication and possible distal embolization due to arterial wall damage. In this situation, the popliteal artery often follows an anomalous course below the knee and is trapped by the heads of the gastrocnemius muscle during plantar flexion. The popliteal artery can also be trapped by fibrous bands in this area. To test for popliteal entrapment syndrome, the patient should lie prone with the legs gently flexed and the feet hanging over the end of the examination table. The below-knee popliteal artery should be imaged at the level of the gastrocnemius muscle heads. The patient should point the foot down (plantar flex) against a counterpressure, typically by having a colleague apply moderate pressure against the foot. Narrowing or occlusion of the popliteal artery during this maneuver may indicate popliteal entrapment syndrome. However, there is evidence to suggest that significant compression of the popliteal artery can occur in normal volunteers during this investigation, casting some doubt on the usefulness of this test (Erdoes et al. 1994).

Cystic adventitial disease of the popliteal artery

This rare disease is caused by cystic swelling of the arterial wall, which impinges into the lumen of the popliteal artery, leading to eventual occlusion. The location of the lesion is often found across the knee joint. It should be considered as a potential cause of symptoms in the young patient, especially in the absence of any other pathology. Treatment is by excision and local repair or bypassing.

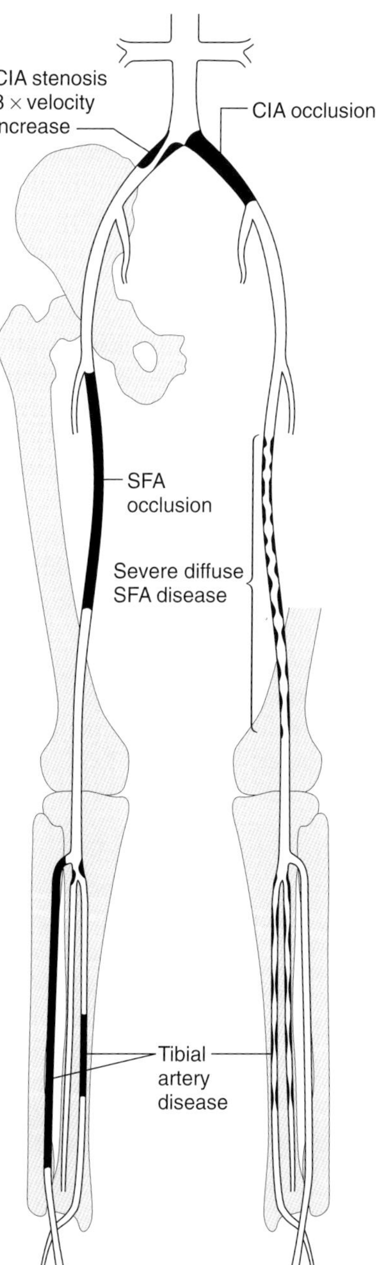

Figure 9.21 • The easiest method of reporting lower-limb scans is by the use of diagrams. Areas of narrowing can be drawn on to the map and the corresponding velocity recordings indicated. Occlusions are demonstrated by blocking out the appropriate regions. CIA, common iliac artery; SFA, superficial femoral artery.

REPORTING

In our experience, the use of diagrams demonstrating the position of disease and corresponding velocity measurements and ratios is the simplest method of reporting results, as shown in Figure 9.21. Areas that were impossible to assess due to bowel gas or calcification can be hatched out on the diagram. Surgeons and physicians also find this method of reporting helpful when reviewing results in a busy outpatient clinic, as reading pages of text can be very time-consuming. Copies of the report can be sent to the radiology department with a request card if the patient requires an angiogram or angioplasty, thus allowing the radiologist to pre-plan puncture sites. In many situations an angioplasty can be performed without a diagnostic arteriogram.

References

AbuRahma A F 2000 Segmental Doppler pressures and Doppler waveform analysis in peripheral vascular disease of the lower extremities. In: AbuRahma A F, Bergan J J (eds) Noninvasive vascular diagnosis. Springer, London, pp 213–229

Cossman D V, Ellison J E, Wagner W H et al. 1989 Comparison of contrast arteriography to arterial mapping with color-flow duplex imaging in the lower extremities. Journal of Vascular Surgery 10: 522–529

Egglin T K, O'Moore P V, Feinstein A R et al. 1995 Complications of peripheral arteriography: a new system to identify patients at increased risk. Journal of Vascular Surgery 22: 787–794

Erdoes L S, Devine J J, Bernhard V M et al. 1994 Popliteal vascular compression in a normal population. Journal of Vascular Surgery 20: 978–986

Fowkes F G, Housley E, Cawood E H et al. 1991 Edinburgh Artery Study: prevalence of asymptomatic and symptomatic peripheral arterial disease in the general population. International Journal of Epidemiology 20: 384–392

Hennerici M, Neuerburg-Heusler D 1998 Vascular diagnosis with ultrasound. Thieme, Stuttgart, pp 179–180

Jager K A, Ricketts H J, Strandness D E Jr 1985 Duplex scanning for the evaluation of lower limb arterial disease. In: Bernstein E F (ed.) Noninvasive diagnostic techniques in vascular disease. C V Mosby, St Louis, pp 619–631

Legemate D A, Teeuwen C, Hoeneveld H et al. 1989 The potential of duplex scanning to replace aortoiliac and femoropopliteal angiography. European Journal of Vascular Surgery 3: 49–54

Legemate D A, Teeuwen C, Hoeneveld H et al. 1991 Spectral analysis criteria in duplex scanning of aortoiliac and femoropopliteal arterial disease. Ultrasound in Medicine and Biology 17: 769–776

McCarthy M J, Nydahl S, Hartshorne T et al. 1999 Color-coded duplex imaging and dependent Doppler ultrasonography in the assessment of cruropedal vessels. British Journal of Surgery 86: 33–37

Norgren L, Hiatt WR, Dormandy MR et al. 2007 Inter-Society consensus for the management of peripheral arterial disease (TASC II). European Journal of Vascular and Endovascular Surgery 33: S1–S75

Pemberton M, London N J 1997 Color flow duplex imaging of occlusive arterial disease of the lower limb. British Journal of Surgery 84: 912–919

Rutherford R B, Baker J D, Ernst C et al. 1997 Recommended standards for reports dealing with lower extremity ischemia: revised version. Journal of Vascular Surgery 26: 517–538

Sensier Y, Hartshorne T, Thrush A et al. 1996 A prospective comparison of lower limb color-coded duplex scanning with arteriography. European Journal of Vascular and Endovascular Surgery 11: 170–175

Sensier Y, Bell P R, London N J 1998 The ability of qualitative assessment of the common femoral Doppler waveform to screen for significant aortoiliac disease. European Journal of Vascular and Endovascular Surgery 15: 357–364

Further reading

AbuRahma A F, Bergan J J 2000 Noninvasive vascular diagnosis. Springer, London

Hennerici M, Neuerburg-Heusler D 1998 Vascular diagnosis with ultrasound. Thieme, Stuttgart

Polak J F 1992 Peripheral vascular sonography. Williams & Wilkins, Baltimore

Zwiebel W J, Pellerito J S 2005 Introduction to vascular ultrasonography 5th edn. Elsevier Saunders, Philadelphia

Duplex assessment of upper-limb arterial disease

10

CONTENTS

INTRODUCTION

In contrast to lower-limb arteries, atherosclerotic disease in the upper extremities is rare and accounts for approximately 5% of all extremity disease (Abou-Zamzam et al. 2000). The most commonly affected sites are the subclavian (SA) and axillary arteries. The disorder is sometimes associated with extracranial carotid artery disease. Radiotherapy in this region, resulting in fibrosis and scarring, can also cause damage to the SA and axillary arteries. Compression of the SA in the area of the thoracic outlet, known as thoracic outlet syndrome (TOS), can produce significant upper-limb symptoms.

Acute obstruction of the axillary or brachial arteries may also occur due to embolization from the heart or SA aneurysms. In this situation, duplex scanning is useful for demonstrating the length and position of the occlusion. Microvascular disorders, such as Raynaud's phenomenon, can produce significant symptoms in the hands, which may be confused with atherosclerotic disease.

ANATOMY OF THE UPPER-EXTREMITY ARTERIES

The anatomy of the upper-extremity arteries is illustrated in Figures 10.1 and 10.2. The left SA divides directly from the aortic arch, but the right SA originates from the innominate or brachiocephalic artery. The thoracic outlet is the point where the SA, subclavian vein, and brachial nerve plexus exit the chest. The SA runs between the anterior and middle scalene muscles and passes between the clavicle and first rib to become the axillary artery. The diameter of the SA ranges from 0.6 to 1.1 cm. The SA has a number of important branches, including the vertebral artery and internal thoracic artery (also referred to as the mammary

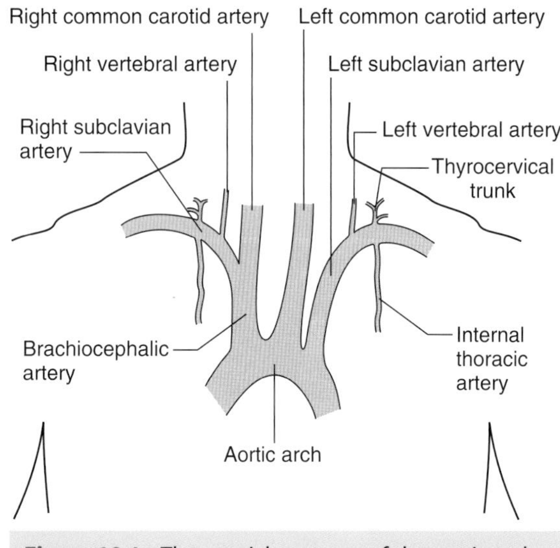

Figure 10.1 • The arterial anatomy of the aortic arch and subclavian artery.

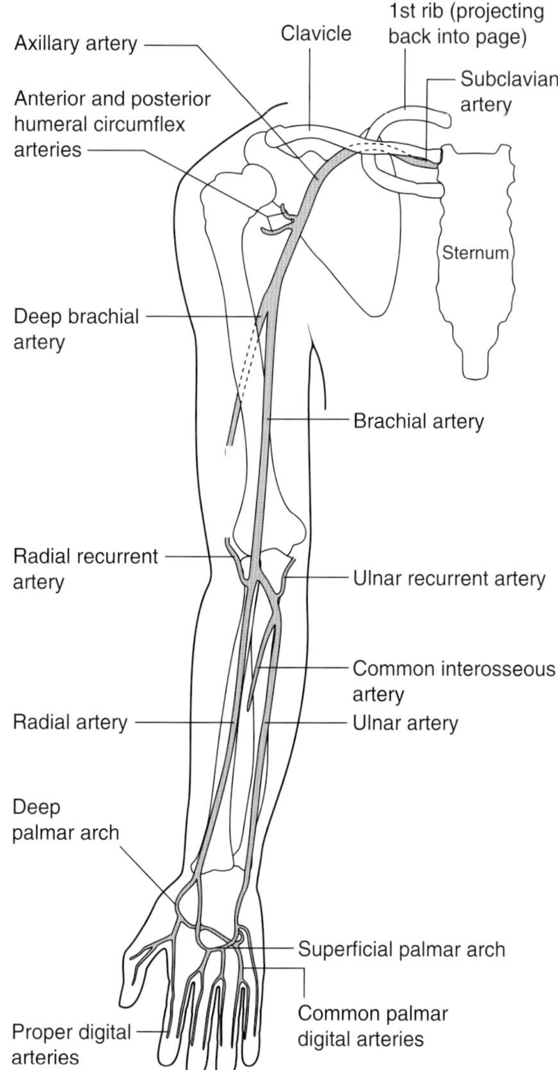

Figure 10.2 • The arterial anatomy of the arm and hand.

artery), which is frequently used for coronary artery bypass surgery.

The axillary artery becomes the brachial artery as it crosses the lower margin of the tendon of the teres major muscle, at the top of the arm. The diameter of the axillary artery ranges between 0.6 and 0.8 cm. The brachial artery then runs distally on the medial or inner side of the arm in a groove between the triceps and biceps muscles. The deep brachial artery divides from the main trunk of the brachial artery in the upper arm and acts as an important collateral pathway around the elbow if the brachial artery is occluded distally. The brachial artery runs in a medial to lateral course over the inner aspect of the elbow (cubital fossa) and then divides, 1–2 cm below the elbow, into the radial and ulnar arteries. However, the bifurcation can be quite variable in position and can sometimes be seen in the upper arm. The ulnar artery dives deep beneath the flexor tendons in the upper forearm. The radial artery runs along the lateral side of the forearm toward the thumb and is palpable at the wrist. The ulnar artery runs along the medial side of the forearm and is sometimes the dominant vessel of the forearm. The common interosseous artery is an important branch of the ulnar artery in the upper forearm as it can act as a collateral pathway if the radial and ulnar arteries are occluded. The radial artery supplies the deep palmar arch in the hand, and the ulnar artery supplies the superficial palmar arch. There are usually communicating arteries between the two systems. In some people only one of the wrist arteries will supply the palmar arch system. The fingers are supplied by the palmar digital arteries. There are a number of anatomical variations in the arm that are shown in Table 10.1. The arms normally develop good collateral circulation around diseased segments. The major collateral pathways of the arm are summarized in Table 10.2.

ARTERY	VARIATION
Left subclavian artery	Common origin with common carotid artery from aortic arch
Brachial artery	High bifurcation of brachial artery
Radial artery	High origin from axillary artery
Ulnar artery	High origin from axillary artery

Table 10.1 Anatomical variations of the upper-limb arteries

DISEASED SEGMENT	NORMAL DISTAL ARTERY	POSSIBLE PATHWAYS
Proximal subclavian artery	Distal subclavian artery	Vertebral artery, internal thoracic artery, and thyrocervical trunk
Distal subclavian or proximal axillary artery	Distal axillary artery	Collateral flow to the circumflex humeral arteries
Brachial artery	Distal brachial artery or proximal radial and ulnar arteries	Deep brachial artery to the recurrent radial and ulnar arteries
Radial and ulnar arteries	Distal radial and ulnar arteries	Interosseous artery and branches of the recurrent radial and ulnar arteries

Table 10.2 Major collateral pathways of the upper arm

SYMPTOMS AND TREATMENT OF UPPER-LIMB ARTERIAL DISEASE

The main causes of upper-limb disorders are shown in Box 10.1. Many patients with chronic upper-limb arterial disease experience few symptoms because of the development of good collateral circulation in the arm. However, some patients complain of aching and heaviness in the arm following a period of use or exercise. Patients with significant chronic symptoms can be treated by angioplasty, provided that the lesion is suitable for dilation. Arterial bypass surgery is rarely performed in the upper extremities. Acute obstructions can produce marked distal ischemia, and the forearm and hand may be cold and painful. In many cases of acute ischemia the condition of the arm and hand improves with appropriate anticoagulation. However, embolectomy, thrombolysis, or bypass surgery may be performed if there is persistent distal ischemia. Trauma, due to injury or stab wounds to the arm or shoulder, can result in arterial damage, requiring local repair or bypass surgery. SA or axillary artery aneurysms can be bypassed with grafts, although in some cases endovascular repair can be performed by deploying a covered stent across the aneurysm to exclude flow in the aneurysm sac. Occasionally, patients with arteriovenous malformations will be encountered. These malformations range in size and distribution and can affect the fingers, hands, or arm.

BOX 10.1 Common causes of symptoms involving the arterial and microvascular circulation of the arms and hands

- Atherosclerotic disease
- Acute obstruction due to emboli from the heart
- Aneurysms
- Fibrosis of the subclavian and axillary arteries due to radiotherapy
- Shoulder and arm dislocation
- Trauma or stab wounds
- Damage caused by arterial access and invasive blood pressure lines
- Thoracic outlet syndrome
- Raynaud's phenomenon
- Reflex sympathetic dystrophy
- Vibration white-finger disease
- Takayasu's arteritis
- Giant cell arteritis

PRACTICAL CONSIDERATIONS FOR DUPLEX ASSESSMENT OF UPPER-EXTREMITY ARTERIAL DISEASE

The objectives of an upper-limb arterial scan

- Locate, identify, and grade the severity of arterial disease
- Identify aneurysms, including false aneurysms caused by arterial access
- Assess for arterial thoracic outlet syndrome

A minimum of half an hour should be allocated for an upper-limb examination.

There is no special preparation required prior to the scan, although the patient will have to expose the shoulder and upper arm for scanning of the distal SA and axillary arteries. The examination room should be at a comfortable ambient temperature (>20 °C) to prevent vasoconstriction of the distal arteries. It is possible to scan the arm vessels with the patient in a sitting position or lying supine. When scanning the patient in a supine position the head can be supported on a thin pillow for comfort and the SA and proximal axillary artery scanned with the operator sitting behind the patient. This is usually a more comfortable position than scanning from the side of the patient. To image the distal axillary and brachial arteries, the patient should be examined from the side of the examination table and the arm should be abducted, externally rotated, and resting on an arm board or a suitable rest. The distal brachial, radial, and ulnar arteries are imaged with the hand in a palm-up position (supination), resting on a support. Scanning the patient in the sitting position is particularly useful for thoracic outlet examinations, as this enables full freedom of arm movement during provocation maneuvers. The scanner should be configured for a peripheral arterial examination, and in the absence of a specific upper-limb preset, a lower-limb arterial option should be selected.

SCANNING TECHNIQUES

A mid-frequency linear array transducer is the most suitable probe for scanning the SA and axillary arteries. A high-frequency linear array transducer produces the best images of the brachial, radial, and ulnar arteries, particularly as the radial and ulnar arteries are very superficial at the wrist. Imaging of the digital arteries is easier with the use of a small high-frequency 'hockey stick'-type probe. In addition, a mid-frequency curved linear array transducer can be useful for imaging the proximal SA at the level of the supraclavicular fossa, as it fits more easily into the contour of this region. The transducer positions for imaging the upper-extremity arteries are shown in Figure 10.3.

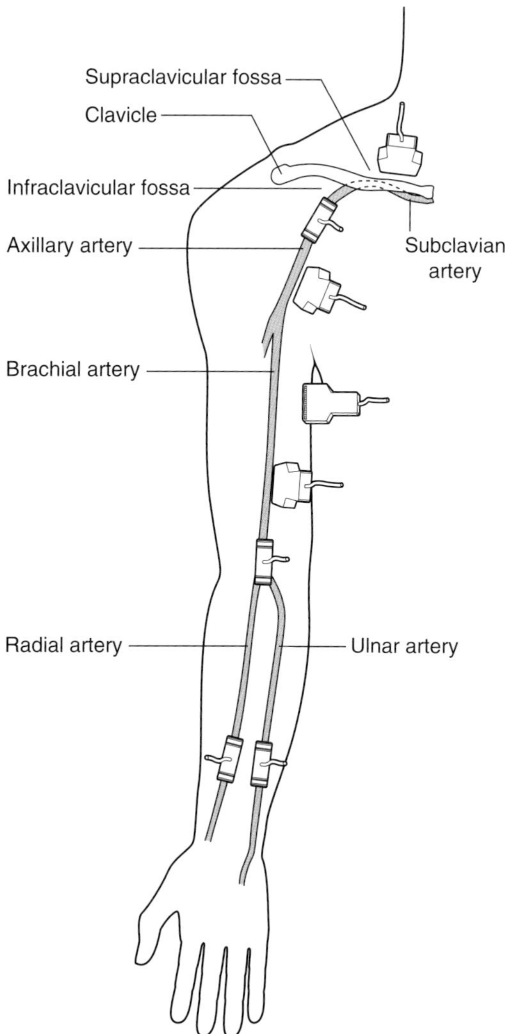

Figure 10.3 • Transducer positions for scanning the upper-extremity arteries.

A color flow montage of the upper-extremity arteries is shown in Figure 10.4.

Subclavian and axillary arteries

The SA is initially located in a transverse plane in the supraclavicular fossa, where it will lie superior to the subclavian vein. The transducer is turned to image the artery in longitudinal section and followed proximally toward its origin. The left SA origin is usually impossible to image, as the vessel arises from the aortic arch. It can sometimes be tracked toward its origin with a low-frequency phase array transducer. This type of transducer can also be useful for imaging the brachiocephalic artery as it has a small footprint which allows access to the limited window. Sometimes the origin of the right SA can be difficult to image, especially if the patient has a large or short neck. Extra gel may be needed to fill the depression of the supraclavicular fossa to enable good contact with a linear array transducer. The SA should then be followed laterally in longitudinal section, where it will disappear underneath the clavicle. There will be a large acoustic shadow below the clavicle (see Fig. 10.13). A mirroring artifact of the SA is often seen due to the chest wall beneath the artery (see Fig. 7.7).

The SA reappears from underneath the clavicle and is followed distally, where it becomes the axillary artery. Two positions may be used to image the length of the axillary artery. The first is the anterior approach, in which the axillary artery will be seen to run deep beneath the shoulder muscles. A low-frequency curved array transducer can sometimes be useful for following the distal axillary artery from this position as the axillary artery can lie quite deep at this point. The second approach images the axillary artery from the axilla (armpit), where it can be followed distally to the brachial artery.

It is worth noting that the proximal segment of the internal thoracic artery, a branch of the SA, can often be imaged from the supraclavicular fossa. This artery is frequently used in coronary bypass surgery and is surgically grafted to the heart. It divides at a 90° angle from the inferior aspect of the SA to run down the chest wall. Beyond its origin it runs behind the upper ribs and is only visible in the spaces between them. It is possible to confirm graft patency by identifying flow in the proximal thoracic artery just beyond its origin. The flow pattern in the artery supplying the heart will exhibit an unusual waveform shape, as most of the flow occurs in the diastolic phase of the cardiac cycle (Fig. 10.5).

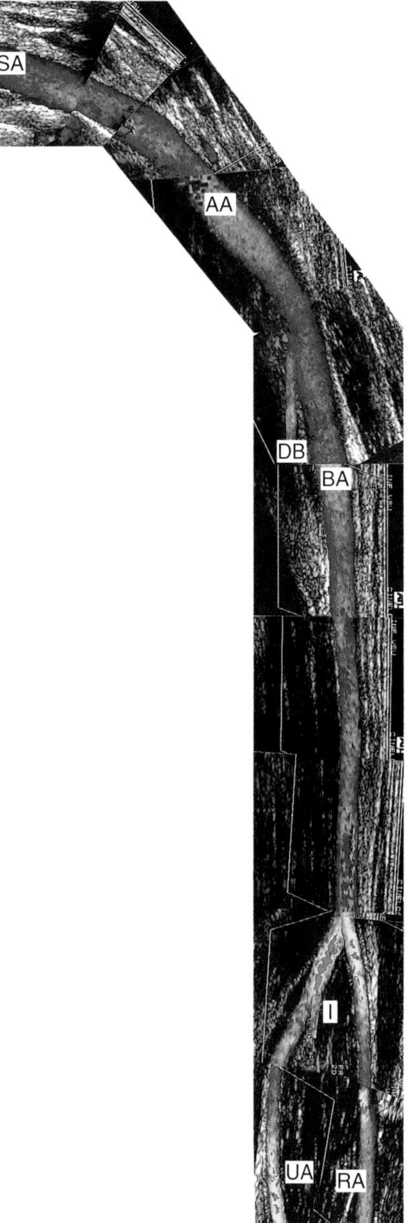

Figure 10.4 • A color flow montage of the left upper-extremity arteries demonstrating the subclavian artery (SA), axillary artery (AA), brachial artery (BA), deep brachial artery (DB), radial artery (RA), common interosseous artery (I), and ulnar artery (UA).

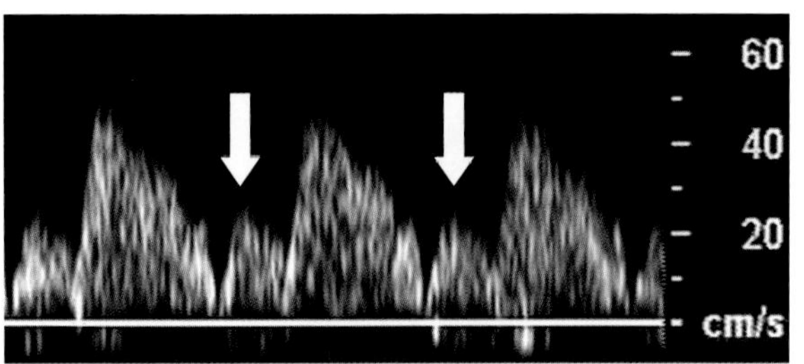

Figure 10.5 • A Doppler waveform recorded from a left thoracic artery grafted to a coronary artery following heart bypass surgery. The systolic phase is shown by the arrows.

Brachial artery

The brachial artery is followed as a continuation of the axillary artery along the inner aspect of the arm to the elbow, where it curves around to the cubital fossa and lies in a superficial position. The distal brachial artery is scanned across the elbow to the point where it divides in the upper forearm into the radial and ulnar arteries.

Radial and ulnar arteries

> **Caution**
>
> Cold rooms or cold ultrasound gel applied to the hand can cause significant peripheral vasoconstriction leading to high-resistance flow signals in the radial ulnar and digital vessels that may not be detected with standard machine settings

The bifurcation of the brachial artery into the radial and ulnar arteries is easier to locate in a transverse plane. The two arteries are then followed distally to the wrist in a longitudinal plane. In its proximal segment, the ulnar artery runs deep to the radial artery before becoming more superficial in the mid-forearm. It is often easier to locate the radial and ulnar arteries at the wrist and then to follow them back to the elbow.

Palmar arch and digital arteries

Duplex scanning can be used to image the palmar arch and digital vessels, although continuous-wave Doppler can be considerably quicker and easier to use for the detection of arterial signals, especially in the digital arteries. The radial artery is sometimes harvested to be used as a graft for coronary artery bypass surgery. To ensure that the ulnar artery will maintain perfusion to the hand, it is possible to listen to arterial flow signals in the hand with continuous-wave Doppler whilst the radial artery is being manually compressed. If the arterial signals disappear, removal of the radial artery could result in hand ischemia. Alternatively, an Allen's test can be performed. The hand is clenched tight and then the radial and ulnar arteries are simultaneously compressed at the wrist with finger and thumb pressure to occlude them. The hand is then opened whilst maintaining pressure on each artery. At this point, pressure on the radial artery is released. Rapid "pinking" or reperfusion of the hand confirms flow continuity into the hand. However, if the hand remains blanched for more than 10–20 seconds, this indicates limited or poor perfusion from the radial artery. The test is then repeated with pressure being released from the ulnar artery to assess its contribution.

> **Problems**
>
> - The proximity of a number of veins and arteries in the supraclavicular fossa can present a confusing display and venous signals may appear pulsatile due to the proximity of the right side of the heart
> - Imaging of the axillary artery can be difficult where the artery runs deep under the shoulder muscles. Scanning from the axilla or selecting a lower-frequency probe may help
> - There may be mirroring artifact of the subclavian due to the chest wall (see Fig. 7.7)

ULTRASOUND APPEARANCE

Normal appearance

The normal appearance of upper-extremity arteries is the same as that described for the duplex scanning of lower-limb arteries (see Ch. 9). The spectral Doppler waveform is normally triphasic at rest but becomes hyperemic with high diastolic flow following exercise. Changes in external temperature can have marked effects on the observed flow patterns in the distal arteries. There is a cyclical effect on the appearance of the flow patterns in the distal arteries towards the wrist and hand related to factors such as body temperature control. This cyclical effect can cause the waveform shape to change from high-resistance flow to hyperemic flow within the space of a minute (Fig. 10.6). Peripheral vasodilation will cause a reduction in peripheral resistance and an increase in flow. In this situation, the waveform in the radial and ulnar arteries can become hyperemic. Vasoconstriction increases peripheral resistance, producing a reduction in flow, and the waveform becomes biphasic. The range of normal peak systolic velocities in the SA has been reported as 80–120 cm/s (Edwards & Zierler 1992). It is often assumed that the radial artery is the dominant vessel in the forearm because it is easier to palpate at the wrist, but in many cases there is higher flow in the ulnar artery.

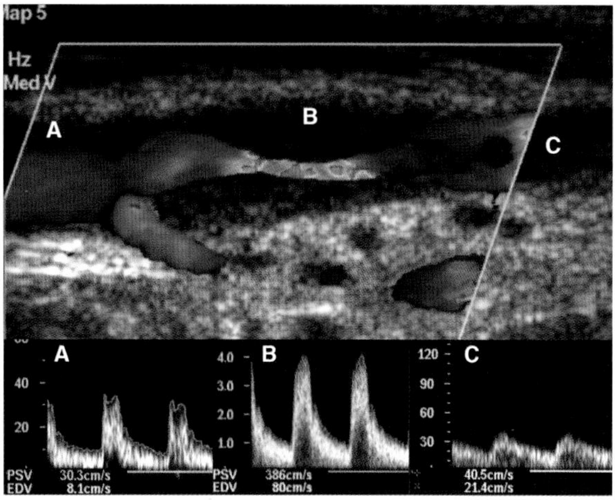

Figure 10.7 • A severe stenosis of the proximal brachial artery with Doppler waveforms recorded proximal to the stenosis (A), across the stenosis (B), and distal to the stenosis (C).

Abnormal appearance

In the absence of any specific criteria for grading upper-limb disease, we would advocate the same criteria as for grading lower-limb disease. Therefore, a doubling of the peak systolic velocity across a stenosis compared with the proximal normal adjacent segment indicates a >50% diameter reduction (Fig. 10.7). However, many upper-limb lesions are located at the origin to the SA, making proximal measurements from the aortic arch or brachiocephalic artery unreliable or impossible due to vessel depth, size, and geometry. In this situation the diagnosis is usually made by indirect signs, such as high-velocity jets, turbulence or poststenotic damping (Fig. 10.8). Peak systolic

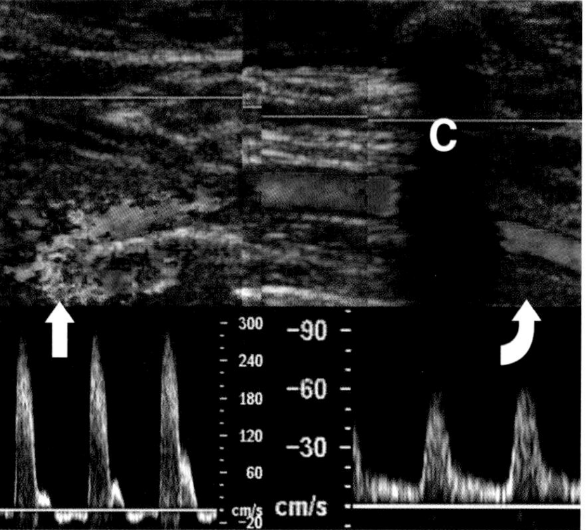

Figure 10.8 • A severe high-grade stenosis of the proximal right subclavian artery (straight arrow) is demonstrated by marked color flow disturbance and aliasing. Mirroring artefact is also seen in the region of the stenosis. The large acoustic shadow is due to the clavicle (C). High peak systolic velocity (280 cm/s) is recorded at the level of the stenosis (straight arrow). An abnormal waveform is recorded at a point distal to the stenosis (curved arrow) with an increased systolic rise time.

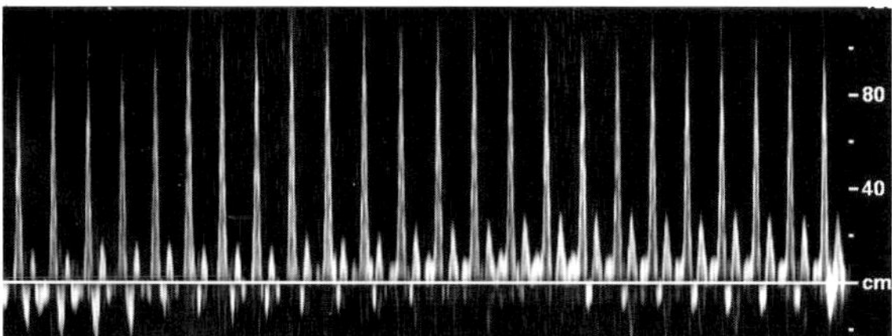

Figure 10.6 • A cyclical change in the appearance of the blood flow patterns in the radial and ulnar arteries can be observed, relating to factors such as the control of body temperature.

velocities in excess of 180 cm/s are considered significantly abnormal. In addition the ipsilateral vertebral artery should be examined for evidence of flow changes, indicated by damping or flow reversal (see Ch. 8). It can also be difficult to visibly identify plaques at the origin to the SA. Occlusions of the proximal SA can be difficult to differentiate from severe stenoses (von Reutern & von Büdingen 1993), and any uncertainty should be highlighted in the report. Dissection of the radial, brachial, or axillary arteries can occur due to trauma of the vessel wall following catheter access. It may be possible to see flaps, dual lumens, or acute obstruction.

Acute occlusions of upper-extremity arteries are frequently caused by embolization from the heart and occur most commonly in the brachial, radial, and ulnar arteries. The arterial lumen may appear relatively clear, but there will be an absence of flow in the vessel, as demonstrated by color flow imaging (Fig. 10.9). Some acute occlusions occur as a result of embolization from the SA due to damage caused by TOS.

Large arteriovenous malformations will be immediately obvious with color flow imaging as a region of high vascularity. Spectral Doppler will demonstrate low-resistance, high-volume flow waveforms within the malformation.

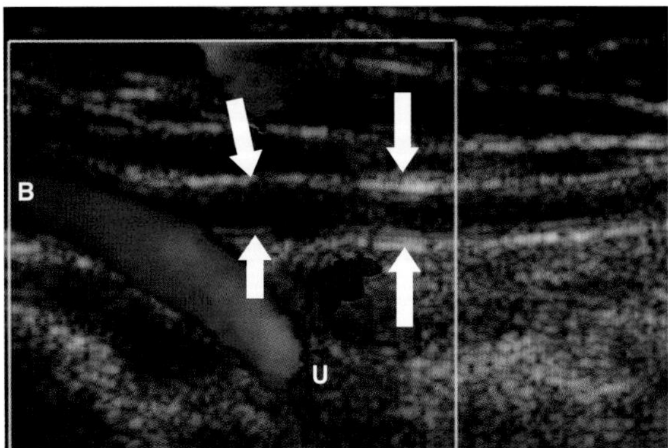

Figure 10.9 • An embolus from the heart has acutely obstructed the radial artery from its origin (arrows) causing an occlusion, as evidenced by an absence of color flow. The arterial lumen appears clear, as the occlusion is acute and has a similar echogenicity to blood. The distal brachial artery (B) and proximal ulnar artery (U) are seen in this image.

THORACIC OUTLET SYNDROME

The vascular laboratory is frequently asked to assess patients with suspected TOS. The thoracic outlet is the region where the SA and brachial plexus leave the chest and pass in between the anterior and middle scalene muscles over the first rib and underneath the clavicle (Fig. 10.10). This is a compact anatomical area, and compression on the nerves or arteries by a number of mechanisms can produce sensory symptoms in both the hand and arm. Compression can occur in three main areas. The first is at the point where the SA passes between the scalene muscles and can be caused by muscle hypertrophy or fibrous bands or may be due to the presence of an additional accessory rib originating from the seventh thoracic vertebra, termed a cervical rib (Fig. 10.11). Accessory ribs occur in less than 1% of the population (Makhoul & Machleder 1992). The second area of compression occurs as the artery runs between the first rib and clavicle. Fibrous bands or fibrosis due to injuries in this region, such as fractures of the clavicle, can also cause compression. The third, less common area of compression occurs in the subcoracoid region, where the axillary artery runs under the pectoralis minor muscle and close to the coracoid process of the scapula.

Typically, the vessels and nerves are compressed when the arm is placed in specific positions. The symptoms include sensory changes, such as pain,

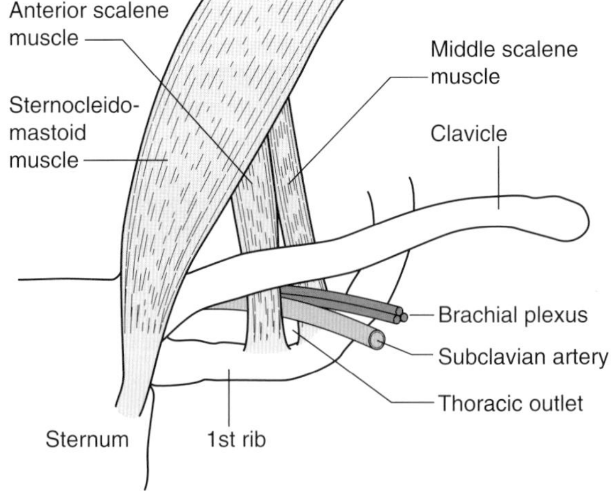

Figure 10.10 • The anatomy of the thoracic outlet.

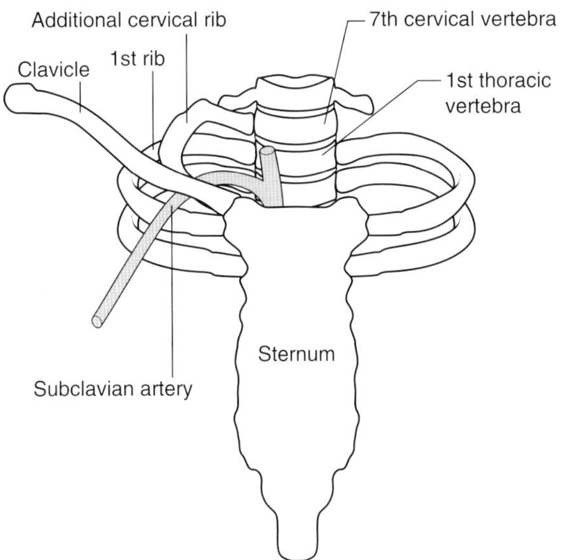

Figure 10.11 • The presence of a cervical rib originating from the seventh thoracic vertebra can cause compression of the brachial nerve plexus and subclavian artery.

"pins and needles" in the hand, hand weakness, and other neurological disorders. TOS can be purely neurogenic, due to compression of the brachial plexus alone (this accounts for approximately 90% of cases). Neurogenic TOS often produces abnormal nerve conduction recordings and can be associated with muscle weakness and wasting in the lower arm or hand.

Arterial and venous TOS is less common and accounts for approximately 10% of cases, although there is sometimes a combination of neurogenic and vascular compression. Aneurysmal dilations of the SA are sometimes seen just distal to the point of compression due to poststenotic dilation. These aneurysms can be the source of distal emboli in the fingers, which can be the initial presentation of a patient with TOS. There is still considerable debate about the assessment and treatment of TOS, which often involves surgical resection of a cervical rib and sometimes the first rib, with the division of any fibrous bands to relieve the compression. Although the majority of patients who have undergone surgery show improvement in symptoms, a few show no signs of improvement and may return to the vascular laboratory for further assessment.

Maneuvers for assessing TOS

Continuous-wave Doppler recording of the radial artery signal, performed with the arm in a range of positions, can be a useful prelude to the duplex examination (Fig. 10.12). There are a range of provocation maneuvers that can be used. Unfortunately, testing can be associated with false-positive and false-negative responses and the maneuvers may need to be repeated a number of times to obtain consistent readings. It should be noted that there appears to be considerable variability in the descriptions of these tests in medical literature and therefore the use of specific names such as Adson's and Roos test has been avoided.

Hyperabduction test

The patient should be sitting comfortably, and the arm should then be slowly extended outward (abducted). With the arm fully abducted, the forearm is rotated so that the palm faces upward and the elbow downward (external rotation). The arm should be raised and lowered in this position and the patient's head turned away from the side under investigation. This test can indicate compression between the clavicle and first rib or coracoid region.

Costoclavicular maneuver

The patient is asked to push the chest outward while forcing the shoulders backward with deep inhalation, the so-called military position, as this may reveal arterial compression between the clavicle and first rib.

Deep inspiration maneuver

During deep inspiration the patient is asked to extend the neck and rotate the head to the affected side and then to the other side while the pulse is checked at the wrist. A positive test indicates possible compression between the scalene muscles or the presence of a cervical rib.

Traction test

Locate the radial pulse. Apply firm traction on the arm for several seconds, checking for diminishing pulse. A positive sign indicates cervical rib pressure on the tested side.

Finally, the patient should also be asked to place the arm in any position that provokes symptoms,

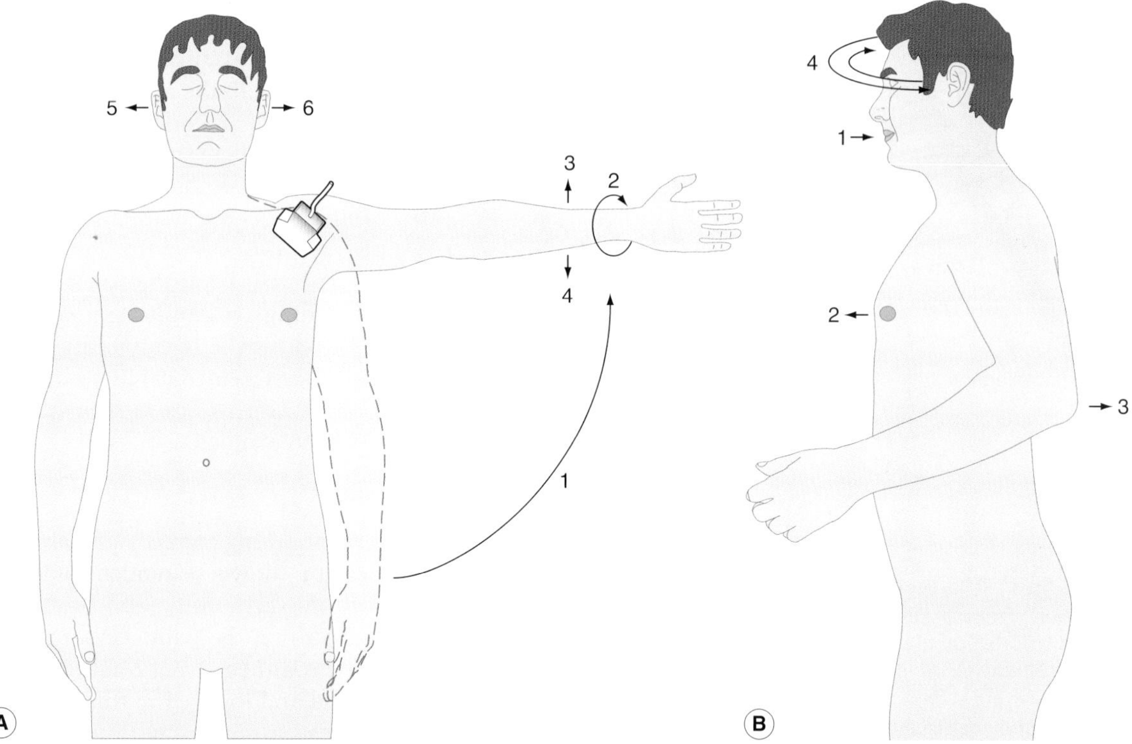

Figure 10.12 • Provocation maneuvers used for the assessment of thoracic outlet syndrome. (A) Hyperabduction test. The arm is abducted (1) and the arm externally rotated (2). The arm can also be raised or lowered during this test (3 and 4) and the head rotated to either side (5 and 6). The position for placing the duplex transducer to assess blood flow during these maneuvers is shown on this illustration. (B) Costoclavicular maneuver. During deep inspiration (1) the chest is pushed forward (2) and the arms backward (3). The head is turned from side to side (4).

such as raising it above the head. In some cases this will result in a positive result although the maneuvers above may have been negative. Any change to, or loss of, the Doppler signal during these maneuvers suggests compression of the SA. The patient should also be asked to indicate any symptoms that occur during arm maneuvers, as a normal Doppler signal in the presence of symptoms may indicate a nonvascular cause for the complaint.

Duplex assessment of TOS

It is generally easier to image the arteries with the patient in a sitting position so that certain provocation tests can be performed. The SA is initially imaged from the supraclavicular and infraclavicular positions. The flow velocities are recorded and any abnormalities, such as tortuosity or aneurysmal dilations, noted. The SA can then be imaged using any of the provocation maneuvers that were found to reduce or obliterate the radial artery signal with pencil Doppler. One useful maneuver involves scanning of the SA from the infraclavicular position while the arm is fully abducted. Any changes in the flow pattern or areas of significant velocity increase along the SA during provocation tests should be recorded. Typically, most high-velocity jets are recorded in the region of the clavicle (Fig. 10.13). There are no clearly defined criteria as to the point at which TOS is indicated, but a doubling of the peak systolic velocity at one location is indicative of a significant hemodynamic effect. Patients with severe vascular symptoms show complete occlusion of the SA during provocation maneuvers, posing less of a diagnostic

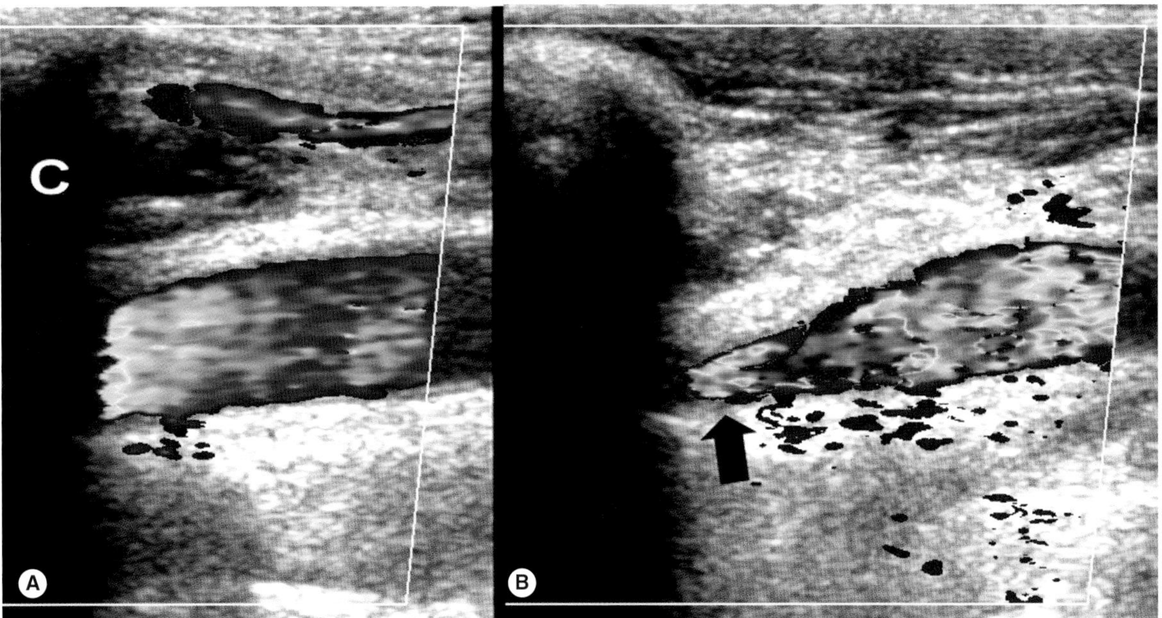

Figure 10.13 • (A) A normal color flow image of the subclavian artery as it passes underneath the clavicle (C) with the arm at rest. (B) Following arm abduction there is marked compression of the subclavian artery associated with color aliasing (arrow), indicating thoracic outlet syndrome. Note the large acoustic shadow below the clavicle.

dilemma. Many clinicians request examination of both arms, as both sides could be positive but only one symptomatic, and this may suggest that treatment of the symptomatic side may be less beneficial.

ANEURYSMS

Aneurysms involving the upper extremities are rare and are most frequently seen in the SA, associated with TOS. False aneurysms or pseudoaneurysms are most commonly seen in the radial, brachial, or axillary artery following arterial puncture for catheter access. Some patients present to the clinic with visible pulsatile swelling in the supraclavicular fossa, which is usually on the right side of the neck. This is invariably due to tortuosity of the distal brachiocephalic artery, proximal common carotid artery, and proximal SA. Occasionally, pulsatile swellings are seen in the area of the radial or ulnar artery at the wrist, and this can be due to a ganglion lying adjacent to the artery and distorting its path. The ganglion can be surgically removed.

OTHER DISORDERS OF THE UPPER-EXTREMITY CIRCULATION

Some hand and arm symptoms are due to microvascular or neurological disorders. Duplex scanning can exclude large-vessel disease, but patients suffering from these types of abnormalities are best evaluated in specialist microvascular units.

Raynaud's phenomenon can be a primary disorder related to vasospasm in the fingers or a rarer and more serious secondary disorder associated with connective tissue diseases such as scleroderma. Primary Raynaud's phenomenon produces symptoms of digital ischemia in response to changes in ambient temperature and emotional state. This is observed as color changes of the fingers, causing blanching, or bluish discoloration due to cold. The blanching is followed by a period of rubor (redness) caused by hyperemia as the fingers warm. These signs may be mistaken for the presence of atherosclerotic occlusive disease, but pencil Doppler recordings will detect pulsatile flow signals in the radial and ulnar arteries, and the brachial systolic pressure should be equal in both arms. Secondary Raynaud's causes more persistent symptoms and in extreme cases can result in amputation of one or more fingers.

Vibration white-finger disease is a disorder caused by the use of drills and other vibrating machinery over a long period of time, leading to damage to the nerves and microvascular circulation in the fingers and hand. It can result in blanching of some or all of the fingers, loss of sensation, and loss of dexterity. Again, Doppler signals may be normal to wrist level. However, Doppler recordings may demonstrate high-resistance flow patterns in the digital arteries due to the increased resistance to flow caused by the damaged arterioles and capillary beds. If the damage is severe, no flow may be detected with Doppler interrogation.

Reflex sympathetic dystrophy (RSD) is a poorly understood condition that usually occurs after local trauma, sometimes minor, to the hand or arm and results in severe pain, sensitivity, and restricted movement of the affected area. Patients often report pain that is out of proportion to the severity of the injury, which might be a simple sprain or bruise. The condition can persist for many months, and intensive treatment is sometimes required to restore full use to the limb. This condition can affect young adults and children. The hand or arm may feel cold to the touch and appear discolored or cyanosed. However, Doppler recordings usually demonstrate pulsatile arterial signals in the brachial, radial, and ulnar arteries. RSD can also affect the lower extremities.

REPORTING

The simplest form of reporting upper-extremity investigations is with the use of diagrams, similar to the method used for lower-limb investigations. This can be associated with a brief report. In the case of TOS, a written report may suffice.

References

Abou-Zamzam A M Jr, Edwards J M, Porter J M 2000 Noninvasive diagnosis of upper extremity disease. In: AbuRahma A F, Bergan J J (eds) Noninvasive vascular diagnosis. Springer, London, p 269

Edwards J M, Zierler R E 1992 Duplex ultrasound assessment of upper extremity arteries. In: Zwiebel W J (ed.) Introduction to vascular ultrasonography, 3rd edn. W B Saunders, Philadelphia, p 228

Makhoul R G, Machleder H I 1992 Developmental anomalies at the thoracic outlet: an analysis of 200 consecutive cases. Journal of Vascular Surgery 16: 534–545

von Reutern G M, von Büdingen H J 1993 Ultrasound diagnosis of cerebrovascular disease. Thieme, Stuttgart, pp 249–250

Further reading

Hennerici M, Neuerburg-Heusler D 1998 Vascular diagnosis with ultrasound. Thieme, Stuttgart

Zwiebel WJ, Pellerito JS 2005 Introduction to vascular ultrasonography 5th edn. Elsevier Saunders, Philadelphia

Duplex assessment of aneurysms and endovascular repair

CONTENTS

INTRODUCTION

True aneurysms are abnormal dilations of arteries. The term ectasia is often used to describe a moderate dilation of arteries. The abdominal aorta is one of the commonest sites for aneurysms to occur. The main risk of abdominal aortic aneurysms (AAA) is rupture, which is fatal in most cases. In the USA rupture of an AAA is the 14th commonest cause of death and is estimated to kill approximately 10 000 people per year (Birkmeyer & Upchurch 2007). In England and Wales, this figure is approximately 5000 people (Office for National Statistics 2006). Men over the age of 65 years are the most common group to be affected. Ultrasound can detect almost all AAAs and, when screening is combined with elective surgery, the mortality associated with the disease is almost halved (Ashton et al. 2002). A recent analysis of four large, randomized clinical trials has also confirmed that population-based screening substantially reduces AAA-related mortality in selected patient groups (Fleming et al. 2005) In the USA, the US Preventive Services Task Force (2005) and a consortium of leading professional organizations recommend one-time screening with abdominal ultrasonography for all men aged 65–75 years who have ever smoked. In the UK, a national screening program should be under way by the time this edition is published.

Ultrasound is the obvious modality for screening as it is a rapid, cheap, and simple noninvasive method of detecting aneurysms and can be used for serial investigations to monitor any increase in size of small aneurysms. However, if surgical intervention is being considered, other imaging techniques, such as computed tomography (CT) and magnetic resonance imaging (MRI), are required to demonstrate the relationship of an aneurysm to major branches and other structures within the body. In the past, treatment of AAA was by open surgery but nowadays approximately 50% of patients are treated by the less invasive technique of endovascular aortic aneurysm repair (EVAR), where a stent graft is inserted via the femoral arteries. Endovascular repair can also be used to treat aneurysms in other areas of the body. This chapter concentrates on ultrasound scanning of aortic aneurysms and surveillance of EVAR procedures but also considers the assessment of aneurysms in other areas of the peripheral circulation.

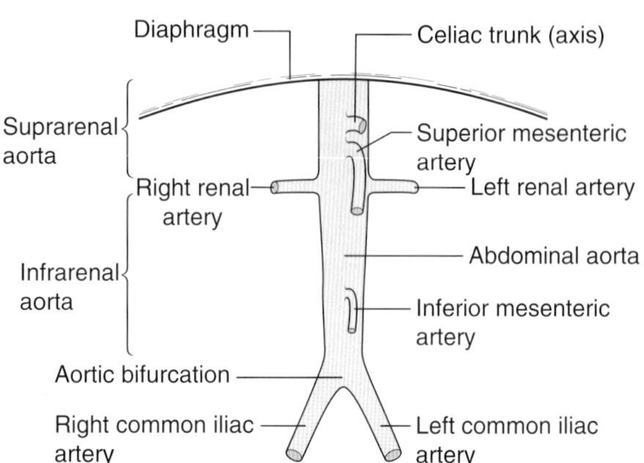

Figure 11.1 • Anatomy of the abdominal aorta and its major branches.

Definition of an aneurysm

It has been suggested that an aneurysm is a permanent localized dilation of an artery having at least a 50% increase in diameter compared to the normal expected diameter (Johnston et al. 1991). Ectasia is characterized by a diameter increase <50% of the normal expected diameter. It is worth remembering that there is considerable variability in the normal diameter of arteries among individuals, and this will be dependent on factors such as physical size, sex, and age.

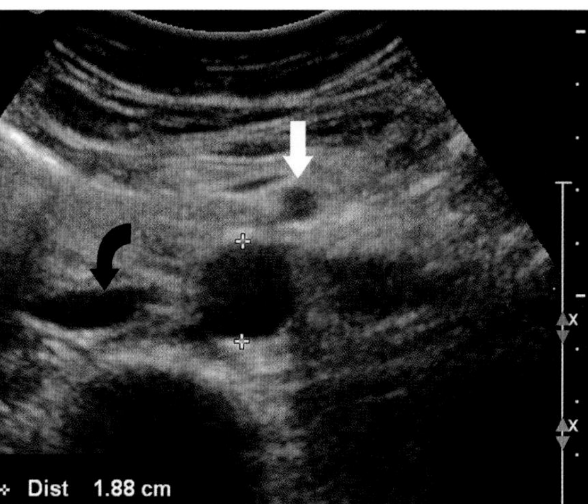

Figure 11.2 • A transverse image of a normal abdominal aorta. The inferior vena cava (curved arrow) is seen to the right of the aorta and the superior mesenteric artery (straight arrow) is seen anterior to the aorta (note that the probe orientation means that the right side of the patient is on the left of the image).

ANATOMY OF THE ABDOMINAL AORTA

The abdominal aorta commences at the level of the diaphragm and lies just in front of the spine. It descends slightly to the left of the midline to the level of the fourth lumbar vertebra, where it divides into the left and right common iliac arteries (Fig. 11.1). It tapers slightly as it descends, owing to the large branches it gives off. Major branches of the aorta that can be easily identified with ultrasound include the celiac axis and superior mesenteric artery (SMA) (Fig. 11.2). These can act as important reference points when determining the upper limit of an aneurysm. Visualization of the inferior mesenteric artery is variable. The vena cava lies to the right of the aorta and may assume a variety of shapes, especially in the presence of an aneurysm, and commonly appears 'flattened' when compared to the circular shape of the aorta.

PATHOLOGY OF ANEURYSMS

The mechanism of aneurysm development is uncertain but may involve a multifactorial process leading to the destruction of aortic wall connective tissue. There is evidence that increased local production of enzymes capable of degrading elastic fibers as well as interstitial collagens is associated with AAA (Wassef et al. 2001). The lumen of an aneurysm is often lined with large amounts of thrombus that can be a potential source of emboli. This is also why arteriograms, which only demonstrate the flow lumen, are not accurate for estimating the true diameter of an aneurysm, as the flow lumen can be significantly smaller than the diameter of the entire vessel. Aortic aneurysms can also extend into the iliac arteries. Some aortic aneurysms are involved in an inflammatory process, with marked periaortic fibrosis surrounding the aorta making surgical resection difficult (see Figure 11.12D). Aneurysms can also be caused by a variety of infections, such as bacterial endocarditis, and are termed mycotic aneurysms. These can occur anywhere in the body.

Popliteal aneurysms may be the source of distal emboli. They can also occlude, leading to symptoms of acute lower-limb ischemia. This should always be considered as a potential cause of the acutely ischemic leg, especially in patients with no other obvious risk factors.

False aneurysms occur predominantly in the femoral artery following puncture of the arterial wall for catheter access. In this situation, blood continues to flow backward and forward through the puncture site into a false flow cavity outside the artery.

ANEURYSM SHAPES AND TYPES

Aneurysms vary considerably in shape and size (Fig. 11.3). Most aneurysms are fusiform in shape and there is uniform dilation across the entire cross-section of the vessel. Saccular aneurysms exhibit a typical localized bulging of the wall. Dissecting aneurysms occur due to a disruption of the intimal lining of the vessel, allowing blood to enter the subintimal space. This can result in the stripping of the intima, and sometimes of the media, from the artery wall. If the aorta partially dissects, large amounts of thrombus may be seen in the subintimal space (Fig. 11.3F). If there is a full dissection, a false flow lumen is created and the dissected layer of intima may be seen flapping freely in time with arterial pulsation (Fig. 11.3G). Some aortic dissections are not associated with aneurysms and can start in the chest, extending through the aorta into the iliac arteries. It is possible for aortic branches, such as renal arteries, to be supplied via either lumen. Occasionally, two aneurysmal dilations may be seen along the length of the abdominal aorta, separated by a normal segment of the aorta, which gives rise to a classic "dumb-bell" shape when viewed in longitudinal section (Fig. 11.3H). As the aorta dilates, it also tends to increase in length, producing tortuosity that often shifts the aorta to the left of the midline or deflects it in an anterior direction.

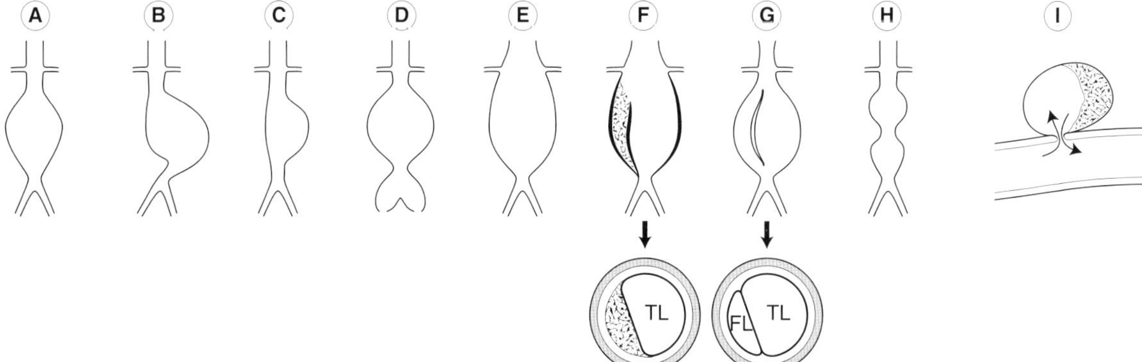

Figure 11.3 • Aneurysms are very variable in shape and type. (A) Fusiform infrarenal aortic aneurysm. (B) Tortuous elongated aortic aneurysm with the sac shifted to the left of the midline. (C) Saccular aortic aneurysm. (D) Infrarenal aortic aneurysm extending into the iliac arteries. (E) Suprarenal aortic aneurysm involving the renal arteries. (F) Dissecting aortic aneurysm with a tear between the intima and media allowing blood into the subintimal space. (G) Dissecting aortic aneurysm in which the intima has fully dissected, creating a false flow lumen. (H) Double aneurysm of the aorta producing a "dumb-bell" appearance. (I) False aneurysm of the common femoral artery following arterial puncture. TL, true lumen; FL, false lumen.

AORTIC ANEURYSMS: SYMPTOMS AND TREATMENT

The normal size of the abdominal aorta varies between 1.4 and 2.5 cm in diameter (Johnston et al. 1991) (Fig. 11.2). An aortic diameter slightly above 2.5 cm is considered mildly abnormal or ectatic. A small aortic aneurysm is generally regarded as an aorta having a diameter of 3 cm, and many surgeons will not request serial screening scans unless the aorta reaches this level. However, some vascular units monitor patients with slightly enlarged aortas, especially if the patient is young (<55 years old). As the aorta increases in size, there is a potential for rupture due to increased tension in the arterial wall. The UK Small Aneurysm Trial Participants (1998) demonstrated that the average annual growth rate of aneurysms measuring between 4 and 5.5 cm was 0.33 cm a year. However, rates will vary among individuals and are also dependent on the size of the aneurysm. The prevalence of aortic aneurysms is five to six times greater in men than women (Vardulaki et al. 2000). In addition, there seems to be a strong familial link, with siblings of aneurysm patients having a higher risk of developing an aneurysm compared with the general population.

Clinically, there are usually no symptoms associated with the development of an aortic aneurysm and many are discovered incidentally, during routine examinations or on plain abdominal radiographs. Occasionally, patients present with symptoms of renal hydronephrosis. This is caused by compression of a ureter leading from one of the kidneys by the aneurysm sac and most frequently occurs on the left side. The symptoms associated with aneurysm leakage or rupture include back or abdominal pain and acute shock. Ultrasound is occasionally used to confirm the diagnosis in the emergency room, although the symptoms are usually so acute that emergency surgery is required. However an emergency room scan that excludes an aneurysm can be useful and many emergency physicians have been trained to undertake rapid AAA scanning. The mortality rate for acute rupture of an aortic aneurysm is very high, 65–85% (Kniemeyer et al. 2000), and many patients do not reach hospital alive.

The risk of aortic aneurysm rupture increases with size. The UK Small Aneurysm Trial Participants (1998) found that the mean risk of rupture of aneurysms measuring 4–5.5 cm was 1% per year. However, larger aneurysms carry a higher rate of rupture. A study by Lederle et al. (2002) demonstrated that the average risk of rupture in male patients with a 6–6.9 cm aneurysm was 10% per year and 32% per year for aneurysms measuring more than 7 cm in diameter.

Clearly, there are benefits in detecting aneurysms at an early stage so that serial follow-up can be carried out and elective repair performed if the aneurysm becomes too large. The UK Small Aneurysm Trial Participants (1998) have shown no survival benefit for open repair of aneurysms measuring less than 5.5 cm in diameter compared to ultrasound surveillance and this was also confirmed after a 12-year follow-up analysis of the trial (The UK Small Aneurysm Trial Participants 2007). In the original study, age, sex, or initial aneurysm size did not modify the overall hazard ratio. Therefore, many surgeons will only carry out elective repair if the aneurysm has a diameter of equal to or greater than 5.5 cm, or if there are indications that smaller aneurysms are becoming symptomatic and are at risk of rupturing.

Although aortic aneurysms are much more prevalent in men, there is some evidence that women with aneurysms in the 5–5.9 cm range may be up to four times more likely to undergo rupture compared to men with similar-sized aneurysms (Brown et al. 2003). Further research may prompt a lower threshold for repairing aneurysms in female patients. However, at the present time the mass screening of women does not appear to be cost-effective.

Surgical techniques for aortic aneurysm repair

Open repair

Open repair of aortic aneurysms has been performed for over 30 years and involves a large incision in the abdomen and mobilization of the intestines to expose the aorta. Fortunately, the majority of abdominal aneurysms (approximately 90%) start below the level of the renal arteries (infrarenal aneurysms). This means that surgical clamps, to control the aneurysm, can be positioned below the renal arteries, ensuring that the kidneys are perfused during the operation. Aortic aneurysms that extend above the renal arteries (suprarenal aneurysms) carry a higher rate of perioperative and postoperative complication, as the aorta has to be clamped above the level of the renal arteries and reimplantation of the renal arteries is necessary. Patients can suffer from renal failure following this procedure. This is why it is important that the surgeon be aware of the level of the proximal neck before surgery is performed. Aortic aneurysms are repaired using straight tube grafts unless the aneurysm extends into the iliac arteries, where a bifurcating graft is used. The graft is sutured into position and the sac closed around the graft. Postoperatively, patients normally spend a day or two in intensive care and usually leave hospital 10–14 days after surgery. The elective mortality rate for open repair is in the region of 5%. However, surgically unfit patients have a risk of much higher morbidity and mortality rates.

Endovascular repair

Endovascular repair of aortic aneurysms was described in the early 1990s. There have been significant technical developments in this field since that time, and several types of commercially manufactured grafts are now available. The prosthetic stent graft is introduced through an arteriotomy made in the femoral artery and deployed in the aorta to exclude flow into the aneurysm sac. The grafts are made of a synthetic material such as Dacron and polytetrafluoroethylene (PTFE) and are supported on an expandable metal framework, or skeleton, of nitinol or stainless steel to prevent kinks and twisting.

Nowadays, almost all endovascular grafts are bifurcating devices (Fig. 11.4). These are modular systems with the graft supplied in two parts. The bulk of the graft consists of the main body, one complete limb, and the short stump of the second limb. The remaining modular limb is delivered separately via an arteriotomy in the contralateral common femoral artery. The grafts are prepacked on to the delivery catheter during the manufacturing process and retained in place by an outer sheath until deployed in the aorta. During the procedure the femoral artery is surgically exposed, and the catheter containing the main graft is inserted over a guide wire and positioned with the aid of fluoroscopy so that the top of the graft lies just below the renal arteries in the proximal neck. Many of these devices have uncovered metal stents that extend across the renal arteries (suprarenal fixation) to hold the device in place.

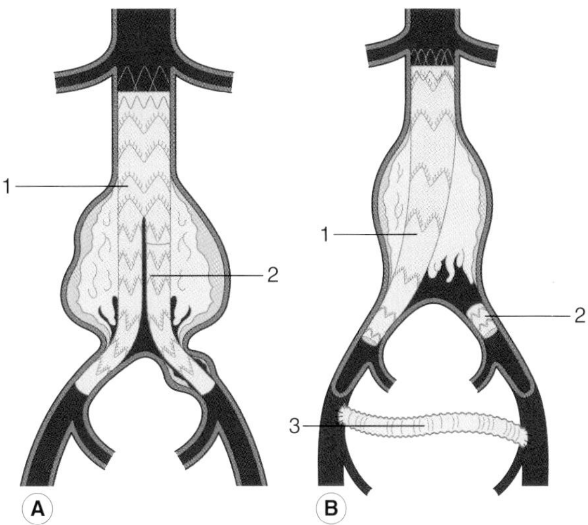

Figure 11.4 • Examples of endovascular aortic aneurysm repair. (A) A bifurcating device. 1 main body, 2 modular limb. (B) An aorto-uniliac device (1) and cross over graft (3). Note the left common iliac artery has been occluded with a covered stopper (2). (Courtesy of WL Gore & Associates.)

The graft is deployed by slowly withdrawing the outer covering sheath. If needed, a soft balloon is inflated to ensure the graft is fully expanded in the proximal neck, just above the sac. Some grafts have hooks at the top that anchor into the aortic wall for further security. The modular limb is then delivered on a separate catheter via the contralateral femoral artery. Under radiographic control it is positioned so that it fits into the stunted limb of the main body and then is fully expanded, using a balloon if necessary, to make a seal. The distal end is then anchored in the common iliac artery. In some cases an aortic uni-iliac device can be inserted if one of the iliac arteries is diseased, occluded, or excessively aneurysmal (Fig. 11.4B).

As the devices are modular, it is possible to add extensions to the limbs to exclude long iliac artery aneurysms. Postoperative recovery is usually very quick, with some patients going home within 2–4 days. However, not all aneurysms are suitable for endovascular repair. This can be due to aneurysm tortuosity, excessive proximal neck diameter, limited proximal neck length, severe iliac artery disease, and marked iliac artery tortuosity. The Endovascular Aneurysm Repair Trial 1 (EVAR 2005) reported a two-thirds reduction in 30-day postoperative mortality compared to open repair. Although endovascular repair appears much less traumatic for the patient, the EVAR 1 trial also found that, by 4 years, 40% of patients who had undergone endovascular repair had suffered a complication and that 20% had required reintervention, including the correction of endoleak. For this reason it has been recommended that patients should undergo lifelong surveillance to detect endoleaks or other graft-related complications (National Institute for Health and Clinical Excellence 2006). An endoleak occurs when blood leaks into the aneurysm sac from the graft or from another source, such as a lumbar or inferior mesenteric artery. In this situation the aneurysm sac can continue to expand and rupture (van Marrewijk et al. 2002; EVAR 2005). The rupture rate in the EVAR 1 trial was 1%. However there is evidence to suggest that some types of endoleak are benign and can be safely left alone unless there is progressive sac expansion. The different types of endoleak and their ultrasound appearances and management are discussed later in this chapter.

PRACTICAL CONSIDERATIONS FOR DUPLEX SCANNING OF AORTIC ANEURYSMS

What information does the physician require?

- The maximum diameter of the aorta
- Any relevant aneurysm features such as shape or position
- Does the aneurysm extend across the iliac bifurcation into the common iliac arteries?
- Indications of thrombus load or mobile areas of thrombus

It is important to note any limitations of the scan and to state clearly what measurements were made and from what positions. Situations have occurred in which the points of measurement have been ambiguously reported and the overall length of an aneurysm has been mistakenly interpreted as its diameter.

The purpose of the scan is to determine if there is an aneurysm involving the aorta or peripheral arterial system and, if appropriate, to monitor the size of the aneurysm on a serial basis. A screening scan can be performed in less than 5 min, but more detailed scans of endovascular grafts may take up to 20 min.

No special preparation is required, although some units use a bowel preparation to improve visualization of the aorta; however, for screening scans this is rarely necessary. The patient should be lying supine with the head supported on a pillow and the arms resting by the sides. Sometimes the patient may have to roll to one side to improve visualization as this may shift obscuring bowel or gas. The scanner should be configured for an aortic investigation but, in the absence of a specific preset, a general abdominal examination setup should be selected. Ensure that the image depth setting is not too shallow or too deep. A depth setting of 8–12 cm is usually sufficient for the average-sized patient. A low-frequency curvilinear array transducer is the most suitable probe for this investigation. Harmonic imaging can be useful for improving the image quality. In very obese patients a low-frequency transducer can help to identify the aorta.

SCANNING TECHNIQUE

For screening scans the key measurement is the maximum diameter of the aorta. However, the following description is for a comprehensive investigation of the aorta. The shape of the aneurysm and features such as tortuosity or dissection should be documented. The scanning technique for imaging the aorta is demonstrated in Figure 11.5. The procedure is as follows:

1. The aorta is usually easiest to identify by starting with the transducer in a transverse image plane, approximately 3–4 cm above the umbilicus. The aorta is then imaged throughout its visible length and, if possible, from the upper abdomen above the celiac axis, or SMA, to the aortic bifurcation.
2. The abdominal aorta is then imaged in a longitudinal or sagittal plane, from the midline along its length to the aortic bifurcation.
3. The aorta is then viewed from a coronal scan plane throughout its length in a longitudinal

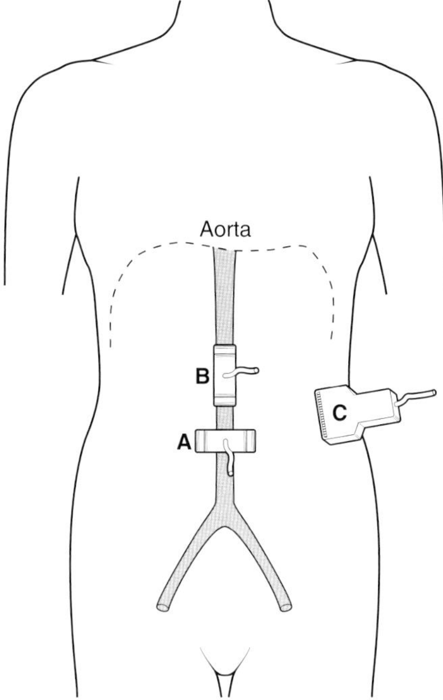

Figure 11.5 • Transducer positions for scanning the abdominal aorta. (A) Transverse. (B) Sagittal or longitudinal. (C) Coronal. The coronal view is used for measuring the lateral diameter of the aorta (i.e., side to side). Examples of the images obtained from these positions are shown in Figure 11.6.

view to obtain more accurate measurements of the lateral diameter of the aorta (side to side).

4 It is good practice to assess the proximal iliac arteries in transverse and longitudinal scan planes (see Ch. 9) to exclude an isolated iliac artery aneurysm or to define the lower limit of an aneurysm if it extends into the iliac arteries (see Fig. 11.17).

ULTRASOUND APPEARANCE

Normal appearance

The aorta should measure less than 2.5 cm at its maximum diameter (Fig. 11.2) and there is usually slight tapering of the aorta from top to bottom. In the longitudinal plane, the aorta is sometimes seen to curve gently in a slight convex direction as it lies on the lumbar spine.

Abnormal appearance

The aorta appears abnormally enlarged, as seen on the B-mode image in Figure 11.6. The shape of the aneurysm can vary (Fig. 11.3). Marked kinking of the posterior wall at the level of the proximal neck can occur due to elongation of the aorta, which can be mistaken as an atherosclerotic stenosis. If the aneurysm deflects in an anterior direction, it can be very difficult to demonstrate the level of the renal arteries, and the proximal segment of the abdominal aorta may become tortuous, which is sometimes described as a 'swan neck' appearance.

Thrombus may be imaged as concentric layers with differing degrees of echogenicity depending on the age and organization. Sometimes localized liquefaction of the thrombus can occur, which appears as hypoechoic areas within the thrombus. This appearance can be confused with a dissection, although there is usually a thick layer of thrombus separating the liquefied region and the flow lumen (Fig. 11.7). A dissection may be undetected, as blood that has leaked into the wall may be mistaken for mural thrombus. In a full dissection, flow will be observed in the false flow lumen, which is separated from the true lumen by a flap of intima and, sometimes, media (Fig. 11.8).

Measurement issues

- Many sonographers measure maximum aortic diameter from the outer edge of the anterior wall to the outer edge of the posterior wall (Fig. 11.6). However, some units measure from the inner edge of the anterior wall to the inner edge of the posterior wall as it is claimed that these are more consistently identifiable points. This was the method used in the Multicentre Aneurysm Screening Study (Ashton et al 2002). When measuring an AAA of approximately 5 cm diameter it is possible to find >3 mm difference between these two measurement methods. It is highly likely that the UK aneurysm screening program will use inner wall to inner was as the measurement protocol.
- Due to the puslatile nature of blood flow, aortic diameter can vary through the cardiac cycle and some sonographers take measurements at peak systole when the aorta is maximally distended to improve reproducibility between serial scans. Scrolling through the cineloop can help to identify this point.

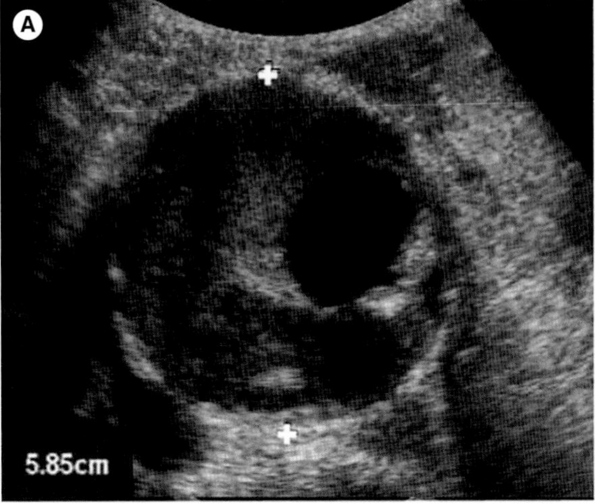

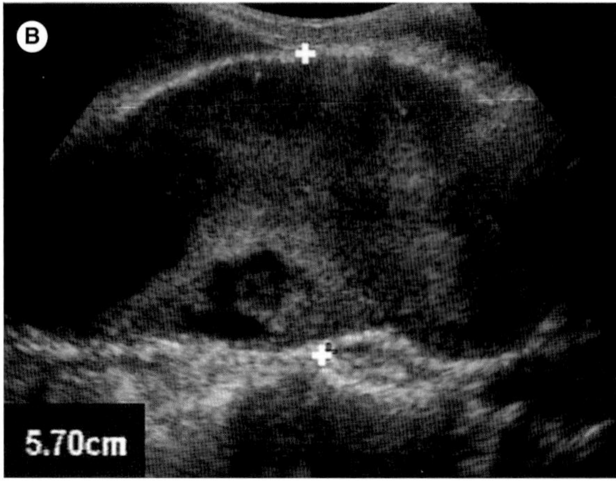

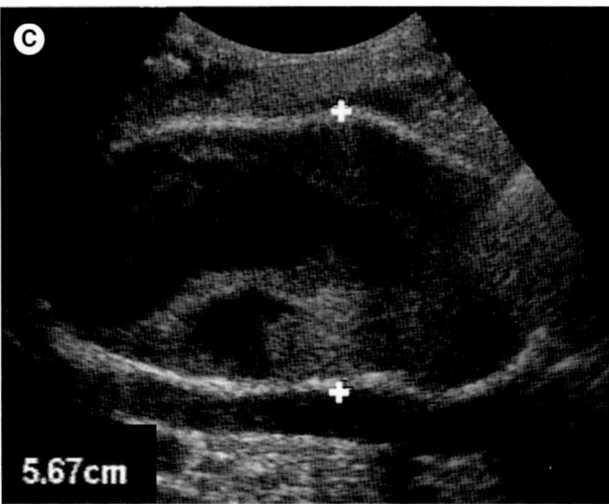

Figure 11.6 • A large abdominal aortic aneurysm is shown from the three different imaging planes demonstrated in Figure 11.5. (A) Transverse image. The anteroposterior (AP) diameter is measured from the outer wall to the outer wall (callipers). (B) A sagittal image, demonstrating the calliper positions to measure the aneurysm in this plane. (C) Image from the coronal position. Note that in this example the diameter measured in the transverse image (A) is slightly larger, due to obliquity (see Fig. 11.9). The measurement taken from the sagittal position (5.7 cm) would be the most accurate to quote in the report.

Inflammatory aneurysms demonstrate a hypoechoic area of ill-defined fibrosis around the aorta on the B-mode image, but this appearance can be confused with the presence of periaortic lymph nodes. The ultrasound diagnosis of a leaking aneurysm is extremely difficult, although it is sometimes possible to identify areas of fresh blood or hematoma as hypoechoic areas associated with the aneurysm in the retroperitoneal space. This type of assessment should be carried out by an experienced sonographer; however, other imaging techniques, such as CT and MRI, are better suited for excluding leaking aneurysms.

MEASUREMENTS

It is important to make accurate diameter measurements of the aorta, especially if a patient is having serial follow-up scans to monitor the size of an aneurysm. The UK Small Aneurysm Trial Participants (1998) showed that the error between operators was in the region of 0.2 cm for aneurysms measuring 4–5.5 cm in diameter. This section explains how to make diameter measurements of the aorta and identifies the potential pitfalls that may be involved. It should be noted that some of these measurements may not be necessary for screening scans.

Aorta diameter

Transverse scanning plane

The maximum diameter of the aorta can be measured in the anteroposterior (AP) direction from the outer anterior wall to the outer posterior wall

(Fig. 11.6). However, if an aneurysm is present, overestimation of its size can occur if oblique measurements are made, in either the AP or lateral direction (Figs 11.6 and 11.9) and for this reason we recommend measurements in the longitudinal plane. Measurements of the lateral diameter of the aneurysm (i.e., from left to right side walls.) in a transverse scan plane are prone to error as the lateral vessel walls are parallel to the ultrasound beam, which therefore produces a very poor image (see Ch. 2). The thickness of any thrombus can also be measured in the AP plane. It is sometimes possible to assess whether the aneurysm starts below the level of the renal arteries by measuring the diameter of the aorta at this level with the aid of color flow imaging. With the transducer in a transverse plane, positioned at the upper abdomen, the right renal artery is normally seen dividing from the aorta at a 10 o'clock position and the left renal artery from a 4 o'clock position. (see Figures 12.2, 12.3 and 12.9). In practice, they can be very difficult to image in the presence of an aneurysm, especially if the aneurysm is tortuous or projecting upward or kinked, and other imaging modalities such as CT scanning are more appropriate for this measurement.

Longitudinal scan plane, from sagittal and coronal positions

Estimates of aortic diameter in sagittal and coronal scan planes are more accurate than measurements in the transverse plane. This is because it is easier to avoid measurement errors due to oblique views of the aorta. To find the maximum diameter of the aorta, the transducer should be swept laterally across the aorta until the widest point can be seen (Fig. 11.6B). The coronal imaging plane should also be used for measuring the lateral diameter of the aneurysm, as some aneurysms are larger in the lateral than in the AP dimension. The length of the aneurysm sac should also be measured in the longitudinal scan plane (Fig. 11.6). The presence and thickness of thrombus can sometimes be difficult to assess on a poor B-mode image. Color flow imaging can be useful for demonstrating the lumen, which may be small in the presence of a large thrombus load.

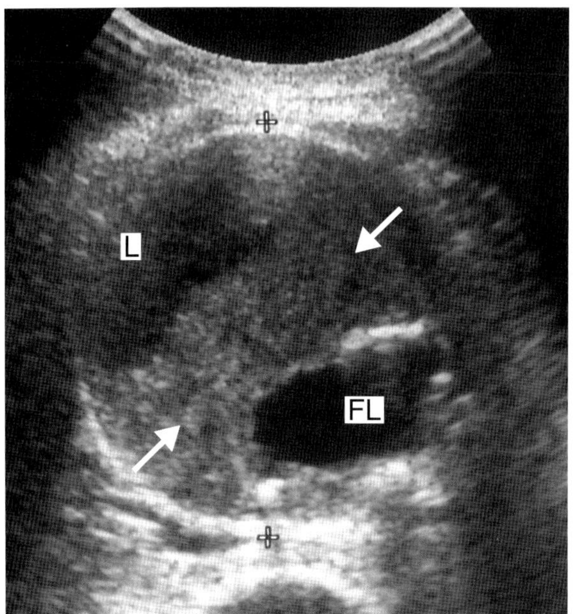

Figure 11.7 • A transverse image of an aortic aneurysm demonstrates a localized area of thrombus liquefaction (L), which may be confused with a dissection. Large areas of thrombus (arrows) separate the area of liquefaction from the flow lumen (FL).

Aortic aneurysm screening programs

Abdominal aortic aneurysm (AAA) screening can be performed using portable hand-held ultrasound scanners. These scans can be performed in the community or at centralized locations dependent on local requirements. The protocol below is used by our unit and is included as an example of a screening program.

AORTA DIAMETER	FOLLOW-UP AND COMMENTS
<2.9 cm	No further follow-up
≥3–4.4 cm	Yearly
≥4.5–5.4 cm	3-monthly
≥5.5 cm	Refer to vascular surgeon
AAA GROWTH RATES	**ACTION**
>5 mm in 6 months	Refer to vascular surgeon
>1 cm in 1 year	Refer to vascular surgeon
ILIAC ANEURYSM	**ACTION**
<3 cm diameter	Surveillance interval to be advised by physician
>3 cm diameter	Refer to vascular consultant

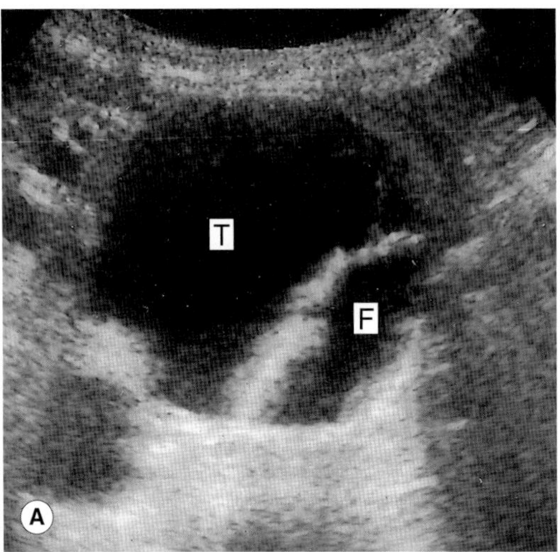

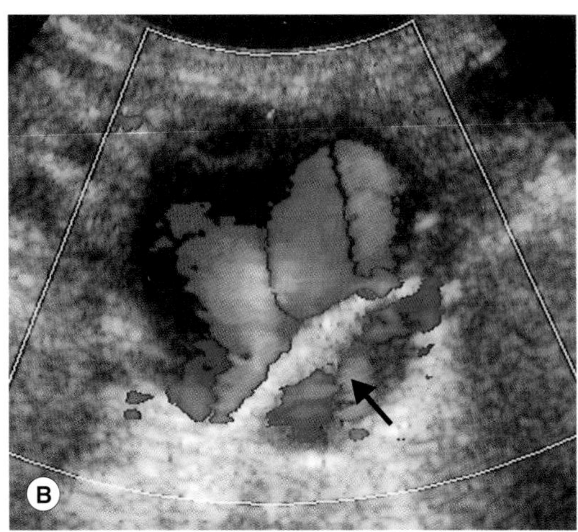

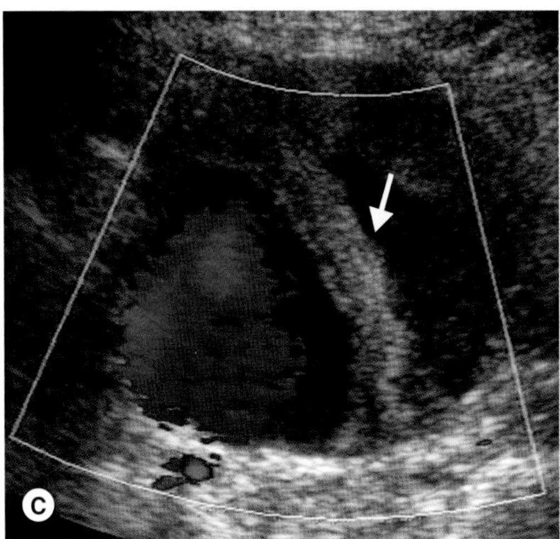

Figure 11.8 • (A) B-mode image of a dissecting aortic aneurysm. In this example the true (T) and false (F) lumens are seen. (B) Color flow imaging demonstrates flow in the false flow lumen (arrow). (C) The appearance of some aneurysms can be inconclusive, as this image gives the appearance of an occluded false lumen but in this case was due to mixed echogenicity of the thrombus (arrow).

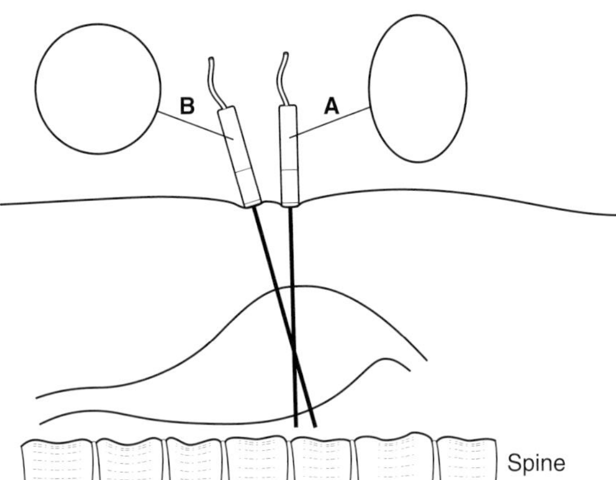

Figure 11.9 • The anteroposterior diameter of a tortuous aorta may be overestimated because of measurement in the wrong scan plane. In this example, the aorta is deflecting in an anterior direction. Scanning in a transverse plane along line A will result in an oblique image of the aorta, and the anteroposterior diameter will be overestimated. The transducer should be tilted to obtain the correct line of measurement along line B. An example of this problem is shown in Figure 11.6.

Limitations, errors, and comparative imaging

The main limitation of aortic scanning is poor visualization due to bowel gas or obesity. It can sometimes be difficult to define the posterior wall of an aneurysm, when the tissue between the lumbar spine and posterior wall appears to merge, making placement of the calliper difficult. Any limitations or doubts should be documented. A major pitfall is to set the image depth too deep when scanning thin patients and misinterpret the lumbar spine as the aorta (Fig. 11.10).

COMMENT

There are often discrepancies between the reported diameter of an aneurysm measured by computed tomography (CT) scanning and ultrasound, with CT scanning normally reporting a larger diameter as the aorta may lie in an oblique orientation, as shown in Figure 11.9. Remember that the aneurysm surveillance trials used ultrasound as the method of measuring aneurysms and therefore the management of small abdominal aortic aneurysms <5.5 cm in diameter is probably more reliable based on ultrasound diameters than CT.

SURVEILLANCE OF ENDOVASCULAR ANEURYSM REPAIR

Rationale

Duplex ultrasound has been shown to be an accurate method for the detection of endoleaks following endovascular repair (McLafferty et al. 2002). Ideally, ultrasound should be used in conjunction with CT scanning in the surveillance program (Sandford et al. 2006) (Fig. 11.11). An example of a surveillance protocol is shown in Table 11.1. Apart from cost-effectiveness and convenience, another major advantage of ultrasound is that the patient is exposed to fewer CT scans and associated contrast injections over the surveillance period, especially as a single abdominal CT scan is roughly equivalent to the radiation dose of over 300 chest X-rays.

Technique

This test should be performed on a top-range scanner. It is important to optimize the scanner

TIME	SCAN TYPE	COMMENT
Predischarge from hospital	Duplex	Bowel gas can be a problem
1 month	Duplex*	
3 months	CT	
6 months	Duplex*	
9 months	Duplex*	
1 year	CT	
Then 6-monthly	Duplex*	CT if significant problem detected

*If there is an increase in sac size ≥0.5 cm, alternative imaging such as computed tomography (CT) may be required.

Table 11.1 A suggested surveillance protocol for the surveillance of endovascular aortic aneurysm repair patients

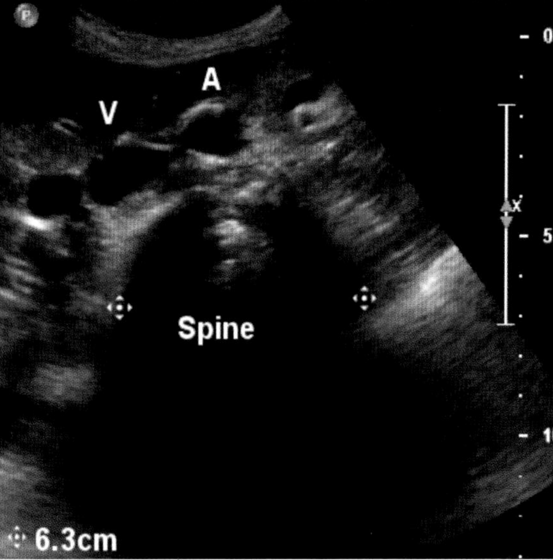

Figure 11.10 • In this image, the scanning depth has been set too deep in a thin patient, and the lumbar spine (S) has been mistaken for an aneurysm. The aorta (A) is of normal diameter. The vena cava (V) can be seen to the right of the aorta.

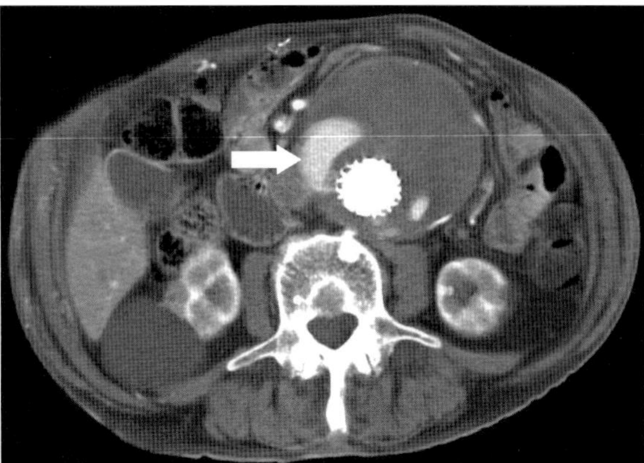

Figure 11.11 • A computed tomographic scan demonstrating a large endoleak (arrow) adjacent to the main body of the graft.

controls so that the system is sensitive to detecting low-velocity flow. This can be achieved by reducing the pulse repetition frequency or color scale to 1–1.5 kHz and increasing color sensitivity. The wall filter should be set to a minimum level and write zoom used to image the area of interest to maintain frame rate. This can produce a noisy color image, but without optimization it is possible, in our experience, to miss endoleaks. This is demonstrated on the DVD.

Scanning technique

1. It is easiest to start the scan by imaging the aorta in transverse section in the middle of the sac using B-mode imaging alone. At this level it is usual to see the two limbs of the graft, which usually lie adjacent to each other (Fig. 11.12C). In some circumstances they can be seen to spiral around each other as the probe is moved in a superior or inferior direction. If poor images are obtained the patient may need to be rolled on to the side into a lateral decubitus position.
2. The graft is then followed proximally through the sac in transverse section. The bifurcation of the graft should be clearly seen, and it is usually possible to see the upper extent of the graft and sometimes the aorta at the level of the renal arteries.
3. Next, the aneurysm and graft are followed distally to the aortic bifurcation, where the two graft limbs should be seen to run down the common iliac arteries. Anechoic areas in the aneurysm sac should be noted, as these could represent areas of blood flow, and should be scrutinized carefully with color flow imaging.
4. The aorta is then scanned in transverse section using color flow imaging. There should be color filling of the graft but no flow visible in the sac outside the device (Fig. 11.13). When using color flow imaging in the transverse plane, the transducer should be tilted with respect to the graft and aneurysm sac as this will improve color filling by creating a Doppler angle. The maximum diameter of the aneurysm sac should be recorded so that any changes in size can be assessed on serial scans. A progressively expanding sac could indicate an undetected endoleak or endotension. A variety of scan planes, including a coronal plane, may be required to obtain the maximum diameter. Some units also measure proximal neck diameter to monitor any increase in size due to progression of aneurysmal disease.
5. Color flow imaging in longitudinal section using sagittal and coronal planes is used to examine flow through the device and to identify any areas of flow disturbance or stenosis that could be caused by kinking of the graft, especially of the limbs as they run into the common iliac arteries or at the distal attachment sites (Fig. 11.12D). Spectral Doppler can then be used to assess the flow in the graft limbs and any abnormal areas or shown on the color flow image. The sac should also be examined for endoleaks in the longitudinal orientation as this may help to identify leaks or the source of leaks not seen in the transverse plane.

Types of endoleak

Endoleaks have been categorized into the following types (Veith et al. 2002) and are demonstrated in Figure 11.14. The ultrasound appearance of

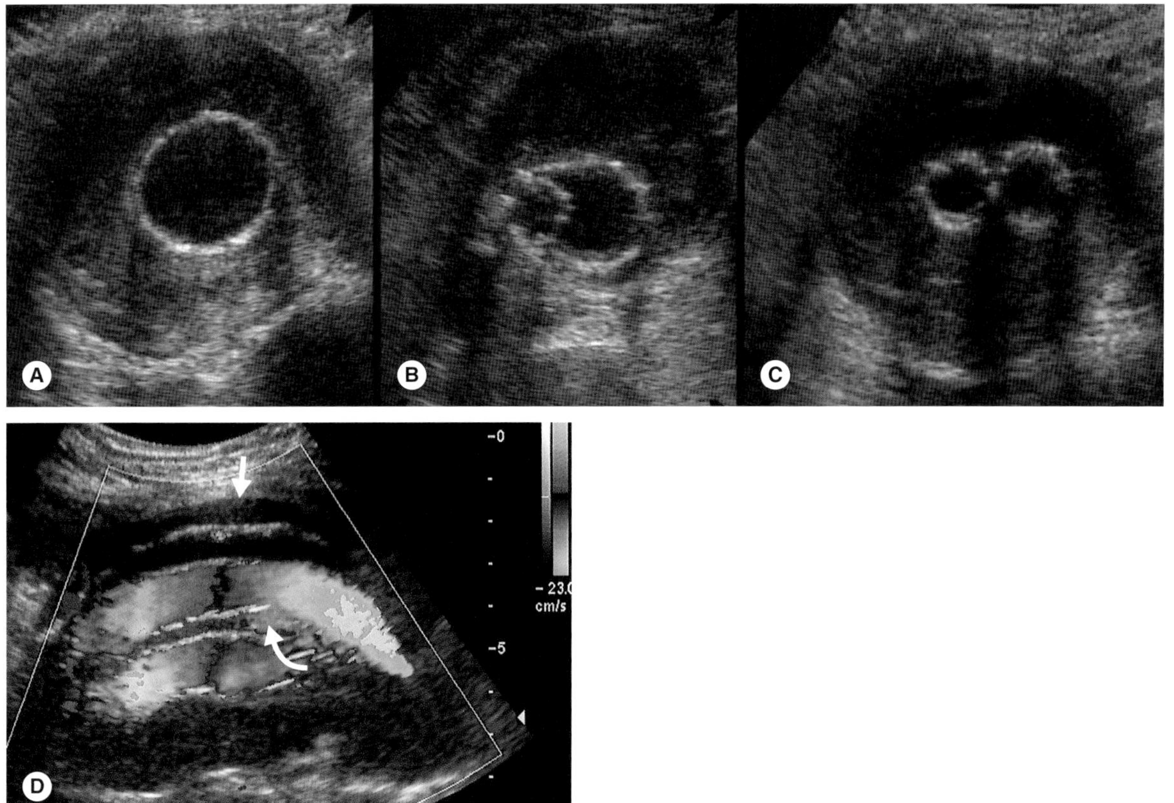

Figure 11.12 • Images of a successfully deployed aortic endovascular graft. (A) A transverse B-mode image of the main body. (B) A transverse image at the device bifurcation. (C) A transverse image showing both graft limbs. (D) Longitudinal image. In this example the limbs are lying on top of each other, but in many cases they lie side by side, as shown in example C, where use of a coronal scan plane would be needed to demonstrate both limbs in the same image. Note that mirroring artifact can sometimes be seen below the graft walls, as shown by the curved arrow. This aneurysm also had an inflammatory component, as demonstrated by the outer cuff (straight arrow).

some types is shown in Figure 11.15. Remember that it may be possible for a patient to have more than one type of endoleak.

Type Ia and Ib: Attachment site leaks. These occur at the proximal (Ia) or distal attachment sites (Ib) when there is an inadequate seal between the device and the aortic or iliac artery wall, respectively. Color flow imaging demonstrates evidence of flow, often in the form of a jet at the point of the leak, filling part of the aneurysm sac (Fig. 11.15A). The amount of flow in the sac can be variable and in some cases a large proportion of the sac may be perfused.

Type II. Collateral endoleaks involve some filling of the sac via lumbar vessels or the inferior mesenteric artery or accessory renal arteries (Fig. 11.15B and C). They may have an inflow only or can have an outflow via a second branch. Many type II endoleaks will seal spontaneously after a month or two (Veith et al. 2002).

Type III. Leaks between the modular limb and main body of the graft or tears in the graft (Fig. 11.15D). These types of leaks are rare.

Type IV. Thought to occur due to graft porosity or 'sweating' of graft material, leading to progressive increase in sac size within the first month. It is not possible to image this type of leak in real time, but serial surveillance scans may show a progressive increase in the diameter of the aneurysm sac. This type of leak

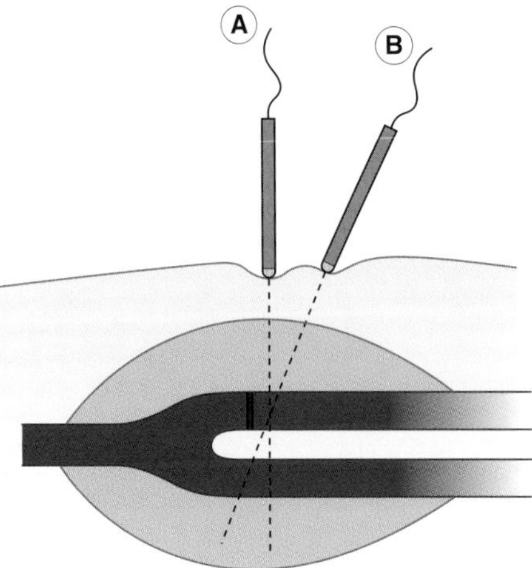

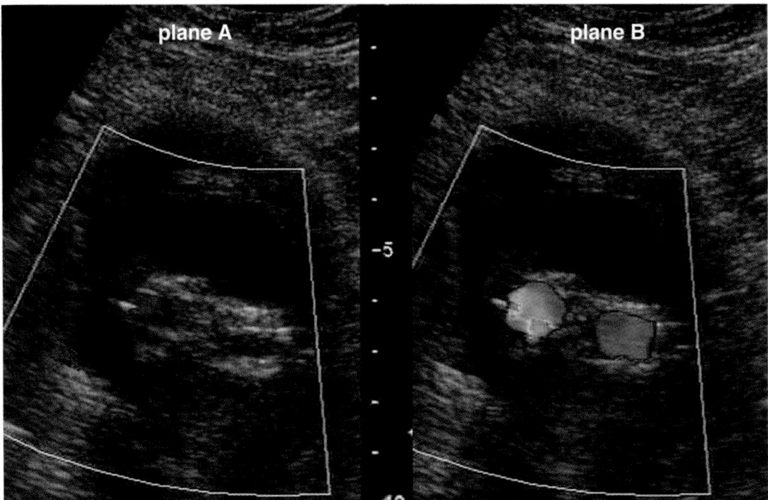

Figure 11.13 • To demonstrate flow in the graft or detect an endoleak with color flow imaging in the transverse plane, it is usually necessary to tilt the transducer from position (A) to (B), so that an angle of insonation of <90° is created relative to the device and sac. Optimum imaging (plane B) does not demonstrate any evidence of endoleak.

is though to be less common in the new generation of grafts.

Endotension has been classed as a fifth type of leak. This is described as a persistent or recurrent pressurization of the sac without a visualized endoleak. This can lead to expansion of the sac and potential rupture. The causes of endotension are uncertain, but it has been suggested that the sac is pressurized by mechanisms such as excessive pulsation of the graft, osmosis into the sac, or transmission of pressure through the thrombus. In practice, some cases of endotension could be due to a very small, undetected endoleak.

Current practice suggests that type I and III endoleaks should be investigated carefully with other imaging modalities. They may require intervention such as a stent cuff extension to occlude the leak as these types of endoleak are more closely associated with increasing sac size and potential

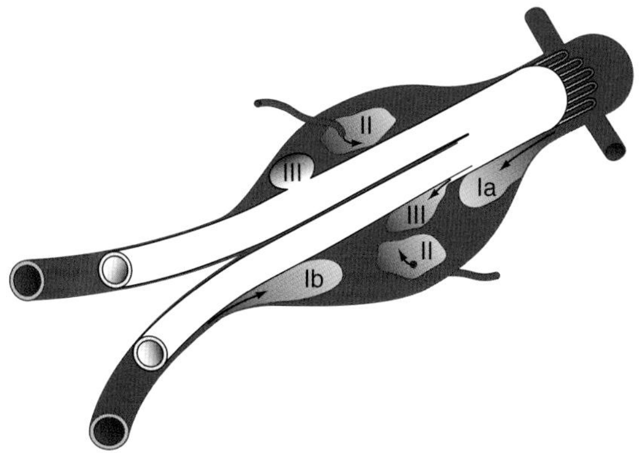

Figure 11.14 • A diagram of the different types of endoleak that can occur following endovascular repair of an aortic aneurysm (see text for description). Type Ia and Ib, failure of proximal or distal anastomotic seals respectively. Type II, perfusion of the sac via patent lumbar or inferior mesenteric arteries. Type III, failure of the modular limb seal or perforation and tears in the graft material. Type IV endoleak cannot be demonstrated in this example.

rupture. In contrast, most type II leaks are simply monitored unless there is a significant or persistent increase in sac size. Other device complications are shown in Table 11.2, but not all of these can be detected with ultrasound.

Doppler flow patterns and endoleaks

Although there is little reference in medical literature, it is possible to observe different spectral Doppler waveform patterns associated with endoleaks.

Firstly, to and fro or reverberant spectral waveforms, similar to the type seen in false aneurysm (Fig. 11.16A), are usually observed when there is a blind ending in the aneurysm sac, i.e., there is only one point of communication with no outflow. This pattern is often recorded in type II branch leaks but can occur in type I and III leaks. Close inspection of the color flow image may show forward and reverse flow across the entry point to the leak in the systolic and diastolic phases respectively.

Secondly, it is possible for a separate entry point and an exit point to exist, so that there is net flow across the sac. Color flow and spectral Doppler can be used to determine the flow direction; for example, if it is from inferior mesenteric artery to lumbar artery or vice versa (Fig. 11.16B).

In addition, with type II endoleaks the timing of the systolic phase observed on the color flow image may be slightly out of phase with the systolic pulse in the graft, lagging slightly behind the graft pulse as the blood flow may have had further to travel.

Long-term surveillance

In the absence of any significant complications, many aneurysm sacs slowly shrink in size and may disappear altogether. Some remain a similar size to the original AAA. It is less common to see an increase in sac size when there is no obvious cause. If a number of sonographers are involved in the surveillance program it is important that they all follow the same protocol for measuring the maximum diameter of the sac size, using sagittal and coronal planes, otherwise significant discrepancies may be recorded between sequential scans.

Surveillance of aneurysms excluded by covered stents

Flow can be excluded in aneurysms involving other areas of the arterial circulation by inserting a covered stent across the region of the aneurysm. The proximal and distal ends of the stent are positioned above and below the aneurysm. These types of stents are most commonly used in the iliac arteries to exclude true aneurysms. They can also be used to exclude flow into false aneurysms following vessel perforation or rupture during angioplasty. They are occasionally used in the subclavian arteries.

The stent is usually visible on the ultrasound image. Flow should be assessed across the stent and then the aneurysm should be scanned, using low-flow settings, to detect any possible filling of the aneurysm sac.

OTHER TRUE ANEURYSMS

Iliac aneurysms

The normal diameter of the common iliac artery ranges between 1.1 and 1.4 cm (Johnston et al. 1991). Iliac aneurysms usually occur as an extension of, or in association with, aortic aneurysms.

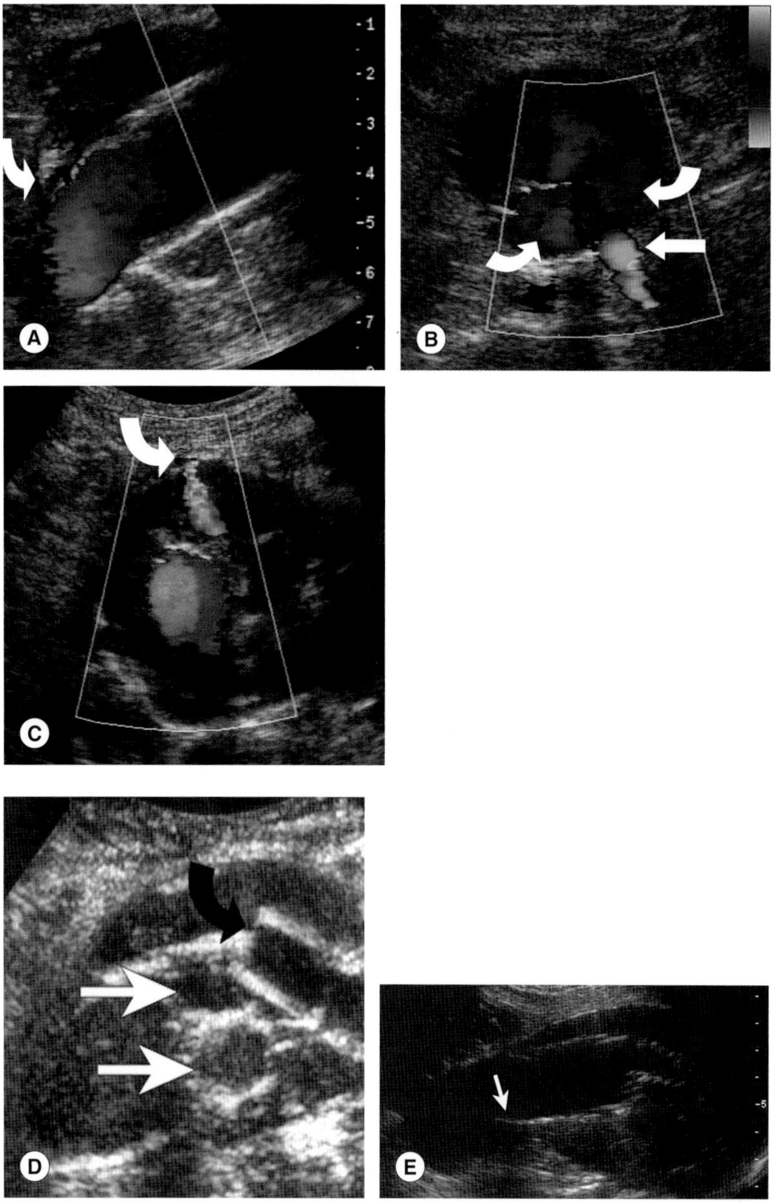

Figure 11.15 • Color flow and B-mode images of different types of endoleak. (A) Longitudinal image showing a type Ia endoleak (arrow) from the proximal end of the graft into the sac. (B) A transverse image of a type II endoleak demonstrating perfusion of the sac via a patent lumbar artery (straight arrow). The two graft limbs are demonstrated by the curved arrows. (C) A transverse image of a type II endoleak from the inferior mesenteric artery (arrow). (D) There is failure of the junction between the modular limb (curved arrow) and main body of the graft (arrows), indicating a type III endoleak. (E) An example of graft migration. The proximal end of the graft (arrow) is now in the sac and not making contact with the posterior aortic wall, which resulted in a type Ia endoleak.

COMPLICATION	COMMENT
Graft limb occlusion or stenosis	Easy to assess with ultrasound
Graft migration	Difficult to assess with ultrasound unless there has been a significant migration (Fig 11.15E).
Stent strut failure	Assessed with plane X-ray

Table 11.2 Other endovascular aortic aneurysm repair device complications

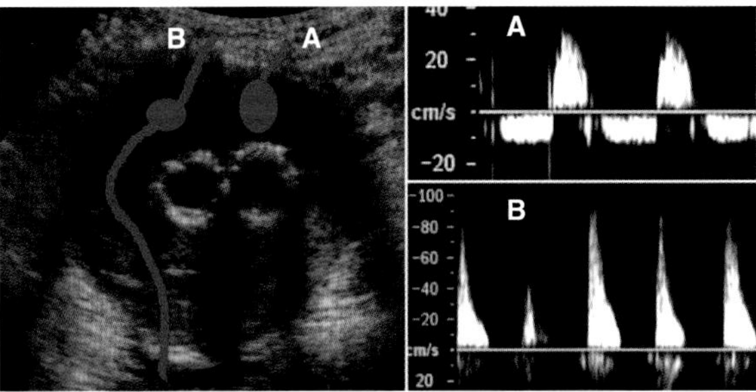

Figure 11.16 • It is possible to observe different spectral flow patterns associated with endoleaks. In example A, there is blind ending in the sac and a reverberant waveform similar to the type observed with false aneurysms is seen. In example B, there are separate entry and exit points and the Doppler waveform demonstrates net flow from a lumbar artery to the inferior mesenteric artery.

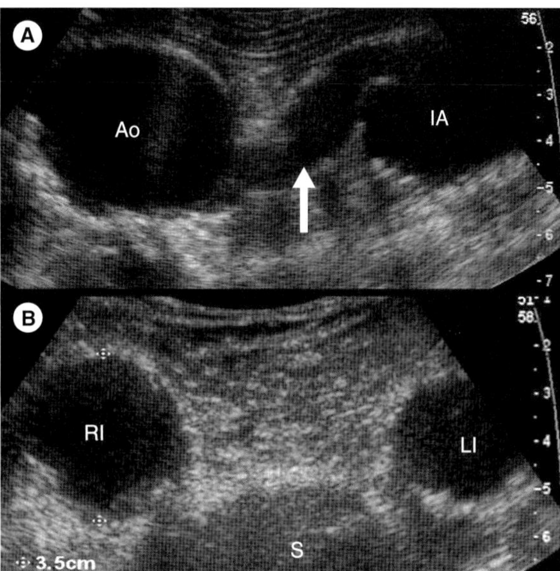

Figure 11.17 • (A) A longitudinal image of a distal aortic aneurysm (Ao) and large iliac artery aneurysms (IA). Note there is a relatively normal segment of common iliac artery (straight arrow) between the aneurysms. (B) Transverse image of right (RI) and left (LI) aneurysms. The spine (S) is visible.

Isolated iliac aneurysms are relatively rare, but rupture can be fatal, and elective repair may be considered for aneurysms measuring 3.5 cm or larger (Santilli et al. 2000) (Fig. 11.17). The technique for scanning the iliac arteries is described in Chapter 9. The measurement of iliac aneurysms is more accurate in a longitudinal plane, as it is difficult to avoid oblique planes if imaging in transverse section. Iliac aneurysms are clinically difficult to diagnose, and ultrasound, CT, and MRI are the methods used for diagnosis.

Popliteal aneurysms

Patients with an aortic aneurysm have a higher incidence of popliteal aneurysms compared to patients without such aneurysms. Popliteal aneurysms are bilateral in about half of patients and for this reason it is worth scanning the opposite artery when a popliteal aneurysm is detected. The normal diameter of the popliteal artery ranges between 0.4 and 0.9 cm, and a popliteal aneurysm is frequently classified as a vessel diameter of greater than 1.5 cm (Fig. 11.18). The complications associated with popliteal aneurysms include embolization, acute occlusion, or, occasionally, rupture. The symptoms of popliteal aneurysms can include pain or a feeling of fullness in the popliteal fossa. Sometimes patients present with a deep-vein thrombosis due to compression of the popliteal vein by the aneurysm. Ultrasound is the primary technique for the diagnosis of popliteal aneurysms.

Scanning of popliteal aneurysms

Using a mid-frequency linear array transducer, the popliteal artery is examined in transverse and longitudinal planes from the popliteal fossa and from the medial aspect of the lower thigh in the adductor canal, as some aneurysms can be located above

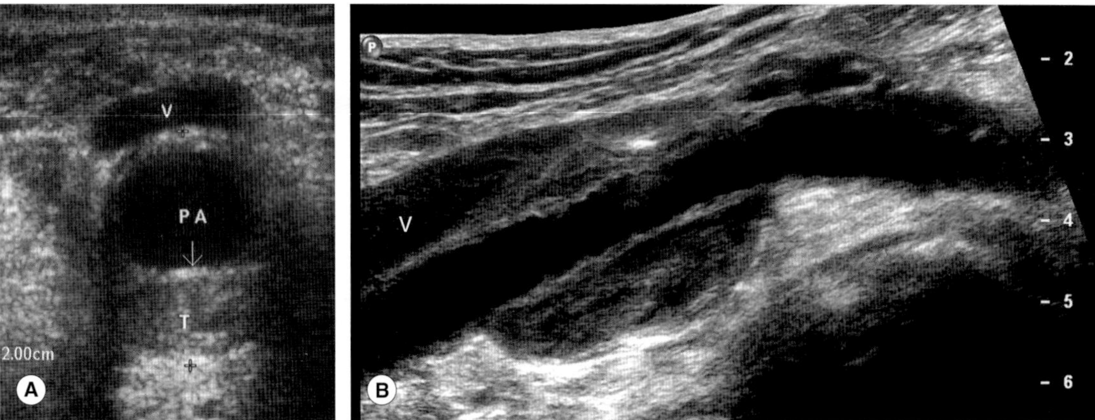

Figure 11.18 • (A) A transverse image of a popliteal artery aneurysm (PA) containing thrombus (T) below the arrow. The popliteal vein (V) is compressed in this example. (B) A longitudinal panoramic image of a popliteal aneurysm. The popliteal vein (V) is seen superficial to the artery.

the knee. B-mode imaging is used to assess the diameter and length of the aneurysms and amount of thrombus within the aneurysm. Color flow imaging is used to demonstrate the size of the flow lumen if the B-mode imaging is poor. Occluded popliteal aneurysms are demonstrated by an absence of color flow in the lumen. The popliteal vein should also be assessed for patency. Baker's cysts have a typical appearance of a neck trailing from the main body of the cyst to the joint capsule, and they have a hypoechoic appearance due to the synovial fluid inside (see Ch. 14). A major diagnostic pitfall is the misdiagnosis of a Baker's cyst as an occluded popliteal aneurysm.

Femoral artery aneurysms

True femoral artery aneurysms occur less frequently and are usually associated with aneurysmal disease elsewhere. Approximately 2–3% of patients with an aortic aneurysm have femoral artery aneurysms. Aneurysmal dilations can occur where graft anastomoses have been performed.

FALSE ANEURYSMS

False aneurysms, also known as pseudoaneurysms, primarily occur following arterial puncture for catheter access, due to poor control of arterial bleeding following the procedure. This is usually due to insufficient pressure being applied over the puncture site or pressure being applied for too short a time. They may also occur following trauma. Blood flows backward and forward through a hole in the arterial wall into the surrounding tissue, forming a flow cavity in the tissue adjacent to the artery. The false lumen often contains thrombus, which may be layered. False aneurysms can increase in size over time and may have multiple chambers. Color flow imaging should be used to confirm flow in the false lumen. The color flow image typically demonstrates a high-velocity jet originating from the defect in the artery wall, which is associated with a swirling pattern inside the false lumen, similar to the yin–yang sign. Spectral Doppler usually demonstrates strong forward and reverse flow components within the arterial jet as flow enters the false aneurysm during systole and exits during diastole (Fig. 11.19). The audible Doppler signal is very characteristic, with high-frequency Doppler shifts heard in the forward phase.

The common femoral artery is the main vessel in which false aneurysms occur, as it is the commonest site for catheter access. False femoral aneurysms may be very large, and bleeding into the retroperitoneal cavity can be a serious complication, leading to shock and death.

Scanning false femoral aneurysms

The patient should lie as flat as possible. The procedure should be started by scanning the common

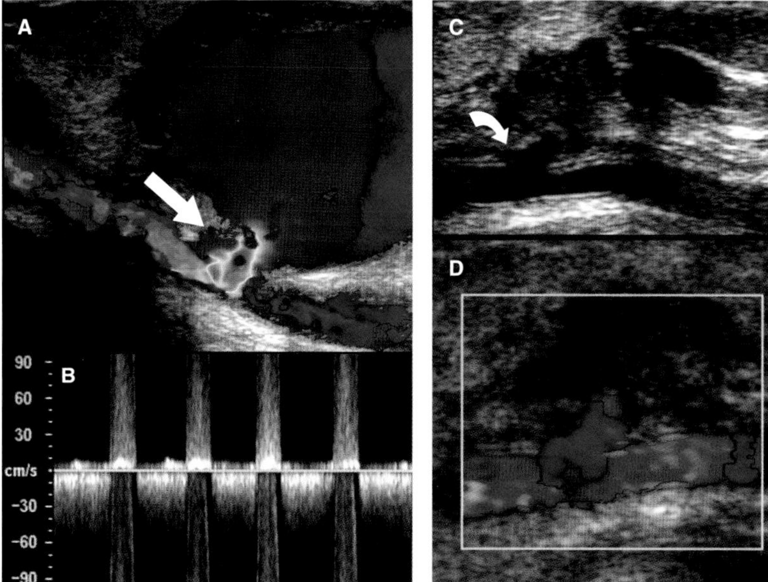

Figure 11.19 • (A) A longitudinal image of a false femoral artery aneurysm and corresponding spectral Doppler waveform (B) from the communicating jet (arrow). (C) A longitudinal image of the brachial artery shows a defect in the anterior wall (arrow) following catheter access. (D) A color flow image of C indicates a very small false aneurysm flow lumen; this would not be suitable for thrombin injection as it is small (<5 mm) with a wide neck.

femoral artery in transverse section. A mid-frequency linear array transducer will usually provide an adequate image. However, in some cases an abdominal curved array transducer may be required, especially if the patient is obese or if the puncture has been very high. In addition, areas of hematoma lying over the vessel, associated with the puncture site, can make the imaging difficult. The common femoral artery should be identified and scanned along its length in transverse section using color flow imaging. The proximal few centimeters of the superficial femoral artery and profunda femoris artery should also be examined, as low punctures can result in false aneurysms of these vessels. A potentially confusing situation can occur if the superficial epigastric artery, a superficial branch of the common femoral artery, runs close to an area of hematoma or swelling, as this might be mistaken for a small leak. Spectral Doppler recordings taken from the superficial epigastric artery will demonstrate a peripheral arterial-type waveform with overall flow in the forward direction as opposed to the high forward and reverse flow components seen in the necks of false aneurysms (Fig. 11.19). The report should include the overall dimensions of the false aneurysm, the diameter of the false flow lumen, and, if possible, an estimation of the size of the neck or communication to the artery.

Treatment of false femoral aneurysms

Traditionally, false aneurysms were repaired surgically. Ultrasound compression of pseudoaneurysms has also been demonstrated as a safe and effective technique for thrombosing false aneurysms. However, more recently ultrasound-guided thrombin injection into the false lumen has proved to be a highly effective method of treating false aneurysms and is considerably easier and less time-consuming, offering higher success rates than compression (Krueger et al. 2005; Webber et al. 2007). Blood in the false lumen clots within 1–2 seconds of the injection, and this can be observed on the ultrasound image. The injection should be away from the point of communication between the artery, to avoid any thrombin entering the systemic circulation.

References

Ashton H A, Buxton M J, Day N E et al. 2002 The Multicentre Aneurysm Screening Study (MASS) into the effect of abdominal aortic aneurysm screening on mortality in men: a randomised control trial. Lancet 360: 1531–1539

Birkmeyer J D, Upchurch G R Jr 2007 Evidence-based screening and management of abdominal aortic aneurysms. Annals of Internal Medicine 146: 749–750

Brown P M, Zelt D T, Sobolev B 2003 The risk of rupture in untreated aneurysms: the impact of size, gender, and expansion rates. Journal of Vascular Surgery 37: 280–284

EVAR Trial Participants 2005 Endovascular repair versus open repair in patients with abdominal aortic aneurysm (EVAR trial 1): randomised controlled trial. Lancet 365: 2179–2186

Fleming C, Whitlock E P, Beil T L et al. 2005 Screening for abdominal aortic aneurysm: a best-evidence systematic review for the US Preventive Services Task Force. Annals of Internal Medicine 142: 203–211

Johnston K W, Rutherford R B, Tilson M D et al. 1991 Suggested standards for reporting on arterial aneurysms. Subcommittee on Reporting Standards for Arterial Aneurysms, Ad Hoc Committee on Reporting Standards, Society for Vascular Surgery and North American Chapter, International Society for Cardiovascular Surgery. Journal of Vascular Surgery 13: 452–458

Kniemeyer H W, Kessler T, Reber P U et al. 2000 Treatment of ruptured abdominal aortic aneurysm, a permanent challenge or a waste of resources? Prediction of outcome using a multi-organ dysfunction score. European Journal of Vascular and Endovascular Surgery 19: 190–196

Krueger K, Zaehringer M, Strohe D et al. 2005 Postcatherization pseudoaneurysm: results of US-guided percutaneous thrombin injection in 240 patients. Radiology 236: 1104–1110

Lederle F A, Johnson G R, Wilson S E et al. 2002 Rupture rate of large abdominal aortic aneurysms in patients refusing or unfit for elective repair. Journal of the American Medical Association 287: 2968–2972

McLafferty R B, McCrary B S, Mattos M A et al. 2002 The use of color-flow duplex scan for the detection of endoleaks. Journal of Vascular Surgery 36: 100–104

National Institute for Health and Clinical Excellence 2006 IPG 163 Stent-graft placement in abdominal aortic aneurysm – guidance. Available online at: www.nice.org.uk

Office for National Statistics 2006 Mortality statistic: cause. ONS, London

Sandford R M, Bown M J, Fishwick G et al. 2006 Duplex ultrasound is reliable in the detection of endoleak following endovascular aneurysm repair. European Journal of Vascular and Endovascular Surgery 32: 537–541

Santilli S M, Wernsing S E, Lee E S 2000 Expansion rates and outcomes for iliac artery aneurysms. Journal of Vascular Surgery 31: 114–121

The UK Small Aneurysm Trial Participants 1998 Mortality results for randomised controlled trial of early elective surgery or ultrasonographic surveillance for small abdominal aortic aneurysms. Lancet 352: 1649–1655

The UK Small Aneurysm Trial Participants 2007 Final 12-year follow-up of surgery versus surveillance in the UK small aneurysm trial. British Journal of Surgery 94: 702–708

US Preventive Services Task Force 2005 Screening for abdominal aortic aneurysm: recommendation statement. Annals of Internal Medicine 142: 198–202

van Marrewijk C, Buth J, Harris P L et al. 2002 Significance of endoleaks after endovascular repair of abdominal aortic aneurysms: the EUROSTAR experience. Journal of Vascular Surgery 35: 461–473

Vardulaki K A, Walker N M, Day N E et al. 2000 Quantifying the risks of hypertension, age, sex and smoking in patients with abdominal aortic aneurysm. British Journal of Surgery 87: 195–200

Veith F J, Baum R A, Ohki T et al. 2002 Nature and significance of endoleaks and endotension: summary of opinions expressed at an international conference. Journal of Vascular Surgery 35: 1029–1035

Wassef M, Baxter B T, Chisholm R L et al. 2001 Pathogenesis of abdominal aortic aneurysms: a multidisciplinary research program supported by the National Heart, Lung, Blood Institute. Journal of Vascular Surgery 34: 730–738

Webber G W, Jang J, Gustavason S et al. 2007 Contemporary management of postcatheterization pseudoaneurysms. Circulation 115: 2666–2674

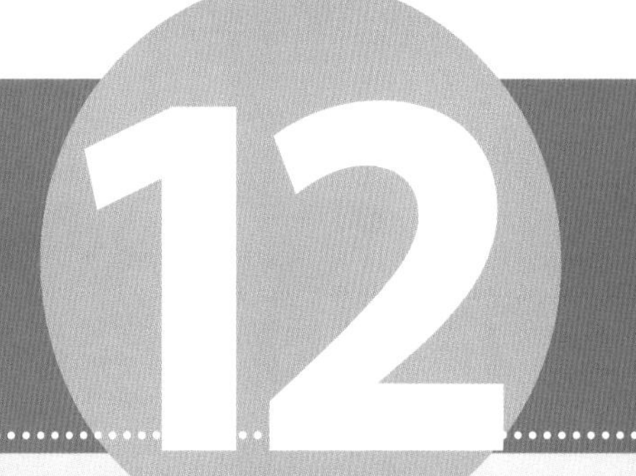

Vascular ultrasound of abdominal aortic branches

Colin Deane

CONTENTS

INTRODUCTION

Doppler investigation of abdominal vessels often forms part of an abdominal ultrasound study. Texts on abdominal ultrasound include details of Doppler investigations, although this is not their main emphasis. For those centers or units whose main interest is vascular ultrasound, there is an increasing requirement to investigate the major aortic branches, particularly the renal vessels, because:

- The staff have skills and equipment to conduct high-quality Doppler studies of renal and other visceral vessels
- Many patients have coexisting arterial disease of leg, carotid, and renal arteries
- Renal and mesenteric arteries are frequently involved in aortic aneurysms; noninvasive examination of the flow in these is useful pre- and postoperatively and can complement computed tomography (CT) investigation.

This chapter mainly covers investigation of renal arteries and the renal circulation which, from our experience, is by far the most commonly requested investigation of abdominal vasculature in a vascular laboratory. There is a brief overview of Doppler investigation of renal transplants and of the celiac axis and mesenteric arteries. Hepatic arteries, portal vein hemodynamics, and liver transplants are not included.

DOPPLER INVESTIGATION OF NATIVE KIDNEYS

Doppler ultrasound of the renal circulation is usually for:

- Investigation of renal artery stenosis (RAS)
- Assessment of chronic changes to the circulation

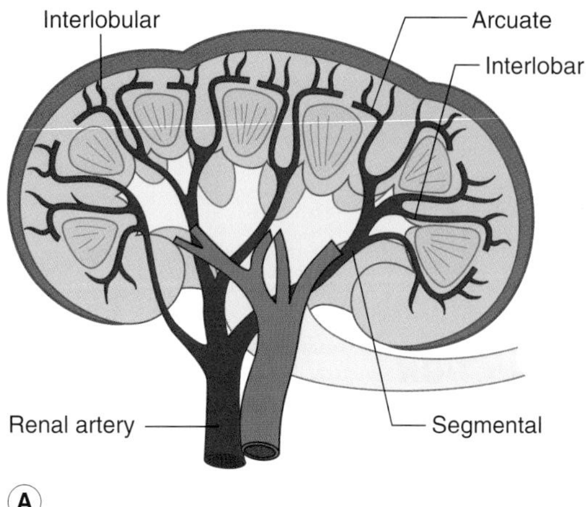

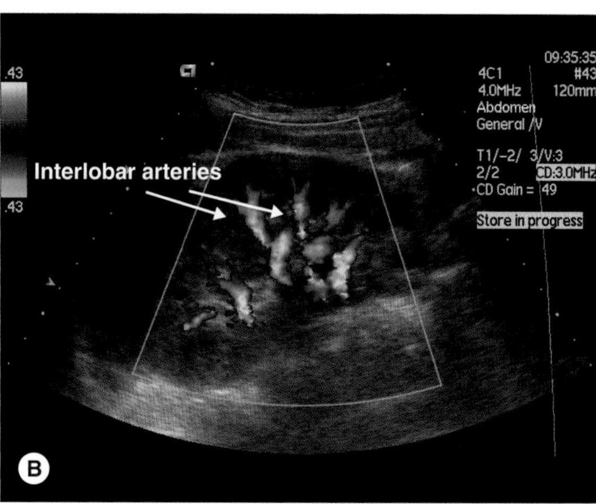

Figure 12.1 • (A) Diagram of renal vasculature indicating the main intrarenal arteries. Intrarenal veins are omitted for clarity. (B) A color flow ultrasound image shows several interlobar arteries.

- Investigation of viability – is there any flow in the kidney, for example following surgery or stenting of abdominal aortic aneurysm?
- Investigation of renal vein thrombosis.

RENAL VASCULAR ANATOMY, HEMODYNAMICS, AND DOPPLER APPEARANCE

The kidneys are supplied most commonly by a single renal artery from the aorta, which arises within 3 cm distal to the superior mesenteric artery. The renal artery divides, usually at the level of the renal hilum into five segmental arteries. These further branch into interlobar arteries which in turn lead to arcuate arteries at the cortex/medulla border (Fig. 12.1). In the cortex, these branch into interlobular arteries from which arise the afferent arterioles to the glomeruli where filtration occurs as part of the renal process. There are no major arterial collateral paths. Venous drainage is similar in pattern, draining to the renal vein which leaves the kidney through the hilum.

In approximately 20% of patients there are multiple renal arteries. The most common variant is a single polar artery proximal or distal to the main renal artery, but three or four arteries are not uncommon. This poses challenges for ultrasound investigation and is often used to question the role of ultrasound in the investigation of RAS.

The right renal artery passes under the inferior vena cava and posterior to the renal vein. The left renal vein passes between the aorta and superior mesenteric artery with the left renal artery posterior to it (Figs 12.2 and 12.3).

The rapid subdivision from renal artery to over 1 million afferent arterioles within a few centimeters means that there is a high density of medium-sized arteries and veins in the kidney, with a corresponding vivid appearance on color flow imaging. In good health kidneys receive approximately 20% of resting blood flow, approximately 1000–1200 ml/min. Flow is fairly constant, with a slight rise following a high-protein meal. The high flow and low resistance lead to flow waveforms with high diastolic flow. Resistance index (RI) at interlobar artery is in the range 0.55–0.7, rising slightly with age. Flow waveforms are slightly more pulsatile in the proximal renal artery and progressively dampen as blood flows to the smaller arteries within the kidney (Fig. 12.4). Blood velocities diminish rapidly as the arteries subdivide. For those with experience of imaging carotid arteries, the flow waveforms and velocities in the renal artery are similar to those in the internal carotid artery. This is a useful aide-mémoire when considering velocity increases to indicate RAS.

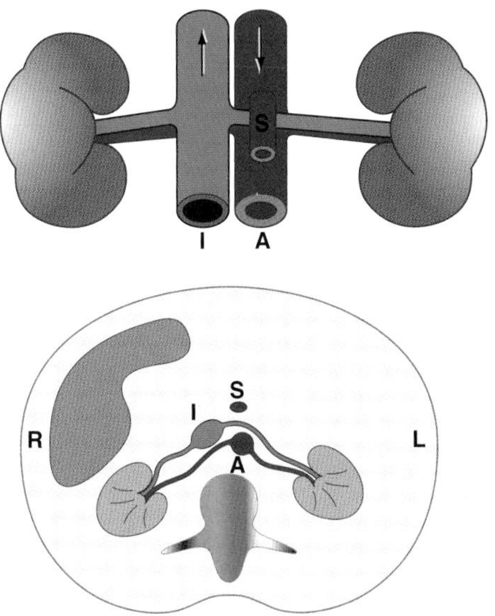

Figure 12.2 • The most common renovascular anatomy. The right renal artery passes deep to the inferior vena cava (I). The left renal vein passes between the superior mesenteric artery (S) and the aorta (A).

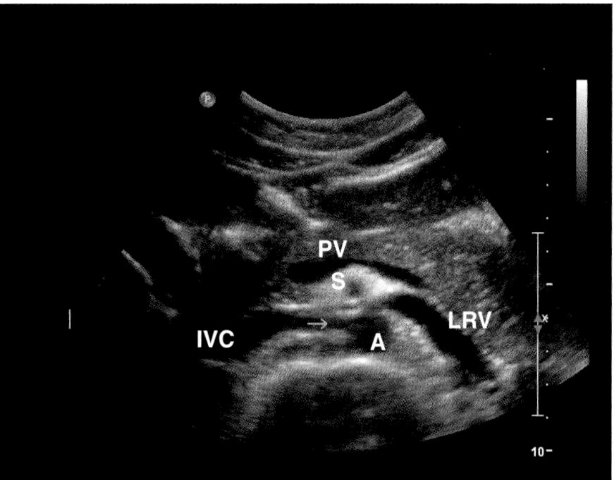

Figure 12.3 • Transverse image from an anterior approach of the right renal artery (arrowed) arising from the aorta (A). Also imaged are the inferior vena cava (IVC), superior mesenteric artery (S), left renal vein (LRV), and portal vein (PV).

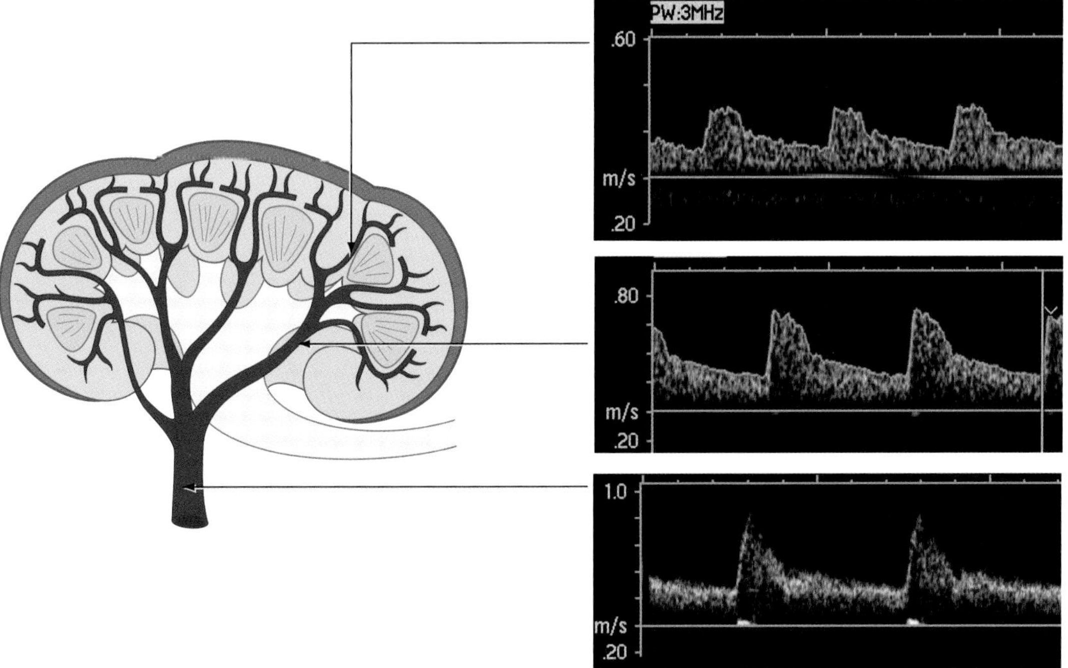

Figure 12.4 • Typical arterial flow waveforms in a healthy kidney. Velocities decrease as arteries subdivide into smaller branches. Flow waveforms become more damped towards the cortex.

SCANNING THE RENAL VASCULATURE

It is imperative to use low-frequency transducers to image the renal arteries. High velocities in deep abdominal arteries produce problems of aliasing and pulse repetition frequency (PRF) limits. Using low color and spectral Doppler transmit frequencies results in low Doppler frequencies, leading to a better chance of unambiguous velocity measurement. Low frequencies also penetrate better and give improved color and spectral sensitivity at large depths. Low-frequency curvilinear arrays (typically 4–1 MHz operating at 2 MHz for Doppler modes) can be used but it may be an advantage to use low-frequency phased array transducers which have good color flow and Doppler sensitivity and are useful when access is limited, for example when the ribs overlie the kidney. However, the phased array B-mode imaging is markedly inferior to its curvilinear counterpart. For imaging intrarenally, higher transducer frequencies give higher Doppler frequencies and improved visualization of the flow waveform for lower velocities in the smaller arteries.

If possible, the patient should be examined in a fasting state. The intrarenal vessels are best imaged by ultrasound from the flank (Figs 12.5 and 12.6). The patient lies in the left (for the right kidney) and right (for the left) decubitus position and the kidneys are imaged with the transducer placed below the ribs. In longitudinal view the large intrarenal arteries in the mid-pole flow towards the transducer, giving good color and spectral Doppler images (Fig. 12.6) adequate for flow waveform analysis. By angling the probe, changing focal position, and reducing transmit frequency, the renal artery can be followed to the origin from the aorta. If images are clear this view may include both renal

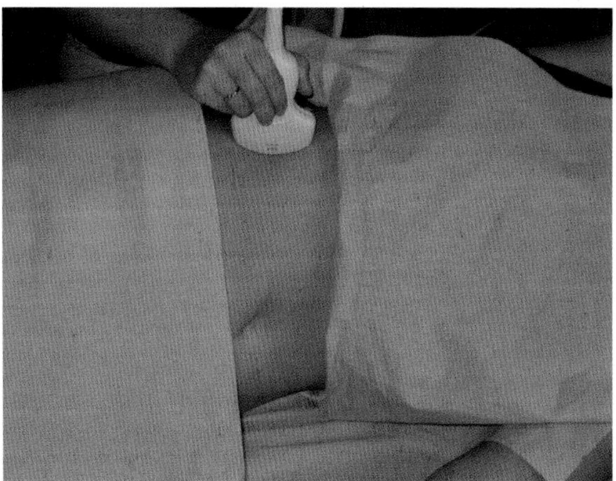

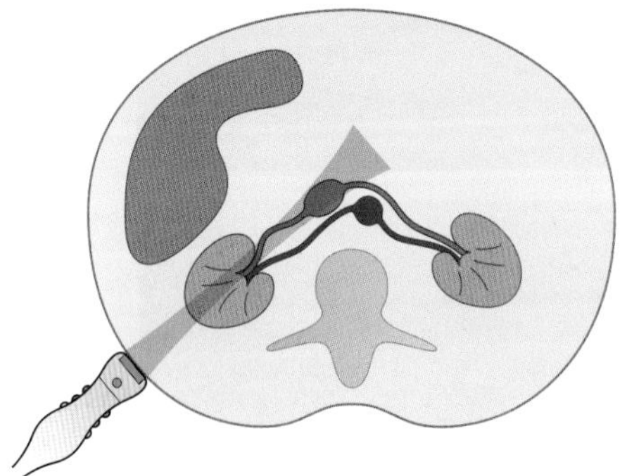

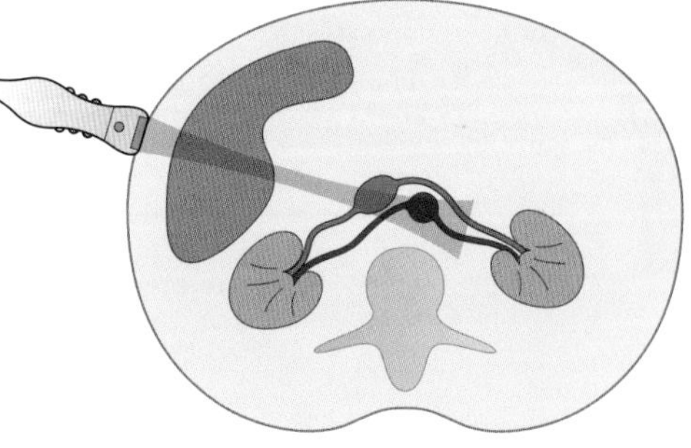

Figure 12.5 • Longitudinal imaging of the kidney from the flank. Different approaches may be necessary to image the kidney (lower left) and the proximal renal artery (lower right).

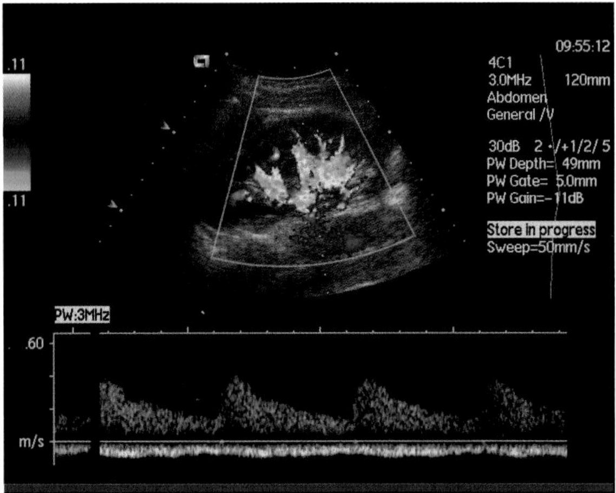

Figure 12.6 • Longitudinal image of the kidney from a flank coronal approach. The color image shows several intrarenal arteries and veins. The sonogram shows low-resistance arterial flow and venous flow with slight fluctuations from vessel at the interlobar level. Note the strength of the venous flow signal in the sonogram; at low-velocity scales, low velocities in intrarenal veins make a large contribution to the color or power Doppler image.

arteries, the classic "banana peel" image (Fig. 12.7), more commonly reproduced in textbooks than in everyday scanning. If there are clear views and if the beam/vessel angle correction is acceptable then it is worthwhile obtaining velocities from the opposite renal artery origin since this may be the clearer view than when scanning from the opposite flank.

The probe can be turned in the transverse plane, which often allows the entire length of the renal artery and vein to be viewed in one plane (Fig. 12.8). There is no standard optimum approach to use from the flank and sometimes the best image of the renal arteries can be obtained from a more anterior approach.

The proximal renal arteries are also usually imaged successfully from an anterior approach. Scanning transversely, the renal arteries are seen in B-mode. From a midline approach the renal arteries are almost perpendicular to the ultrasound beam – good for B-mode images but unsuitable for Doppler imaging (Fig. 12.9). By moving the transducer slightly to the left the beam can image 'down' the right renal artery with Doppler angles suitable for velocity measurement. Similarly, Doppler images of the left renal artery are best if the probe is translated slightly to the right of the midline. Angle correction is usually required for peak systolic velocity (PSV) measurement in this view (Fig. 12.10). Examination of the renal arteries should also include imaging of the aorta, both to exclude unsuspected aortic aneurysm and to measure aortic flow velocities for comparison.

Renal vein flows are seen in the same images as arteries. Intrarenal venous velocities are lower than arterial velocities but veins are larger and at low scales/PRFs can dominate the color image. Renal veins show pulsations dependent on proximal pressure changes from the right heart and from breathing (Fig. 12.11). If venous blood pressure is high, then pulsations in the renal vein may be very high with reverse flow (Fig. 12.12). If arterial flow is difficult to identify, venous fluctuations may mask the arterial signal. This can cause confusion for inexperienced operators.

ABNORMAL RESULTS

High-resistance flow

Reduced diastolic flow is measured as an increase in RI (Fig. 12.13). High RI, typically measured at interlobar artery level, is indicative of raised renovascular resistance (RVR) and decreased renal blood flow (RBF). Elevated intrarenal RIs have been associated with diabetic nephropathy (Platt et al. 1994) and a range of other chronic changes leading to glomerular sclerosis, tubulointerstitial changes, and arteriolosclerosis (Mostbeck et al. 1991; Ikee et al. 2005). The increased direct vascular resistance and reduced compliance that result lead to increased vascular impedance, and studies have shown that markedly elevated RIs are associated with impaired renal function and a poor prognosis (Radermacher et al. 2002). RIs of 1 are associated with severely impaired renal function (Fig. 12.13B).

Increased RI in kidneys has been shown to be indicative of systemic vascular disease and vascular risk factors in addition to intrarenal changes (Heine et al. 2007). This demonstrates that flow waveform indices are influenced by several vascular parameters and changes to indices are not specific to any one factor.

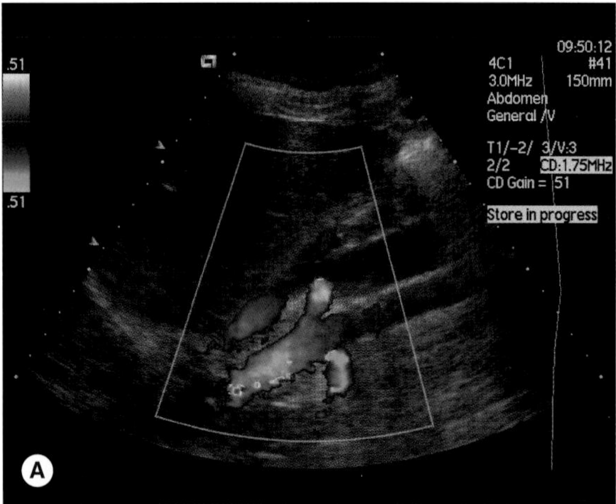

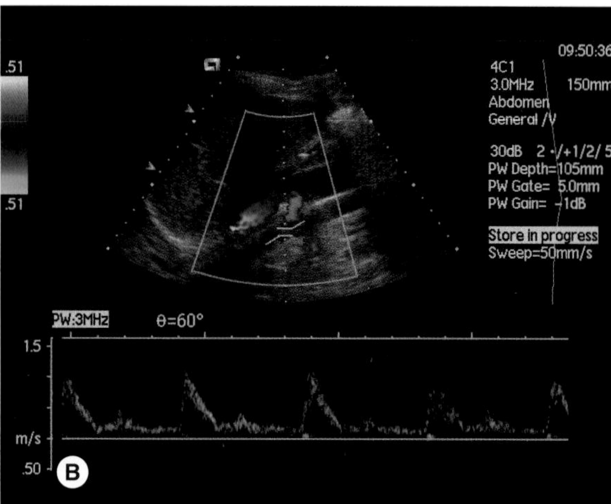

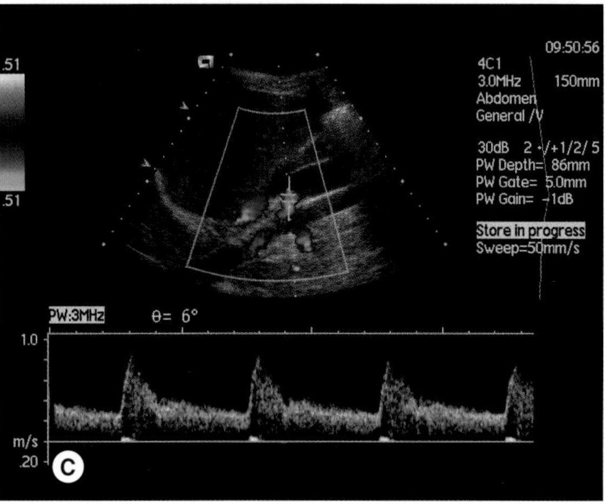

Figure 12.7 • (A) Right (red) and left (blue) proximal renal arteries arising from the aorta from a flank view. Flow waveforms from (B) the aorta and (C) proximal renal arteries. Note the low angle correction required for the renal artery sonogram. In practice, angle correction need not be made if beam/flow angles are low since velocities will be minimally affected between 0 and 20°.

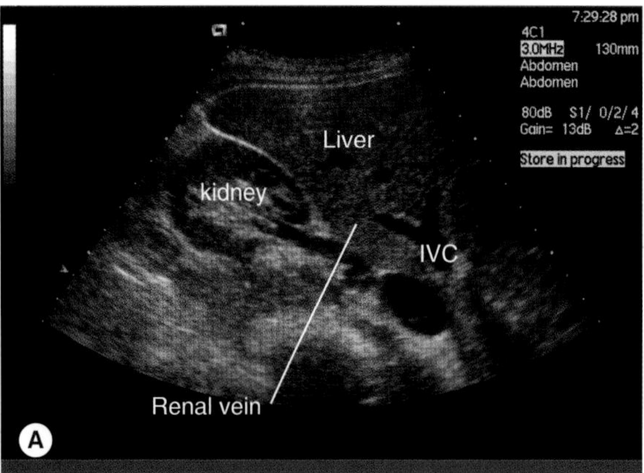

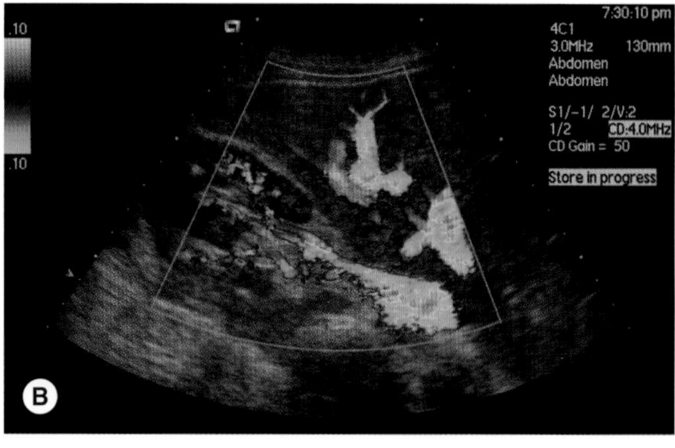

Figure 12.8 • (A, B) Transverse oblique image of the kidney and renal vein in B-mode and with color flow imaging. IVC, inferior vena cava.

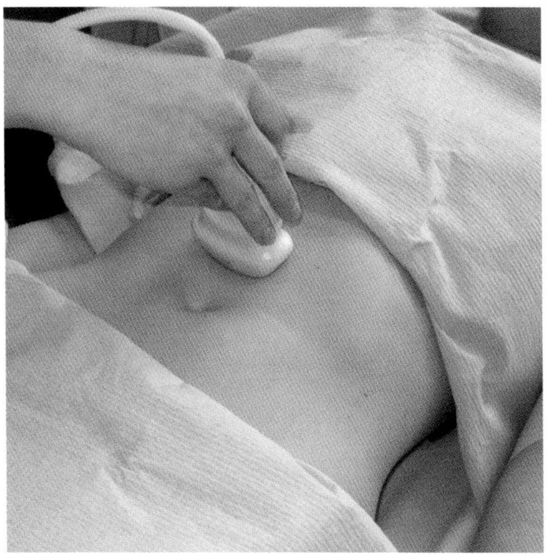

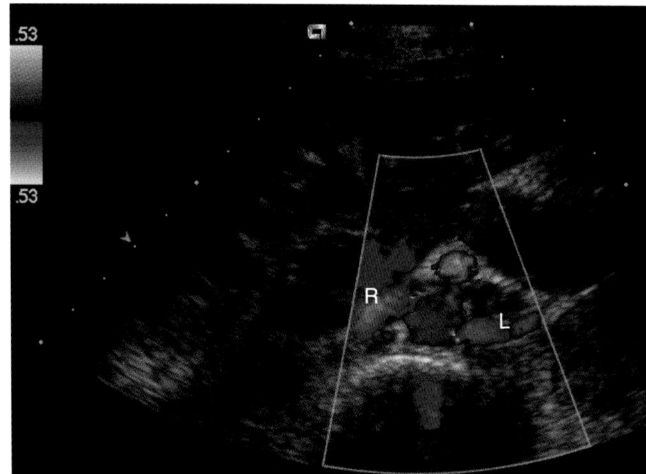

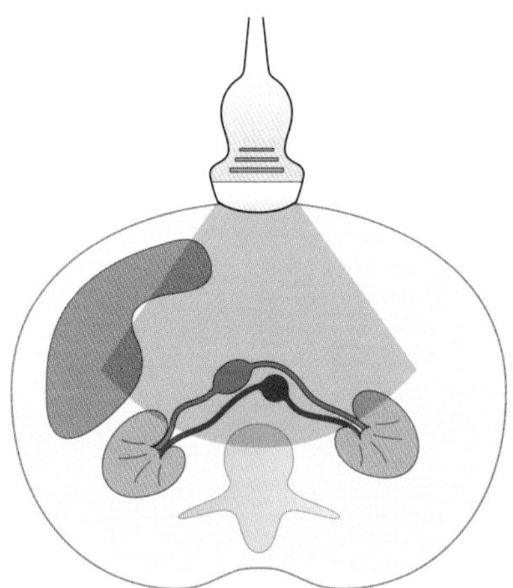

Figure 12.9 • Transverse image from the anterior midline approach. The right (R) and left (L) renal arteries are at a poor angle for spectral Doppler insonation with angle close to 90°, as evidenced by the change in color in the left neral artery.

Renal vein thrombosis

Renal vein thrombosis is evident as absent venous signals and pulsatile arterial flow with reverse flow in diastole matching inflow in systole with no net flow (Fig. 12.14). Thrombus may be evident in the renal vein or inferior vena cava.

Renal artery stenosis

RAS can, if severe enough, reduce flow and blood pressure to the kidney and cause impairment of renal function. RAS can lead to of renovascular hypertension, the cause of approximately 2–4% cases of hypertension in adults. However, hypertension is itself a risk factor for atherosclerotic disease of the renal arteries as it is for other arteries and the presence of a stenosis in a hypertensive patient does not necessarily mean that RAS is causative.

There are two distinct types of RAS referred for imaging:

1 Atheromatous RAS usually affects the renal artery ostium and proximal renal artery. It can lead to hypertension and eventually renal

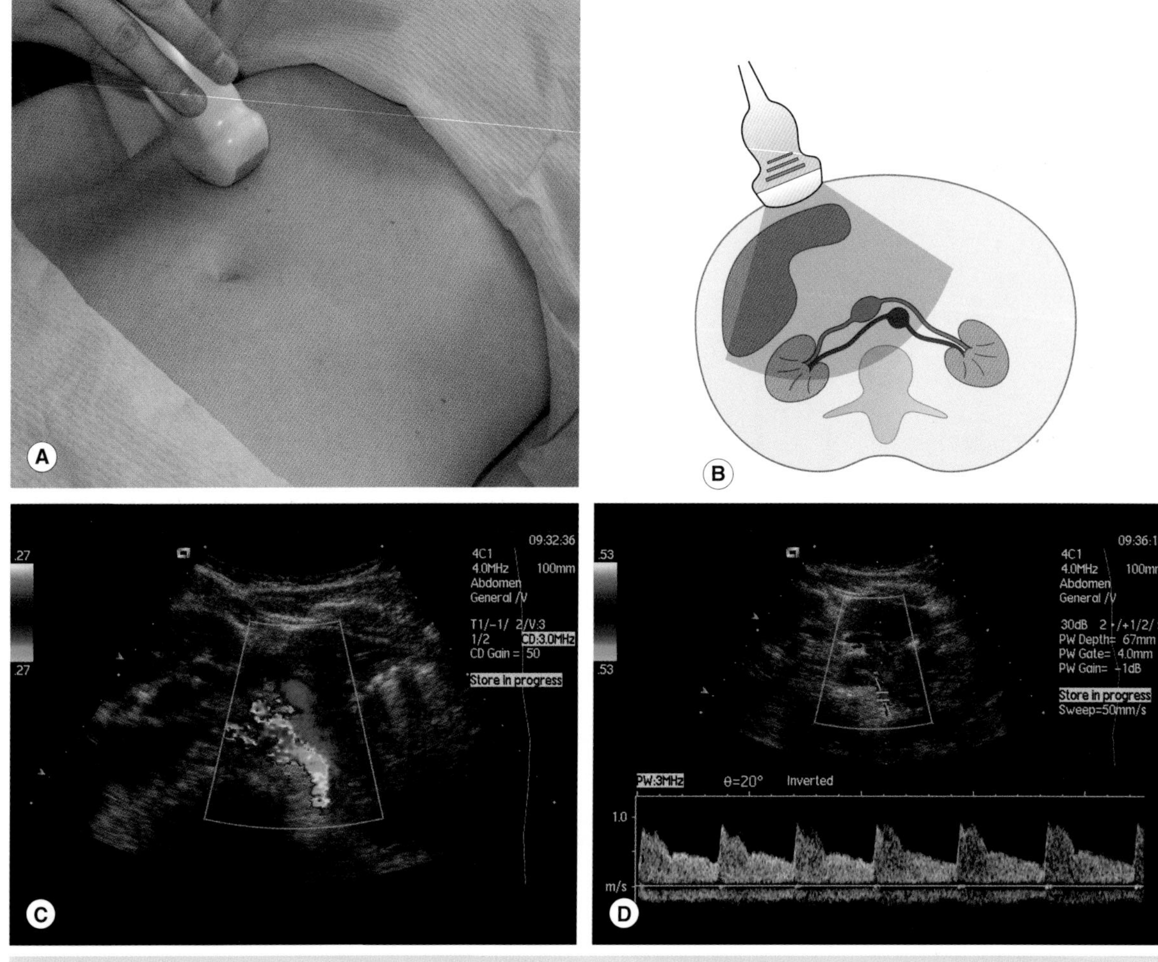

Figure 12.10 • (A–D) By moving slightly to the right of the anterior midline, color and spectral Doppler beam/flow angles in the left renal artery are lower with improved signals and an acceptable angle correction.

failure. Stenosis is more resistant to angioplasty; stenting is usually required.

2 Dysplasia usually affects the mid and distal renal artery and occurs in younger patients and more frequently in women. It causes hypertension with no or little loss of renal function. Dysplasia responds well to angioplasty.

The role of intervention in atheromatous RAS is complex and controversial. For hypertension, nephrologists in this hospital ask for angioplasty and stenting in only a small number of patients with resistant hypertension. They are more willing to use intervention to preserve renal function in chronic renal failure where RAS is the suspected cause in order to postpone the need for dialysis.

Indications for investigation for RAS are given in Box 12.1.

Criteria for renal artery stenosis

There are two main methods for investigating RAS: the direct method, examining velocity changes in the renal artery, and the indirect method, looking at flow waveform changes within the kidney downstream of a stenosis.

In the direct method the arteries are imaged as described above from the aorta to the hilum. The anterior (Fig. 12.15) and flank (Fig. 12.16) approaches should be used; the approach for optimum images is unpredictable. The color

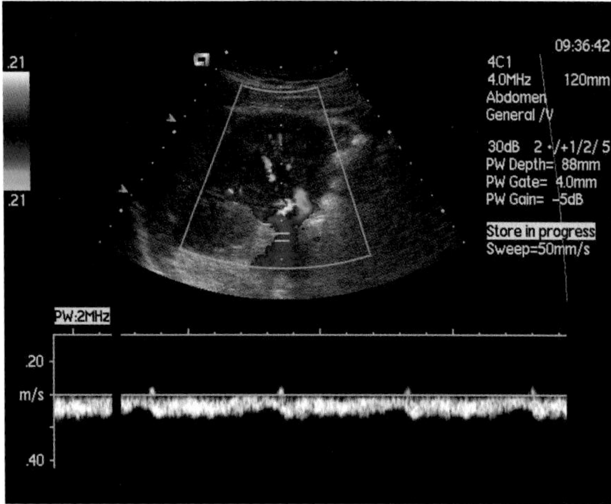

Figure 12.11 • Normal renal vein flow waveform. The slight variation in renal vein velocity is caused by subtle changes in venous pressure which demonstrate that there is no major obstruction to flow between the measurement site and the right heart.

BOX 12.1 Indications of referral for investigation of renal artery stenosis

- Asymmetry of kidney size (>1.5 cm length) without other explanation in elderly (>50) or young patient (<30)
- Significantly impaired renal function (elevated plasma creatinine or estimated low glomerular filtration rate) with significant arterial disease elsewhere
- Significant deterioration in renal function with angiotensin-converting enzyme (ACE) inhibitor or angiotensin receptor blocker
- Resistant hypertension, especially with evidence of arterial disease elsewhere
- Flash pulmonary edema – very rare, pulmonary edema usually other than cause of renal artery stenosis

image is useful in identifying areas of high velocity as changes in color, usually with aliasing. The stenosis may appear as a very small color area; good penetration and color and spectral Doppler sensitivity are essential. If a flank approach is used then little or no angle correction may be required if the renal artery keeps to within a few degrees of the ultrasound beam, since angle corrections between 0° and 20° make negligible differences to the measured velocity. However, renal arteries may be tortuous and angle correction is then required.

Stenosis is determined by the PSV in the stenosis. In studies comparing Doppler with angiographic measurement of RAS, PSVs of 1.8 and 2.0 m/s have been reported to be indicative of a 60% stenosis. This is similar to values for internal carotid artery stenosis and higher values reflect increased stenosis severity in a similar way to the internal carotid artery so that PSVs of 4 m/s can be regarded as approximately 90%. The renal artery to aorta PSV ratio (RAR) is helpful in normalizing the absolute velocity measurements in cases where cardiac output is low. A marked change in velocity locally has also been used as an indicator of stenosis. PSV in the stenosis is compared with that in the artery just distal to this (Souza de Oliveira et al. 2000). This aids in cases where renal artery flow is low, for example in cases where there is a chronic reduction in RBF. Two studies have compared PSV with direct measurement of the pressure gradient at the time of angiography, which can be considered the true gold standard to define a hemodynamically significant stenosis. Values of 219 cm/s (Kawarada et al. 2006) and 212 cm/s (Staub et al. 2007) have been reported as providing optimum accuracy. Kawarada et al. reported that duplex ultrasound had a better correlation with pressure gradient than angiography. Staub et al. recommended criteria of PSV ≥ 200 cm/s and RAR ≥ 2.5, levels which in their study corresponded to 50% stenosis measured angiographically and a mean pressure drop of 23 mmHg.

High velocities result in high Doppler frequencies. If the RAS is deep this can lead to problems of limited PRF. If the scanner has a high PRF (HPRF) override then a signal can usually be obtained, although the Doppler spectrum is usually less clear as a result of noise from the additional unfocused but shallow sample volume that results (Fig. 12.16). It is helpful to use as low a transmit frequency as possible. PRF limitations are less of a problem when stenoses are viewed from an anterior approach as the higher beam/flow angle results in lower Doppler frequencies and the renal artery origin is usually not quite as deep in the image.

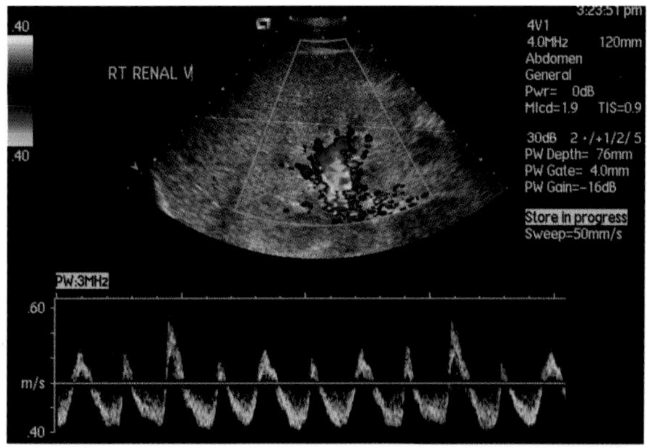

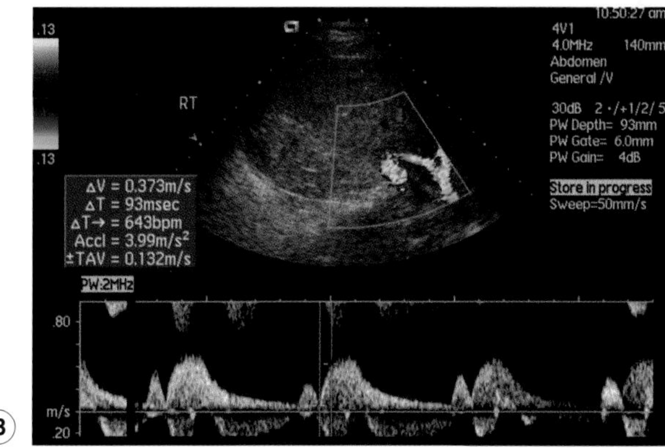

Figure 12.12 • Fluctuations to renal venous velocity. In patients with high venous pressures, changes in right atrial pressure lead to pulsatile flow waveforms. These may exhibit a combination of changes from breathing and right atrial pressure (A). If the sample volume insonates arterial and venous flow then the combined flow may be unclear (B).

However, this approach does suffer from errors of Doppler angle (Fig. 12.15).

The indirect approach uses changes in flow waveform shape from intrarenal arteries. Downstream of a severe stenosis, the waveform shows reduced pulsatility, and slower acceleration and longer acceleration times, sometimes described as tardus parvus (late and weak) (Stavros & Harshfield 1994) (Fig. 12.17). Since acceleration is itself dependent on the velocities in the artery, care should be taken to measure these parameters consistently at a particular level in the kidney. Most authors have used measurement of flow waveform at the interlobar artery level where accelerations of <300 cm/s^2 and acceleration times of > 70 ms are indicative of proximal stenosis. In comparison with direct measurements, indirect measurements are less sensitive but have similar specificity for stenoses >60% (House et al. 1999). This may be because distal flow waveforms are affected at higher level of stenosis and/or because the waveform is also dependent on distal changes in vascular impedance and compliance of the aorta: all of these factors confound simple analysis.

The use of flow waveform shape to predict successful response to angioplasty and stenting has been advocated. A cutoff of RI = 0.8 in the interlobar artery vessels has been shown to be the level above which kidneys showed poor response to angioplasty. Kidneys with an RI ≤0.8 showed

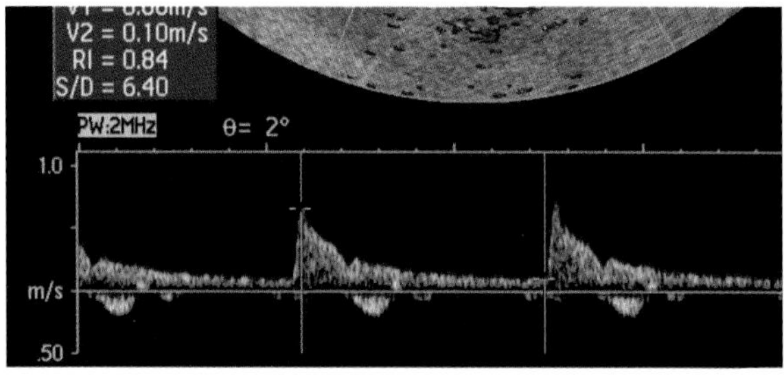

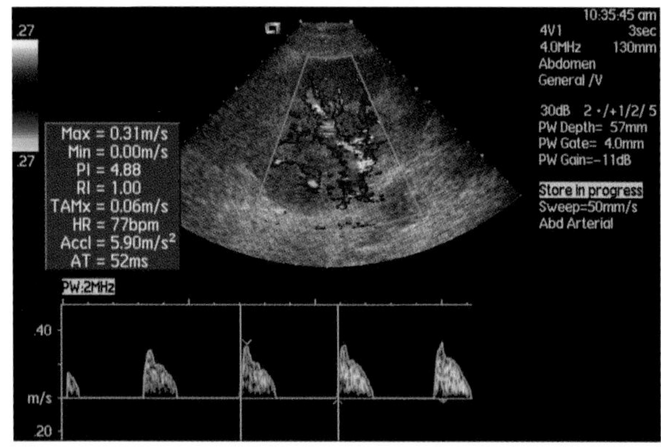

Figure 12.13 • Flow waveforms in raised renovascular resistance (RVR). As RVR increases there is a loss of diastolic flow, evident visually in the sonogram and as measured by resistance index (A). With severely raised RVR, diastolic flow is absent (B).

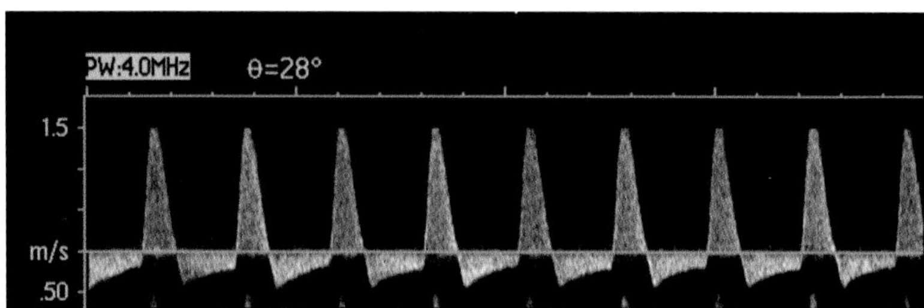

Figure 12.14 • In renal vein thrombosis there is no net flow to the kidney. Arterial waveforms shows flow reversal in diastole.

markedly better improvement in blood pressure and renal function (Radermacher et al. 2001), although other authors have been unable to use this level of RI to discriminate between good and poor outcome to the same degree (Garcia-Criado et al. 2005).

A summary of ultrasound indications for RAS is given in Box 12.2.

Problems when imaging renal artery stenosis

Textbook images of normal renal arteries are usually obtained from healthy, compliant, slim volunteers with good RBF and the ability to hold their breath for several seconds. Not all of these apply to all patients. Problems that occur are:

- Low RBF. Since blood velocities are used for the color flow image and spectral Doppler

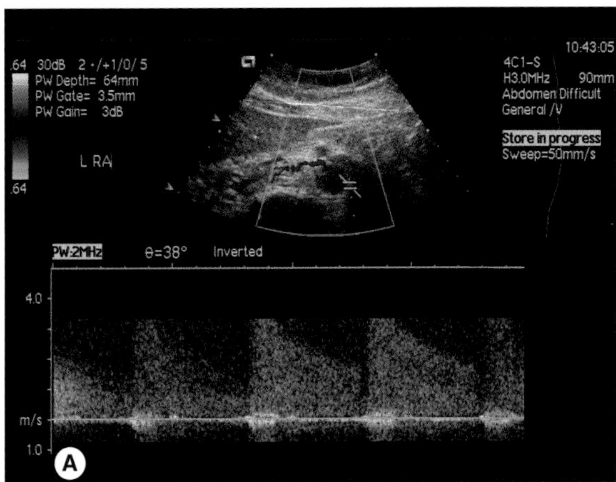

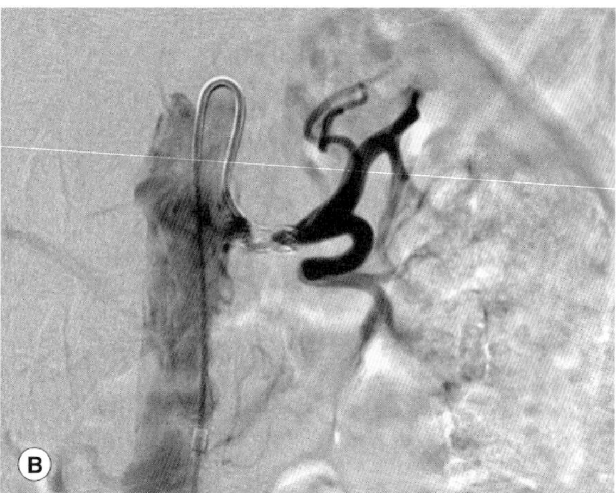

Figure 12.15 • (A) Transverse anterior approach shows high velocities exceeding 3.5 m/s in a renal artery 2 years poststenting. The velocity results in Doppler frequencies exceeding the pulse repetition frequency limits for the depth. The scale is restricted and there is aliasing. (B) Arteriography shows a tight in-stent stenosis.

BOX 12.2 Indications for renal artery stenosis

- Peak systolic velocity (PSV) in renal artery ≥ 180 cm/s
- Renal artery/aortic ratio PSV ≥ 3.5
- Interlobar artery acceleration < 300 cm/s^2
- Interlobar artery acceleration time > 70 ms
- Renal artery/segmental artery PSV ratio ≥ 5

measurements of a stenosis, low RBF prevents accurate measurement. In patients with severely decreased RBF there may be few vessels imaged with the kidney and poor velocities in the renal artery.

- Movement. Many patients present with impaired renal and cardiac function and are unable to hold their breath for very long. In these cases, color flow should be able to show the movement of the renal artery, allowing brief snatches of the spectral Doppler to be obtained for one or two cardiac cycles at a time (Fig. 12.16).
- Depth. Deep arteries may pose problems when imaging high velocities (see above). The lowest-frequency transducer possible is essential for these studies and HPRF facilities should be available.

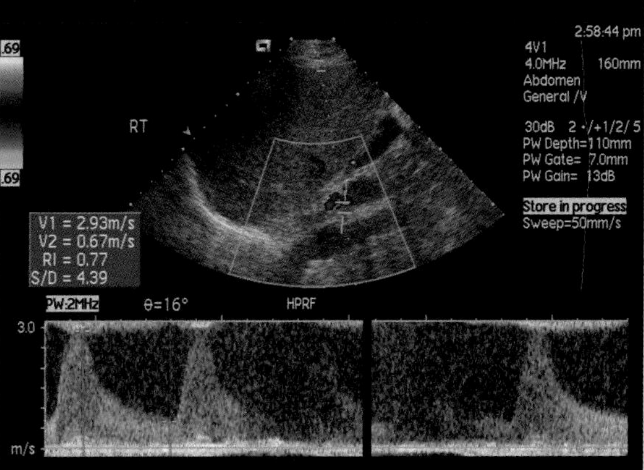

Figure 12.16 • Renal artery stenosis imaged from a flank approach. Flow is towards the transducer, resulting in high Doppler frequencies. The required high pulse repetition frequency leads to an additional superficial sample volume (arrowed). This increases noise in the sonogram. The renal artery moves in and out of the sample volume with breathing motion.

- Poor views. There are occasions when the entire course of the renal artery cannot be imaged. Use several transducer approaches and, if bowel gas obscures a view, move the patient and try again if the gas has moved. The left renal artery may appear to be in close proximity to the splenic artery in large patients and can be misleading. Ensure that the flow

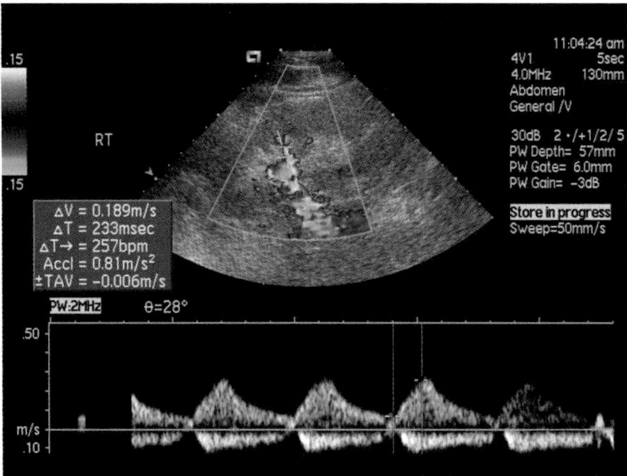

Figure 12.17 • The flow waveform in an interlobar artery downstream of a severe stenosis shows low acceleration and a long acceleration time.

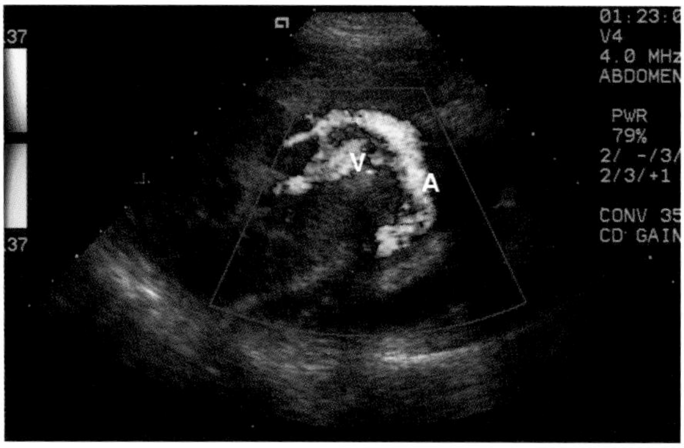

Figure 12.18 • Color flow image of a renal transplant. The renal artery rises superficially (red: A) before turning towards the hilum where it branches (blue). A section of renal vein is evident (V) with flow in the opposite direction. Renal transplant arteries and veins may be tortuous.

waveform in the renal artery matches those in the kidney and follow the renal artery from its insertion to the kidney back to the aorta to ensure continuity.

RENAL TRANSPLANTS

Renal transplants are an excellent target for Doppler ultrasound investigation. The kidney lies in the iliac fossa, is usually superficial, and does not move nearly as much as the native kidneys. In addition, the vascular anatomy, including the presence of multiple arteries, can be obtained from the operation note. Two main arterial surgical anastomoses are used:

1. End-to-side renal artery to external iliac artery anastomosis – usually used in cadaver donor kidneys where a patch of the aorta is used
2. End-to-end renal artery to internal iliac artery – usually used if the kidney is from a living donor.

Doppler ultrasound complements B-mode ultrasound in the investigation of poor function or changes in graft function. It is most useful when investigating vascular causes of poor function, graft artery stenosis, renal vein thrombosis, or arteriovenous fistula. It is helpful, but not specific, when examining flow changes as a result of rejection, drug toxicity, and acute tubular necrosis.

Scanning kidney transplants

Higher-frequency curvilinear arrays (6–2 MHz) are suitable to image the renal transplant and the main arteries and veins. In thin patients, low-frequency linear arrays (3–7 MHz) may be helpful if the iliac arteries are superficial. In a slim patient with a kidney donated from a cadaver, the long length of the extrarenal vessels may result in a tortuous artery and vein. The position and orientation of the kidney may appear unusual (Fig. 12.18).

The intrarenal flow arterial waveforms are measured in the upper, mid, and lower pole. In the early posttransplant period, rapid changes in the vascular resistance can occur. It is advantageous to use the pulsatility index (PI) as a measure of resistance. If there is zero flow at any point in the cardiac cycle, RI = 1. PI discriminates between a waveform with no diastolic flow and one where diastolic flow falls to zero. The range for normal-flow waveforms is wider than for a native kidney. While a normal-flow waveform usually has PIs in the range 0.8–1.5 (RI = 0.6–0.75), there are transplants with good long-term function with higher PIs. A change in flow waveform shape is a more important indication of changing RVR.

Arterial stenosis

The iliac artery should be investigated to ensure there is no proximal stenosis. The normal external

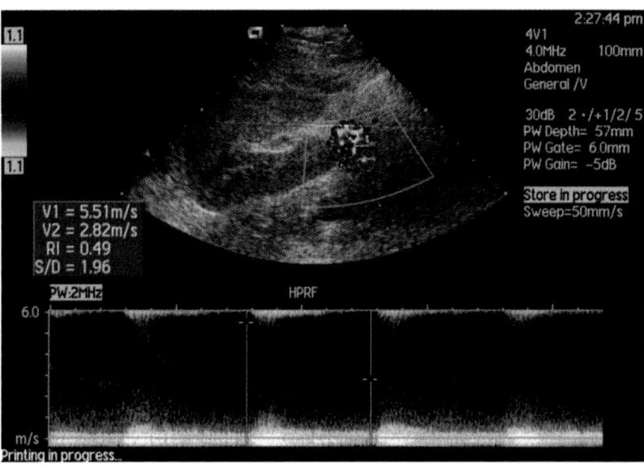

Figure 12.19 • Color noise at high scale settings and high uncorrected peak velocities indicate a renal artery stenosis.

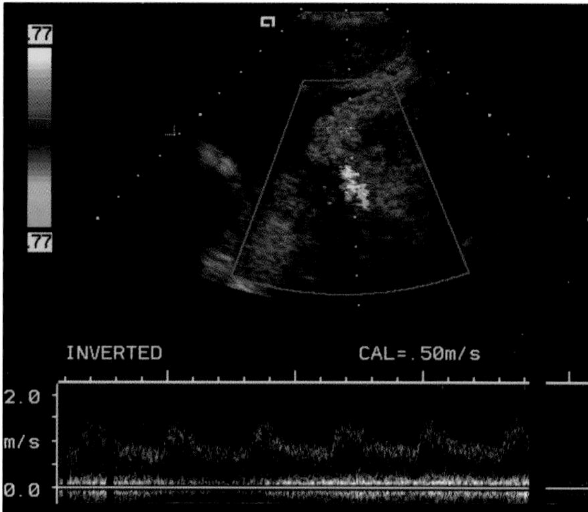

Figure 12.20 • Renal transplant arteriovenous fistula. High velocities and damped flow waveforms in an area with high-scale mixed color flow signals are indicative of a fistula.

iliac artery waveform has high acceleration and a triphasic pattern. Damped flow in the external iliac artery is indicative of proximal disease. This can be quantified by ankle–brachial pressure index measurements and direct imaging of the upstream stenosis.

The renal artery is imaged from anastomosis to hilar level. The range of flow velocities is larger than in native kidneys and local changes at points of tight curvature complicate the overall picture. PSV ratios of ≥2.5 or over are indicative of stenosis, as are PSVs of ≥2.5 m/s (Baxter et al. 1995) (Fig. 12.19). Intrarenal flow waveforms are less helpful than for native kidneys because of the various factors that affect intrarenal flow waveforms. However, severely damped flow waveforms are indicative of upstream stenosis.

Arteriovenous fistula

Arteriovenous fistulas are a common finding postbiopsy. The appearance is of high-velocity disturbed flow at the site of the fistula, with high-velocity low-resistance flow in the artery supplying the fistula and arterial-like pulsations in the vein draining it (Fig. 12.20). Fistulas present a risk if further biopsy is undertaken at the same site. Fistulas are occasionally associated with pseudoaneurysm and can exacerbate the effects of RAS.

Venous thrombosis

Renal vein thrombosis most frequently occurs in the early postoperative period. Doppler flow waveforms show sharp systolic peaks and reversed flow in diastole with no venous flow signals.

Flow changes in rejection

An increase in intrarenal flow waveform resistance between visits as measured by PI or RI is a cause for concern as it is an early sign of rejection (Fig. 12.21). Absolute values vary considerably in the immediate posttransplantation period. High-resistance flow waveforms are also seen in cases of acute tubular necrosis, especially if there has been a comparatively long ischemic period before transplantation. The complex posttransplantation course may also include ciclosporin drug nephrotoxicity, which has also been associated with an increase in PI/RI. Changes in flow waveforms have been shown to lack sensitivity or specificity for rejection but are still useful as an indication of changes in RVR, which merits further investigation. Early acute tubular necrosis is often associated with increases in edema. Changes in arterial flow waveform shape are sometimes accompanied by high intrarenal venous velocities caused by extrinsic compression on the low-pressure veins.

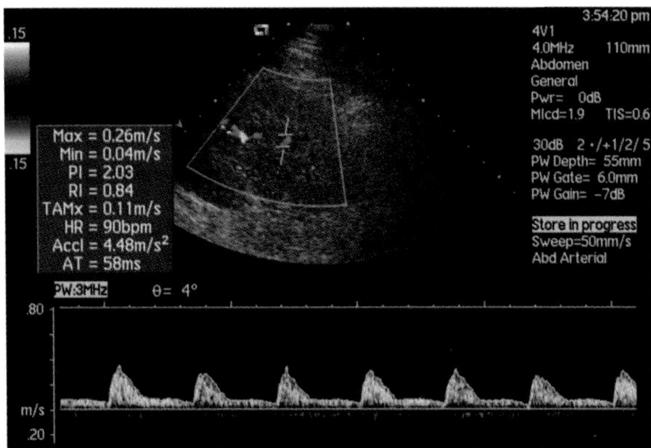

Figure 12.21 • Low diastolic flow reflected in high resistance index and pulsatility index. Rapid increases in resistance between visits may be indicative of rejection but can have other causes.

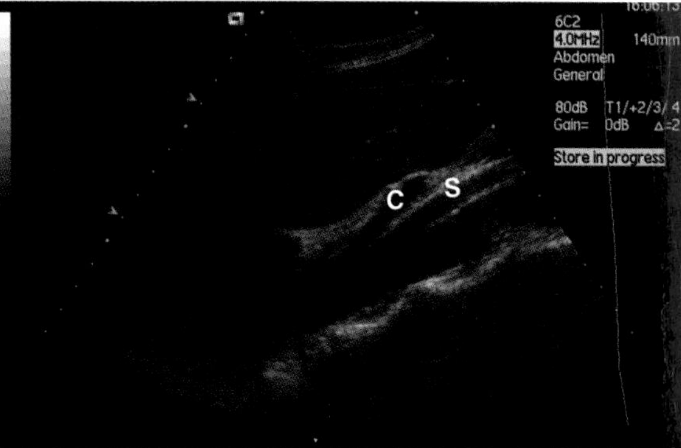

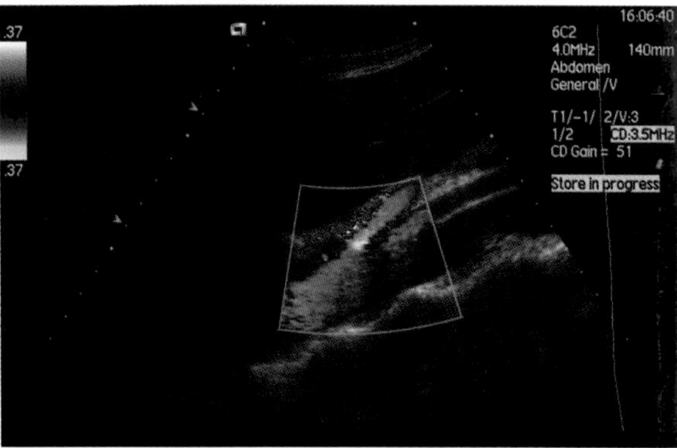

Figure 12.22 • B-mode and color image of the celiac axis (c) and superior mesenteric artery (s) origins seen in a midsagittal plane.

Chronic rejection is manifest by a steady reduction in arterial velocities throughout the kidney, which may be accompanied by a slight rise in PI. These changes are irreversible and are presaged by changes in renal function.

CELIAC AXIS AND MESENTERIC ARTERIES

The celiac axis and superior mesenteric arteries are readily imaged as they rise anterior from the aorta and are usually evident as a close pair of arteries in the longitudinal view (Fig. 12.22). The celiac axis bifurcates into the splenic and common hepatic artery a short distance – 1–3 cm – from its origin. The left gastric artery also branches from the proximal celiac axis but is much smaller. The origin of the inferior mesenteric artery is distal and usually arises slightly left of the anterior midline of the aorta.

Flow waveforms and velocities in the superior and inferior mesenteric artery change markedly after eating. Changes in the celiac axis, which branches into the splenic, hepatic, and left gastric arteries, are less marked. Measurements should be made with the patient fasted (Fig. 12.23).

Doppler examination of these arteries is most commonly requested in the investigation of atherosclerotic disease causing ischemia of the bowel. Elevated velocities in the proximal arteries are indicative of stenosis (Fig. 12.24), as listed in Box 12.3.

BOX 12.3 Indications of stenosis of splanchnic arteries

Celiac axis	peak systolic velocity >200 cm/s
Superior mesenteric artery	peak systolic velocity >270 cm/s
Superior mesenteric artery/aorta ratios	>3.5

In some patients the proximal celiac axis may be compressed by the median arcuate ligament during expiration (Fig. 12.25). In the example shown the highest peak velocity exceeds the criterion for a stenosis; however, by measuring it throughout the breathing cycle, the true cause of the narrowing is evident.

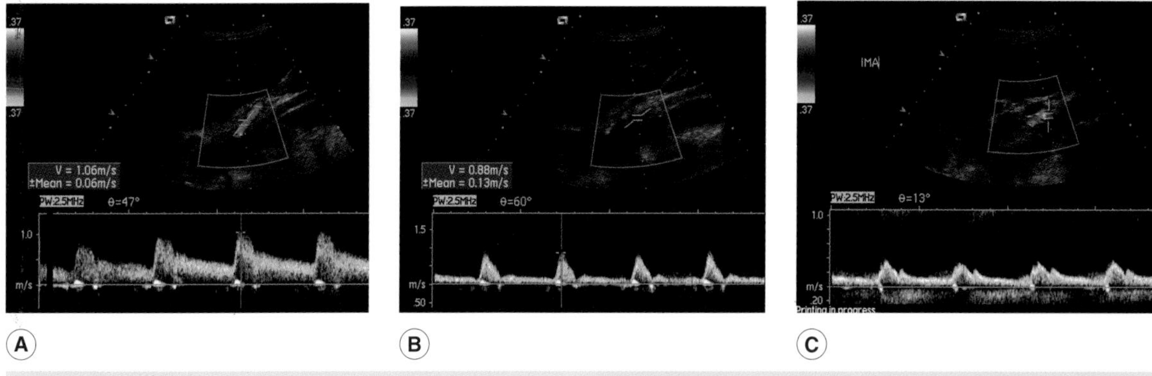

Figure 12.23 • Flow waveforms in the celiac axis (A), superior mesenteric artery (B), and inferior mesenteric artery (C) in a fasted state.

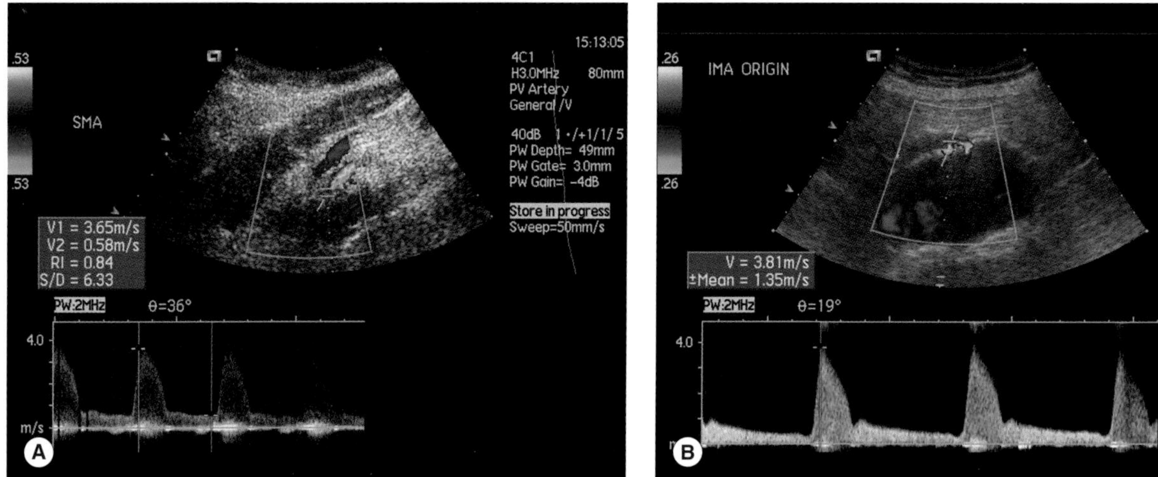

Figure 12.24 • Mesenteric artery stenoses in the superior mesenteric artery (A) and in an inferior mesenteric artery arising from an aortic aneurysm (B).

REPORTING

Reporting should describe major findings, including numerical values for renal artery velocities and mean intrarenal RI (or PI in renal transplants) and an interpretation of these results. Limitations of the test should be described and it is helpful to indicate the clarity with which renal arteries were imaged and measurements were made. For renal transplants with unusual arterial or venous anatomy, a quick sketch can save considerable time at the next visit.

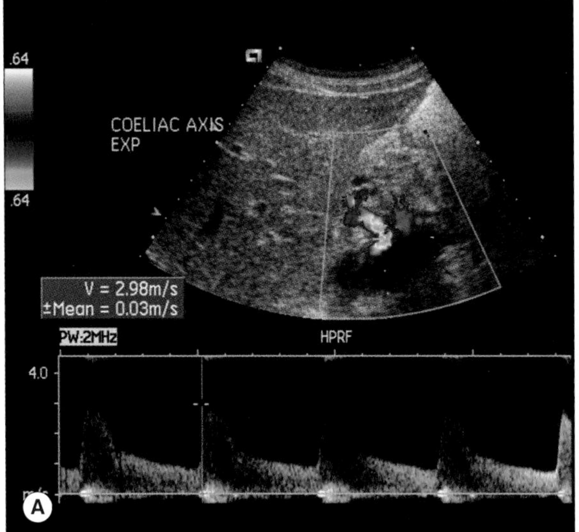

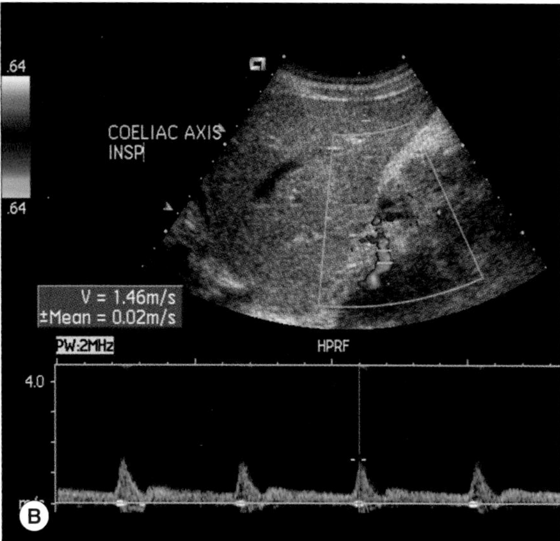

Figure 12.25 • Arcuate ligament compression of the celiac axis origin during expiration (A) causes high velocities which decrease markedly on inspiration (B).

References

Baxter G M, Ireland H, Moss J G et al. 1995 Colour Doppler ultrasound in renal transplant artery stenosis: which Doppler index? Clinical Radiology 50: 618–622

Garcia-Criado A, Gilabert R, Nicolau C et al. 2005 Value of Doppler sonography for predicting clinical outcome after renal artery revascularization in atherosclerotic vascular disease. Journal of Ultrasound Medicine 24: 1641–1647

Heine G H, Reichart B, Ulrich C et al. 2007 Do ultrasound resistance indices reflect systemic rather than renal vascular damage in chronic kidney disease? Nephrology Dialysis Transplantation 22: 163–170

House M K, Dowling R J, King P et al. 1999 Using Doppler sonography to reveal renal artery stenosis: an evaluation of optimal imaging parameters. American Journal of Roentgenology 173: 761–765

Ikee R, Kobayashi S, Hemmi N et al. 2005 Correlation between the resistive index by Doppler ultrasound and kidney function and histology. American Journal of Kidney Disease 46: 603–609

Kawarada O, Yokoi Y, Takemoto K et al. 2006 The performance of renal duplex ultrasonography for the detection of hemodynamically significant renal artery stenosis. Catheterization and Cardiovascular Interventions 63: 311–318

Mostbeck GH, Kain R, Mallek R et al. 1991 Duplex Doppler sonography in renal parenchymal disease. Histopathologic correlation. Journal of Ultrasound Medicine 4: 189–194

Platt J F, Rubin J M, Ellis J H 1994 Diabetic nephropathy: evaluation with renal duplex Doppler u/s. Radiology 190: 343–346

Radermacher J, Chacan A, Bleck J et al. 2001 Use of Doppler ultrasonography to predict the outcome of therapy for renal-artery stenosis. New England Journal of Medicine 344: 410–417

Radermacher J, Ellis S, Haller H 2002 Renal resistance index and progression of renal disease. Hypertension 39: 699–703

Souza de Oliveira I R, Widman A, Molnar L J et al. 2000 Colour Doppler ultrasound: a new index improves the diagnosis of renal artery stenosis. Ultrasound in Medicine and Biology 26: 41–47

Staub D, Canevascini R, Huegli R W et al. 2007 Best duplex-sonographic criteria for the assessment of renal artery stenosis – correlation with intra-arterial pressure gradient. Ultraschall in der Medizin 28: 45–51

Stavros A T, Harshfield D 1994 Renal Doppler, renal artery stenosis and renovascular hypertension: direct and indirect duplex sonographic abnormalities in patients with renal artery stenosis. Ultrasound Quarterly 12: 217–263

Anatomy of the lower-limb venous system and assessment of venous insufficiency

Tim Hartshorne and David Goss

CONTENTS

INTRODUCTION

Venous disorders are a common problem and consume a significant proportion of the resources available to health care systems. A review by Callam (1994) indicated that approximately 20–25% of women and 10–15% of men have visible varicose veins. In contrast, results from the Edinburgh Vein Study found that chronic venous insufficiency and mild varicose veins were more common in men (Evans et al. 1999). Significant venous disease can ultimately lead to venous ulceration, resulting in a marked loss of quality of life. Duplex scanning has had a dramatic impact on the noninvasive assessment of the venous system, and it is now the most commonly performed procedure for the detailed investigation of lower-limb venous insufficiency. Lower-limb venous duplex imaging can be used for the assessment of patients with primary or recurrent varicose veins or for the investigation of patients with skin changes and venous ulceration. Additionally, ultrasound is used to guide endovenous procedures, such as foam sclerosant injection, endovenous laser therapy (EVLT), or radiofrequency ablation (RFA), for the treatment of superficial venous disease. This has had a dramatic impact, as this treatment can be performed under local anesthetic as an office procedure. In comparison with arterial duplex scanning, venous duplex investigations can be technically challenging due to the wide range of anatomical variations in the venous system. This chapter covers the basic anatomy of the venous system and scanning techniques used for the assessment of lower-limb venous insufficiency and also includes a description of ultrasound-guided endovenous procedures.

ANATOMY AND PHYSIOLOGY

In this edition we are using anatomical terminology recommended by the Union Internationale de Phlébologie (UIP) published in a consensus document covering duplex assessment of chronic venous disease of the lower limbs and anatomy (Cavezzi et al. 2006). The description of the anatomy below is not exhaustive and the reader is advised to consult the consensus document.

The lower-limb venous system is divided into the deep and superficial veins. The deep veins lie below the muscular fascia. The superficial veins lie between the muscular fascia and the dermis (Caggiati et al. 2002) (Fig. 13.1). There are numerous interconnections between the deep and superficial veins via perforating veins.

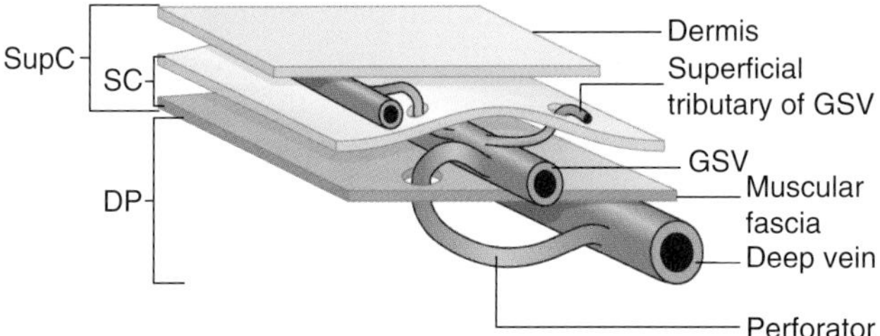

Figure 13.1 • A diagram of the deep and superficial vein compartments. The main trunk of the saphenous vein lies in the saphenous compartment (SC), located within the superficial compartment SupC see text. GSV, great saphenous vein; DP, deep compartment.

Deep venous system

The anatomy of the deep veins is shown in Figure 13.2. Generally, the deep veins are larger than their corresponding artery. The main deep veins of the thigh and calf are the following:

- Common femoral vein
- Deep femoral vein (also called the profunda femoris vein)
- Femoral vein (also called the superficial femoral vein)
- Popliteal vein
- Posterior tibial veins
- Peroneal veins
- Anterior tibial veins
- Gastrocnemius veins
- Soleal veins and sinuses.

Femoral vein nomenclature

The Union Internationale de Phlébologie recommends the use of the term femoral vein instead of superficial femoral vein to describe the vein running between the common femoral vein and popliteal vein. The term superficial is misleading and may be misinterpreted. This vein is part of the deep venous system.

The posterior tibial and peroneal veins are usually paired and are associated with their respective arteries. The paired veins join into common trunks in the upper calf before forming the below-knee popliteal vein. The soleal veins are deep venous sinuses and veins of the soleus muscle that drain into the popliteal vein. They are an important part of the calf muscle pump mechanism (see Ch. 5). The gastrocnemius veins drain the medial and

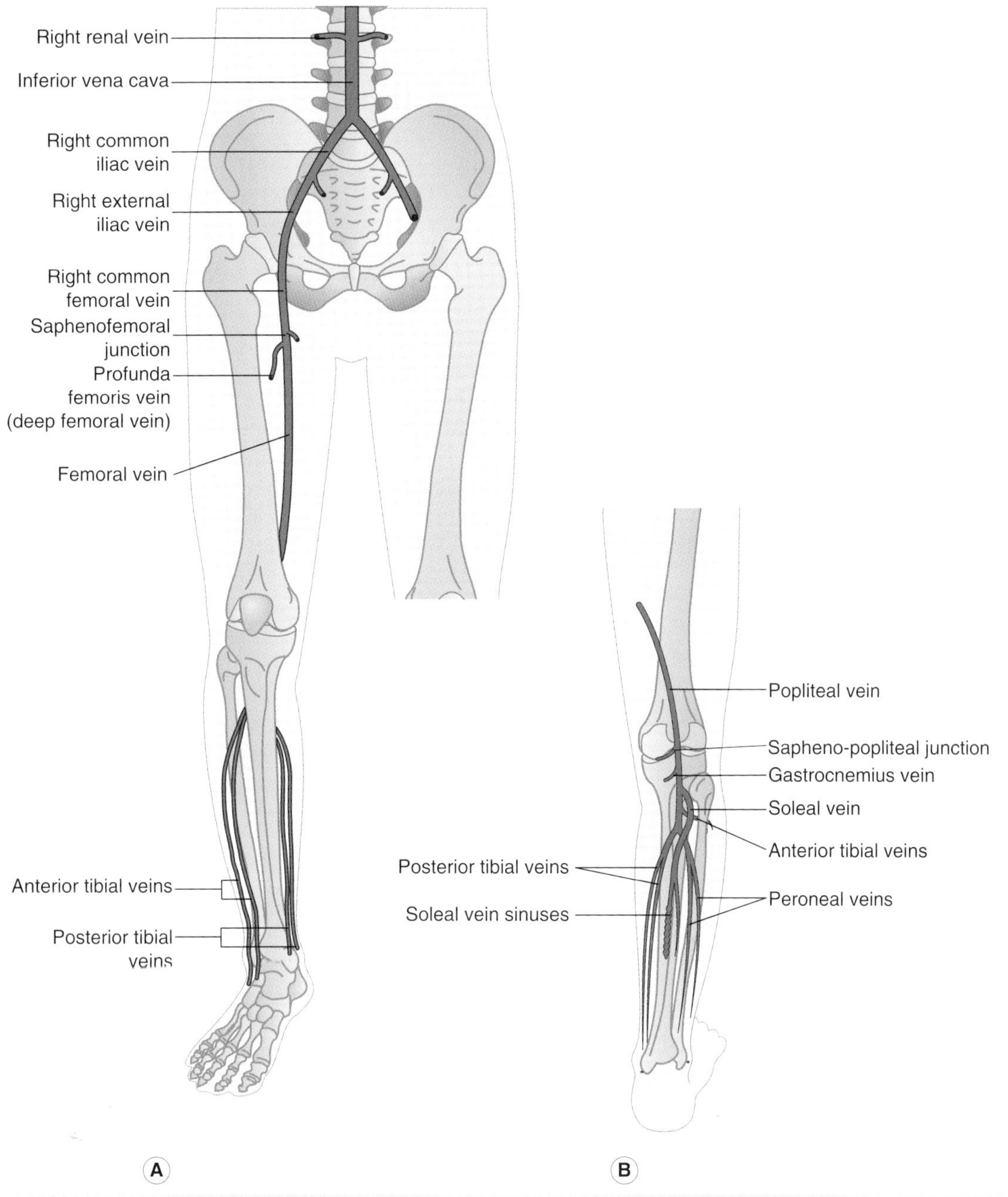

Figure 13.2 • Anatomy of the deep venous system, including the iliac veins and vena cava (A and B).

lateral gastrocnemius muscles. The gastrocnemius veins normally drain into the popliteal vein through single or multiple trunks below the level of the saphenopopliteal junction. The anterior tibial vein is paired and associated with the anterior tibial artery and drains to the popliteal vein. The above-knee popliteal vein runs through the adductor canal and becomes the femoral vein in the lower medial aspect of the thigh. The femoral vein runs toward the groin, where it is joined by the deep femoral vein to form the common femoral vein. This confluence is distal to the level of the saphenofemoral junction (SFJ) and common femoral artery bifurcation (see Fig. 9.8). The common femoral vein lies medial to the artery, becoming the external iliac vein above the inguinal ligament (Fig. 13.2). The external iliac vein runs deep and is joined by the internal iliac vein, which drains blood from the pelvis, forming the common iliac vein. The left common iliac vein runs deep to the right common iliac artery to drain into the vena cava, which lies to the right of the aorta.

Superficial venous system

The main superficial veins are the great saphenous vein (GSV) and small saphenous vein (SSV) (Fig. 13.3) (often referred to as the long saphenous vein [LSV] and short saphenous vein, respectively). The GSV and SSV are contained in a separate saphenous compartment, bounded superficially by the hyperechoic saphenous fascia and deeply by the muscular fascia (Fig. 13.4). Branches, tributaries, and cross-communicating veins lie external to the saphenous compartment (Caggiati et al. 2002) (Fig. 13.1). The saphenous compartment resembles the shape of an Egyptian eye when imaged.

The GSV and saphenofemoral junction

Tributaries and bifid veins

- The anatomically observed image of the main trunk of the great saphenous vein and a large tributary, lying superficial to the saphenous compartment, does not constitute a true bifid or paired system. The term bifid is properly used when both veins are contained in the same saphenous compartment.
- Bifid and duplicated systems are clinically important as either or both veins may be incompetent and either or both may require treatment. They are also clinically important elsewhere, an example being the femoral vein.

The anatomy of the GSV is shown in Figure 13.3A. The distal GSV is located anterior to the medial malleolus (inner ankle bone), runs up the medial aspect of the calf and thigh, and is joined by a number of superficial tributaries. The GSV drains into the common femoral vein approximately 2.5 cm below the inguinal ligament at the SFJ. It is important to have a detailed understanding of the anatomy in this area, as there are at least six other tributaries draining to the GSV at the level of the SFJ (Fig. 13.5). These tributaries can be the source of primary or recurrent varicose veins. It is not usually possible to identify all of these tributaries by ultrasound. The anterior accessory saphenous vein (AASV), sometimes called the anterolateral thigh vein, drains flow from the anterior and lateral aspect of the knee and lower thigh and runs across the anterior aspect of the thigh into the SFJ (Fig. 13.3). However, it can sometimes join the GSV at a variable level below the junction. The AASV is usually easy to identify with ultrasound and it is contained within its own fascial compartment (Figs 13.6 and 13.7). In the upper thigh, it runs in the same line as the femoral vein: this is referred to as the alignment sign and helps to distinguish the AASV from the GSV that lies medial and posterior to the AASV (Fig. 13.7). The posterior accessory saphenous vein also runs in a facial compartment and drains flow from the posteromedial and posterior regions of the lower thigh and usually joins the main trunk of the GSV in the upper thigh. There are sometimes connections between the thigh extension (TE) of the SSV or Giacomini vein, described later in the chapter.

The SSV, saphenopopliteal junction, and Giacomini vein

The anatomy of the SSV is shown in Figure 13.3B.

The distal SSV arises posterior to the outer aspect of the ankle (lateral malleolus) and runs up the posterior calf in an interfascial compartment (Fig. 13.4B). In the upper calf the compartment appears as a triangular shape that is defined by the lateral and medial heads of the gastrocnemius muscle and the superficial fascia that streches over the intermuscular groove (Cavezzi et al. 2006). It drains to the popliteal vein via the saphenopopliteal junction located superior to the insertion of the gastrocnemius vein. Typically the saphenopopliteal junction is located 2–5 cm above the popliteal knee crease. However, the anatomy can be extremely variable. The saphenopopliteal junction may be located proximal to the popliteal fossa, draining to the above-knee popliteal vein or distal femoral vein (Fig. 13.8). The SSV can insert directly into the gastrocnemius vein or share a common

Figure 13.3 • Anatomy of the superficial veins, including the position of commonly located perforators. (A) The great saphenous vein. Posterior tibial perforators (sometimes referred to as Cockett's perforators) are located at distances of approximately 6, 13, and 18 cm above the medial malleolus. Paratibial or Boyd perforators are located in the upper calf, approximately 10 cm below the knee joint. (B) The small saphenous vein.

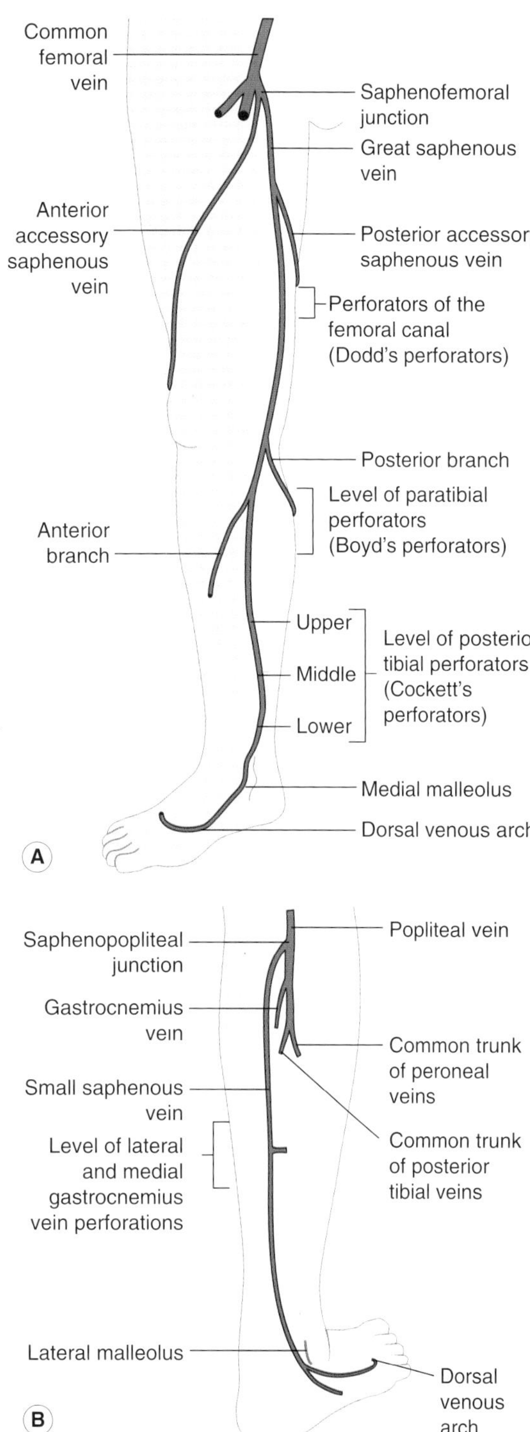

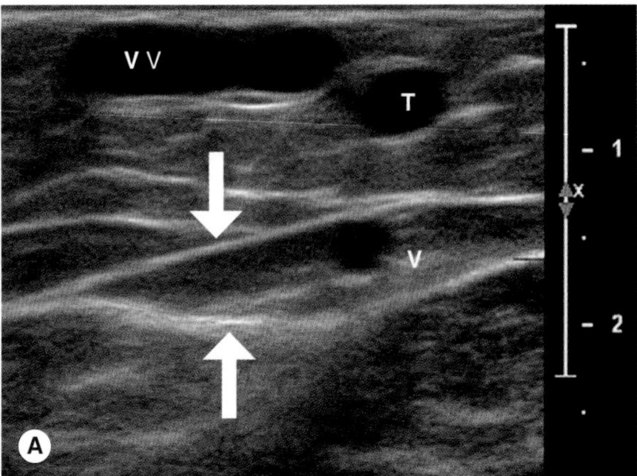

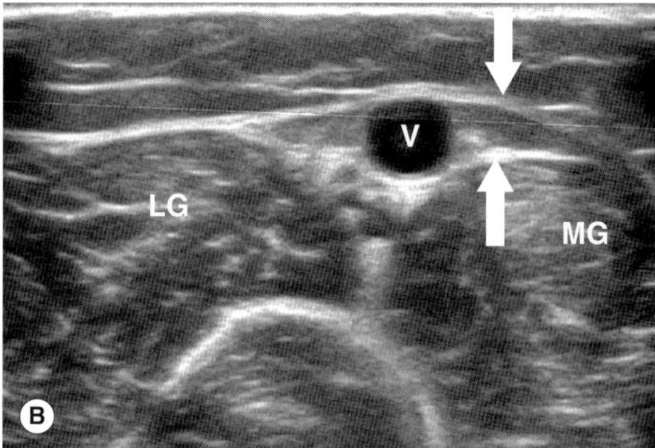

Figure 13.4 • The main trunks of the superficial veins are shown in cross-section. (A) The great saphenous vein (V) lies in the saphenous compartment, bounded by the deep muscular fascia (upward arrow) and the saphenous fascia (downward arrow). Note a superficial tributary (T) and some varicose veins (VV) lying above the saphenous compartment. (B) The small saphenous vein (V) is also bounded by the deep fascia (upward arrow) and saphenous fascia (downward arrow). The medial gastrocnemius muscle (MG) and lateral gastrocnemius muscle (LG) are shown on this image of the right leg.

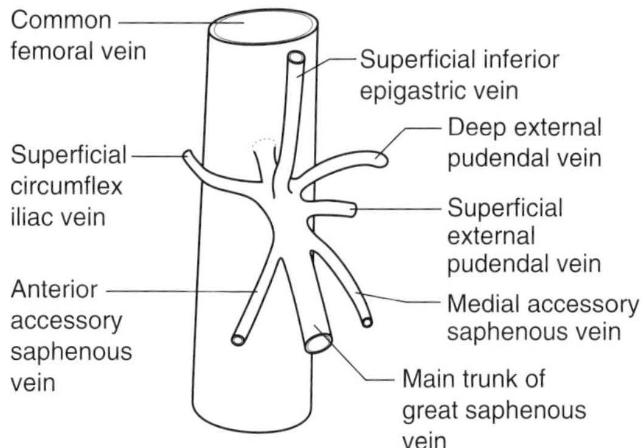

Figure 13.5 • The anatomy of the saphenofemoral junction.

confluence (Fig. 13.8). In addition, it is common to find a TE of the SSV, described by Giacomini in 1873 running in an intrafascial compartment or groove bounded by the semitendinous muscle, long head of biceps, and superficial fascia (Georgiev et al. 2003).

There are a number of terminations for the TE, as shown in Figure 13.8. The TE is often referred to as the Giacomini vein, although strictly this term should only be applied when the vein connects to the GSV. There is sometimes confusion as to whether a posterior thigh vein is the Giacomini vein or merely a superficial posteromedial tributary of the GSV. Generally, the Giacomini vein should appear to run into an intrafascial compartment in the lower thigh before joining the SSV, whereas superficial tributaries of the GSV tend to lie above the superficial fascia. Finally, there are usually intersaphenous veins in the upper calf, running between the GSV and SSV.

Perforators

There are major perforating veins in the GSV and SSV system and these can be variable in their presence, being more numerous below the knee (Fig. 13.3). Large perforators are easy to identify by ultrasound. It is worth noting that some perforators do not connect directly to the main trunks of the GSV or SSV, but communicate via side branches of the main trunks. There are a number of perforating veins associated with the SSV, especially from medial and lateral gastrocnemius veins and soleal veins.

Other superficial veins

There is typically a lateral venous system in the leg but the veins are often very small and difficult to detect. They may represent an embryonic system

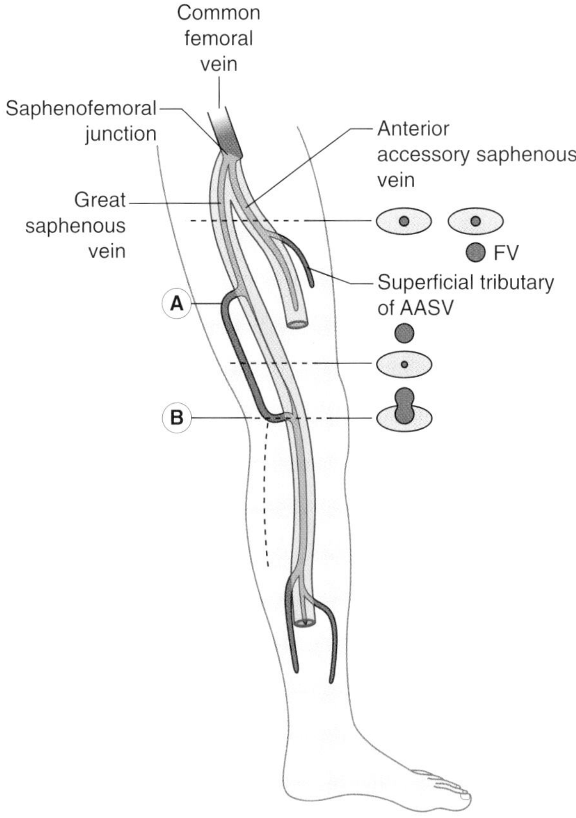

Figure 13.6 • A diagrammatic representation of the saphenous compartments containing the great saphenous vein (GSV) and anterior accessory saphenous vein (AASV). In this example a large incompetent tributary inserts to an incompetent GSV in the mid-thigh (A), with the GSV becoming small and competent beyond this point. The tributary communicates with the main trunk lower in the thigh (B), where the GSV becomes incompetent once more. Alternatively, the large tributary could continue to run down the leg (indicated by the short dashed lines) and the GSV could remain small below point B. There can be many anatomical variations involving the GSV and its tributaries, especially in the knee region and mid to lower thigh. FV, femoral vein.

and are only relevant if there are isolated varicose veins in this area not associated with the GSV or SSV.

Anatomical variations

There are numerous anatomical variations in the lower-limb venous system, and even experienced sonographers will encounter new variations from time to time. Duplicated, or bifid, vein systems are relatively common and mainly involve the femoral vein and popliteal vein (Fig. 13.9). A potentially confusing anatomical variation occurs in patients who have a large deep femoral vein in the thigh running as a large trunk between the popliteal vein and the common femoral vein. In this situation, the size of the femoral vein in the thigh can be small when compared with the size of the superficial femoral artery, and this appearance may be mistaken for evidence of venous obstruction. However, good flow augmentation, with a calf squeeze, will be demonstrated in the common femoral vein just below the SFJ. Careful inspection by duplex will normally reveal the larger deep femoral vein. A low-frequency 2–4 MHz curved linear array transducer may be necessary to identify this vein. A very rare anomaly can occur toward the level of the SFJ, with the GSV running between the superficial femoral artery and profunda femoris artery to drain into the SFJ.

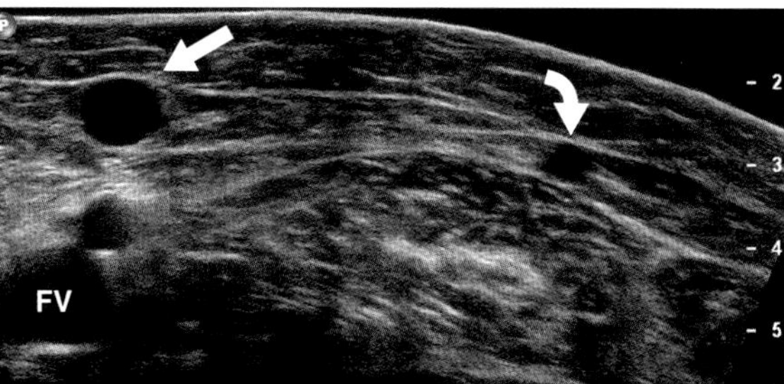

Figure 13.7 • A transverse panoramic view of the right upper thigh showing the anterior accessory saphenous vein (AASV: straight arrow) lying above the femoral vein (FV), indicating the alignment sign. The great saphenous vein (curved arrow) is lying medially in its own saphenous compartment. In this example it is likely that the AASV is incompetent due to its size.

Venous valves

Veins contain bicuspid, valves to prevent the reflux of blood to the extremities. There is often a characteristic dilation of the vein at the valve site that can sometimes be seen on the ultrasound image (Fig. 13.10). Venous valves are able to withstand high degrees of back pressure, typically in excess of 250–300 mmHg. The number of valves in each

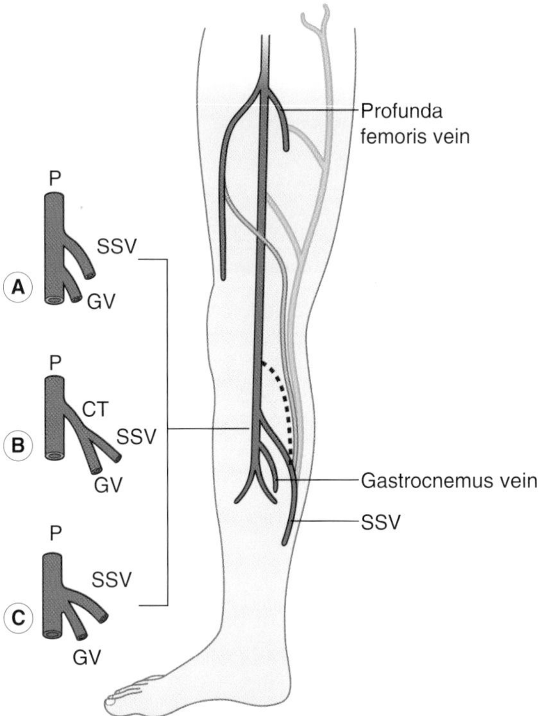

Figure 13.8 • The level of the small saphenous vein (SSV) insertion can be highly variable. Potential positions are shown by numbers and lettered diagrams. The SSV normally drains to the popliteal vein (P) in the popliteal fossa at the saphenopopliteal junction (diagram A). It can share a common trunk (CT) with the gastrocnemius vein (GV) (diagram B). It can share a common junction with the gastrocnemius vein (diagram C). It sometimes has a high junction with the popliteal vein (blue dashed line). The thigh extension vein, when present, runs above the level of the saphenopopliteal junction and has a variable outflow. It may drain to the femoral vein, profunda femoris vein or branches of the internal iliac vein (green lines). It may also drain to the great saphenous vein (GSV) and in this situation the vein is termed the Giacomini vein (orange line). Note that it is possible to confuse the posteromedial tributary of the great saphenous vein with the Giacomini vein; see text.

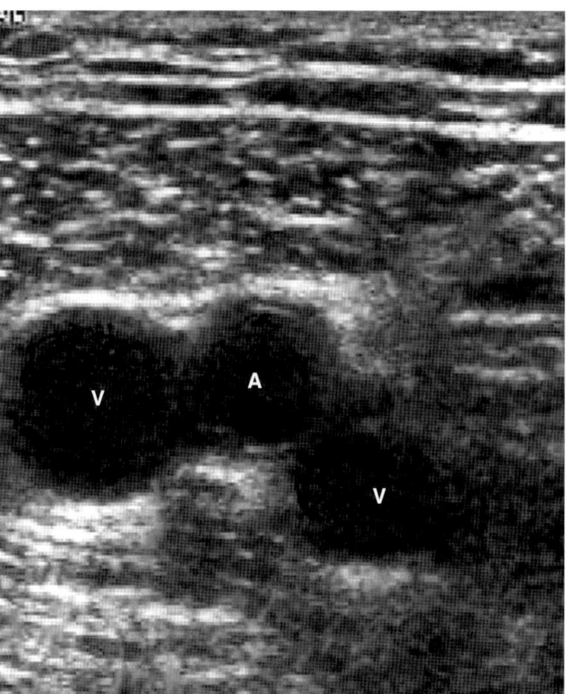

Figure 13.9 • A transverse image of a duplicated or bifid femoral vein with the artery (A) lying between the paired veins (V).

venous segment varies among individuals, but there are more valves in the distal veins than in the proximal veins, as they have to withstand higher hydrostatic pressures. The inferior vena cava and common iliac vein have no valves, and the majority of the population have no valves in the external iliac or common femoral vein. There is usually a valve at the proximal end of the femoral vein and an average of three to four valves along the length of the femoral and popliteal vein to the level of the knee, although the number can be inconsistent. In most people there is a valve in the below-knee popliteal vein that is sometimes referred to as the 'gatekeeper,' as it prevents venous reflux into the proximal calf. The deep veins in the calf contain numerous valves. The GSV and SSV contain approximately 8–10 valves along their main trunks (Browse et al. 1999).

The configuration of the valves at the SFJ is important to consider as there is typically a terminal valve located at the junction and a preterminal valve that is positioned in the GSV, 3–5 cm distal to the terminal valve. Tributaries of the SFJ join between these two points (Fig. 13.11). This explains how it is possible for the junction to be competent but for reflux to occur across the preterminal valve into the proximal GSV due to flow from the tribu-

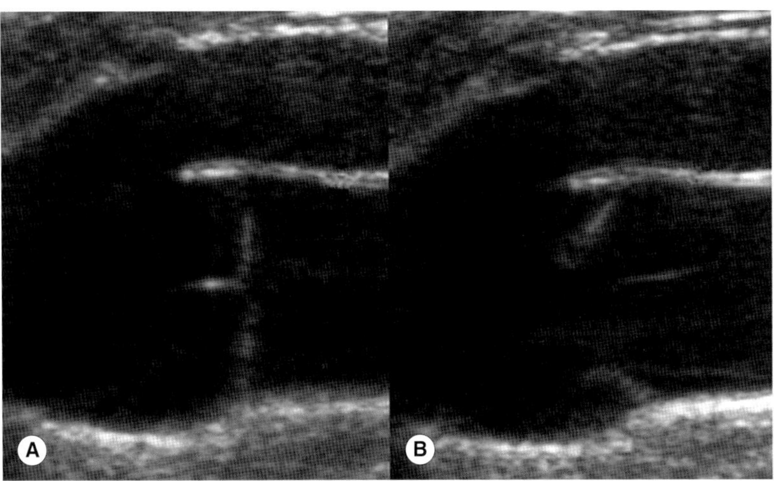

Figure 13.10 • An image of a venous valve site in the popliteal vein just below the gastrocnemius vein. (A) The valve is closed. (B) The valve is open.

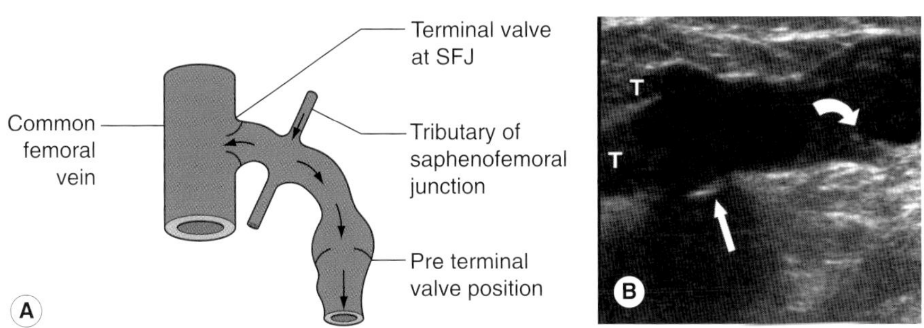

Figure 13.11 • Examples of the saphenofemoral junction (SFJ) and proximal great saphenous vein (GSV) to indicate valve positions. (A) The diagram shows the position of the terminal and preterminal valves. The arrows indicate venous reflux across an incompetent preterminal valve via flow from the tributaries. The terminal valve is competent. (B) An ultrasound example, showing the position of the terminal valve (straight arrow) and preterminal valve (curved arrow) in an incompetent GSV. Two tributaries are shown (T), with one demonstrating marked dilation.

taries (Caggiati et al. 2004) (Fig. 13.11A). A similar pattern can exist in the SSV. In addition, there are normally valves protecting many perforating veins so that flow is directed from the superficial venous system to the deep system. In very rare cases, patients may have absent venous valves due to congenital valve aplasia (Eifert et al. 2000). This can be the cause of deep venous reflux in the very young patient.

Flow patterns in the venous system

The flow patterns in normal deep veins are described in Chapter 5. The venous flow patterns

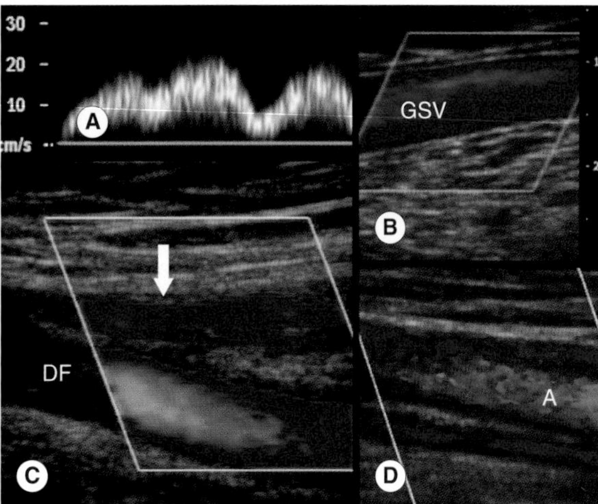

Figure 13.12 • High-volume spontaneous flow is demonstrated in the great saphenous vein (GSV) of a patient with popliteal and femoral vein obstruction due to chronic postthrombotic syndrome. (A) Spectral Doppler recording from the GSV shown in (B) indicating spontaneous flow. (B) A large dilated GSV. (C) The deep femoral vein (DF) is patent but the femoral vein (arrow) is small. (D) An image of the femoral vessels in the mid-thigh demonstrating small collateral veins (blue) adjacent to the artery (A).

in the superficial veins can vary, depending on patient position and external factors, such as ambient temperature. Normally there should be no, or very little, spontaneous flow in the GSV and SSV when the patient is standing or sitting. If the ambient temperature in the room is high, vasodilation may result in increased flow in the superficial veins. Evidence of high-volume spontaneous or continuous flow in the superficial veins at rest should be treated with suspicion, as this may indicate obstruction of the deep veins or could be due to infection, such as cellulitis (Fig. 13.12).

VENOUS DISORDERS AND TREATMENT

Deep-vein thrombosis is covered in Chapter 14.

Classification of chronic venous disorders

The CEAP (Clinical–Etiology–Anatomy–Pathophysiology) classification system for venous disorders was developed by an ad hoc committee of the venous forum (Eklöf et al. 2004). It has been developed to facilitate the use of consistent terminology and diagnosis within the clinical and scientific community. The clinical classes are shown in Table 13.1. Therefore, a patient with a painful venous ulcer due to primary venous disease that included great saphenous and popliteal vein reflux, with perforating vein reflux in the calf would have a basic CEAP classification of $C_{6,s}, E_p, A_{spd}, P_r$. In advance CEAP, the classification would be $C_{2,6,s}, E_p, A_{s,p,d}, P_{r2,3,18,14}$.

Varicose veins

The cause of varicose veins is uncertain, but there is evidence that increased age, female gender, and pregnancy are risk factors (Callam 1994).

Varicose veins appear as dilated, tortuous, elongated vessels on the skin surface, especially in the calf. Abnormal superficial veins can be classified according to their size. Minor cosmetic or intradermal spider veins (telangiectasia) <1 mm in diameter are not visible by ultrasound. Small dilated subdermal veins (reticular veins) 1–2 mm in diameter can also be difficult to image without high-frequency probes. Varicose veins, typically subcutaneous and measuring >3 mm in diameter, often involve, or are associated with, the main superficial trunks and can be easily assessed with ultrasound. Varicose veins most commonly occur due to incompetence of the GSV or SSV, or a combination of both systems.

It is important to identify the supply to the varicose areas and the level of incompetence in the GSV or SSV. This can be highly variable but frequently involves reflux from the saphenofemoral or saphenopopliteal junctions. In some situations varicose veins may be independent of the GSV or SSV systems, such as the lateral thigh. Much debate has surrounded the development of varicose veins, but it appears that incompetence in the main trunks develops distally, in the lower leg, and progresses in a proximal direction over time. This is contrary to traditional teaching, which proposed that incompetence developed at the SFJ, leading to progressive valve failure in a descending direction. The model of progressively ascending valve failure would also explain why it is possible to observe segmental GSV reflux in the lower thigh but com-

CLINICAL CLASSIFICATION	
C0	No visible or palpable signs of venous disease
C1	Telangiectasia or reticular veins
C2	Varicose veins
C3	Edema
C4a	Pigmentation or eczema
C4b	Lipodermatosclerosis or atrophie blanche
C5	Healed venous ulcer
C6	Active venous ulcer
S	Symptomatic, including ache, pain, tightness, skin irritation, heaviness, and muscle cramps, and other complaints attributable to venous dysfunction
A	Asymptomatic
ETIOLOGIC CLASSIFICATION	
Ec	Congenital
Ep	Primary
Es	Secondary (postthrombotic)
En	No venous cause identified
ANATOMIC CLASSIFICATION	
As	Superficial veins
Ap	Perforator veins
Ad	Deep veins
An	No venous location identified
PATHOPHYSIOLOGIC CLASSIFICATION	
Basic CEAP	
Pr	Reflux
Po	Obstruction
Pr,o	Reflux and obstruction
Pn	No venous pathophysiology identifiable
ADVANCED CEAP: SAME AS BASIC CEAP, WITH THE ADDITION THAT ANY OF 18 NAMED VENOUS SEGMENTS CAN BE USED AS LOCATORS FOR VENOUS PATHOLOGY	
Superficial veins	
1	Telangiectasia or reticular veins
2	Great saphenous vein above knee
3	Great saphenous vein below knee
4	Small saphenous vein
5	Nonsaphenous veins
Deep veins	
6	Inferior vena cava
7	Common iliac vein
8	Internal iliac vein
9	External iliac vein
10	Pelvic: gonadal, broad ligament veins, other
11	Common femoral vein
12	Deep femoral vein
13	Femoral vein
14	Popliteal vein
15	Crural: anterior tibial, posterior tibial, peroneal veins (all paired)
16	Muscular: gastrocnemial, soleal veins, other
Perforating veins	
17	Thigh
18	Calf

Modified from Eklöf et al. (2004).

Table 13.1 CEAP (Clinical–Etiology–Anatomy–Pathophysiology) classification

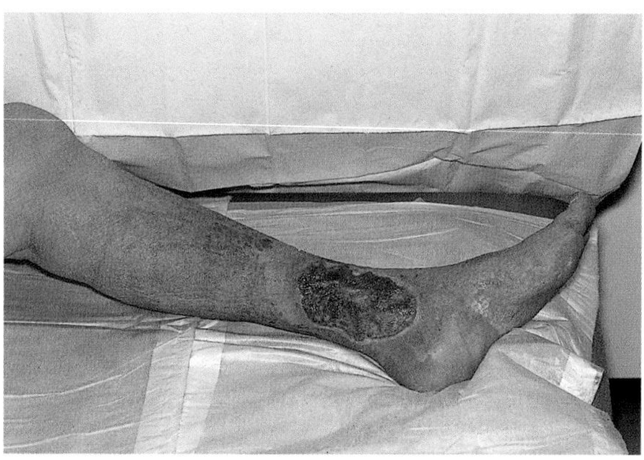

Figure 13.13 • A picture of a venous ulcer involving the lower aspect of the medial calf and ankle. Varicose veins are also seen in the great saphenous vein distribution of the mid-calf.

petence of the vein in the upper thigh and at the SFJ (Abu-Own et al. 1994). Some patients with superficial varicose veins may also have coexisting deep venous insufficiency.

Skin changes and venous ulcers

A serious complication of superficial or deep venous insufficiency is the development of chronic venous hypertension in the lower limb, resulting in venous ulceration (Fig. 13.13). Risk factors associated with ulceration include post-thrombotic syndrome, obesity, immobility, and arthritic conditions, which cause reduced movement of the ankle joint, leading to failure of the calf muscle pump. It is important to note that some ulcers that may appear to be venous in origin are caused by other conditions, such as vasculitis, rheumatoid arthritis, or skin disorders. The underlying cause of ulceration is still unclear but is thought to involve changes in the microcirculation of the skin and subcutaneous tissues in response to local venous hypertension. The venous hypertension causes an increase in venular and capillary pressure, leading to local edema and reduced reabsorption of proteins and fluid from the interstitial tissue spaces. This is combined with damage to the capillary walls, which may cause localized tissue hypoxia. Leakage of red blood cells across the damaged capillary wall and into the interstitial tissue spaces produces the brown pigmentation associated with many ulcers. This is due to hemosiderin deposition caused by the breakdown of the red blood cells. Venous ulcers are usually reasonably shallow and vary in size, and in some cases they may be circumferential around the calf. They frequently become infected with different types of bacteria and can be extremely painful.

Skin changes around the ankle or lower calf are the first physical signs of venous hypertension. This is typically seen as areas of venous eczema and pigmentation, frequently associated with local skin irritation or itching. There is often development of lipodermatosclerosis, typified as hardening of the subcutaneous tissues in the lower calf and ankle, giving a hard, 'woody' feel to the area. The development of an ulcer is sometimes initiated by a minor injury or abrasion that fails to heal. It is important to remember that some venous ulcers are also associated with arterial disease, and patients with mixed venous and arterial ulceration pose a challenging diagnostic problem for the vascular laboratory. It is therefore routine practice to measure the ankle–brachial pressure index (ABPI) in all patients with venous ulceration to exclude a significant arterial component. However, in some situations it may be impossible to measure the ABPI due to pain, and a subjective assessment of the pedal artery waveforms will have to suffice. A layer of cling film or Saran wrap is ideal for wrapping around areas of ulceration to protect the ulcer and to keep the pressure cuff clean.

Historically, it was thought that venous ulceration was primarily due to deep venous insufficiency following valve failure, postthrombotic syndrome, or failure of the calf muscle pump, resulting in deep venous hypertension. However, later studies (Scriven et al. 1997; Magnusson et al. 2001) demonstrated that a significant number of patients with ulceration have superficial reflux alone, with the deep veins being competent. Therefore, ligation of the relevant superficial vein junction, with or without stripping of the superficial vein, results in the healing of the majority of ulcers due to the reduction in venous hypertension. The role of perforator ligation remains controversial, but there is evidence that chronic venous insufficiency is associated with an increase in the number and diameter of medial calf perforators (Stuart et al. 2000). Presurgical marking of incompetent perforators may be performed with the aid of the duplex scanner.

Varicose ulcers caused by superficial incompetence alongside significant deep venous insufficiency are not usually treated by the ligation or stripping of superficial varicose veins, as the underlying deep venous hypertension will not be corrected. Instead, the use of compression bandaging, which reduces edema and venous hypertension, has proved to be an effective method of healing ulcers. Different grades of compression bandaging can be used depending upon the clinical situation (Lambourne et al. 1996). However, an ABPI of ≥0.8 is required for the application of four-layer compression dressings, in order to avoid arterial compromise in the tissues under the bandaging. This can be a serious complication and can lead to limb loss in extreme cases.

Treatment of superficial venous disorders

A range of treatment options is available depending on the severity of the condition (Browse et al. 1999). Conservative treatment is with compression hosiery. Thread veins can be treated by microinjection sclerotherapy, followed by local compression to occlude the vein. They can also be treated by local laser therapy. Larger varicose veins can be treated by a variety of methods, including foam sclerotherapy, open surgery, or endovenous ablation. Some patients undergo combined procedures to achieve optimum results. In the case of open surgery for primary GSV incompetence, the SFJ and tributaries are ligated at the groin, and the main trunk stripped with a vein stripper to knee level or below. Surgery of the SSV normally involves ligation of the saphenopopliteal junction. Some surgeons strip the vein, but others leave it intact to avoid injury to the sural nerve, which is closely associated with the vein. Some surgeons also ligate large perforators, and these can be marked preoperatively with the aid of duplex scanning. Any remaining veins are then removed or avulsed using small microincisions. It is worth observing some varicose vein surgery as it gives a better appreciation of the anatomy seen during duplex examinations.

PRACTICAL CONSIDERATIONS FOR DUPLEX SCANNING OF VARICOSE VEINS

What does the clinician want to know?

- Is there reflux in the great saphenous vein, small saphenous vein, or tributaries and at what level?
- Is there reflux across the saphenofemoral or saphenopopliteal junction or relevant perforators?
- Are there any large localized dilations (varices) present?
- Are there other sources of reflux, such as the lateral thigh system?
- Indication of veins that have been removed or stripped or are not present
- Unusual anatomy of the saphenopopliteal junction, including the presence of thigh extension or Giacomini vein
- Is there deep venous reflux or obstruction?
- Are the veins suitable for endovenous therapy (i.e., assessment of diameter and tortuousity)
- Abnormal anatomy

The purpose of the scan is to assess the competency of the superficial and deep veins and identify the cause of the varicose veins. At least half an hour should be allocated for a bilateral vein scan. Adopting a logical approach to the examination is useful, as this reduces the length of time required for the assessment. The patient should be asked the following questions before starting the examination:

- *Have you had any previous varicose vein treatment, either by surgery, endovenous therapy or by injection sclerotherapy?* It is not uncommon to find that the request card has omitted previous clinical details, and the patient may have undergone some form of treatment in the past. This may be evident on the duplex scan.
- *Have you ever had a deep-vein thrombosis or severe leg swelling?* If the patient has had a deep-vein thrombosis, there may be chronic

damage of the deep venous system, causing deep venous insufficiency or obstruction, which may be the cause of the current symptoms.

The sonographer should also visually examine the position and distribution of the varicose veins, as this can provide a clue to their supply. No preparation is required before the scan, but the legs should be accessible from the groin to the ankle. It is necessary to position the patient so that the feet are substantially lower than the heart in order to generate sufficient hydrostatic pressure to assess the competency of the venous valves. If the patient is lying completely flat, there is very little pressure differential between the central venous system and the legs. Therefore, any reflux occurring after a distal calf squeeze may be of such low velocity that it is not detected. Many units perform the examination with the patient in a standing position. When standing, partial weight should be on the examined limb with the knee slightly flexed, but most weight-bearing should be on the contralateral limb. The patient can use a hand rail, or suitable alternative, for support. Other common positions in which to assess a patient include the supine position on the examination table with the whole table tilted feet-down by an angle of at least 30° (reverse Trendelenburg position). Alternatively, the patient can sit on the edge of the examination table, and partial weight-bearing is achieved by placing the foot of the examined limb on a stool. It is not uncommon for patients, especially younger ones, to feel faint during the examination due to the calf compressions. Let the patient lie down immediately if he or she feels unwell, and, if necessary, appropriate medical advice should be sought.

AUGMENTATION MANEUVERS AND VENOUS REFLUX

Before considering the practical techniques used for scanning the venous system, it is important to have an understanding of the methods most commonly employed for assessing venous valve competency (Coleridge-Smith et al. 2006). These are calf compression, to augment flow toward the heart, and the Valsalva maneuver for examining the competency of the veins in the groin. In addition, proximal compression can be used to assess flow in perforators.

Valsalva maneuver

Caution

It is possible for enthusiastic patients performing a very strong Valsalva maneuver to generate pressures beyond the normal physiological range, leading to reflux.

The competency of the proximal deep veins and SFJ can be assessed with a Valsalva maneuver. The patient is told to inhale deeply and then to push out and expand the cheeks without breathing out, while at the same time bearing pressure down on the abdomen. This produces an increase in intra-abdominal pressure, thus increasing the venous blood pressure in the iliac and femoral veins. It is usual to see the common femoral vein distending during a Valsalva maneuver. Provided that the venous valves are competent, there should be no reflux across the SFJ or proximal superficial femoral vein during Valsalva testing (Fig. 13.14). There

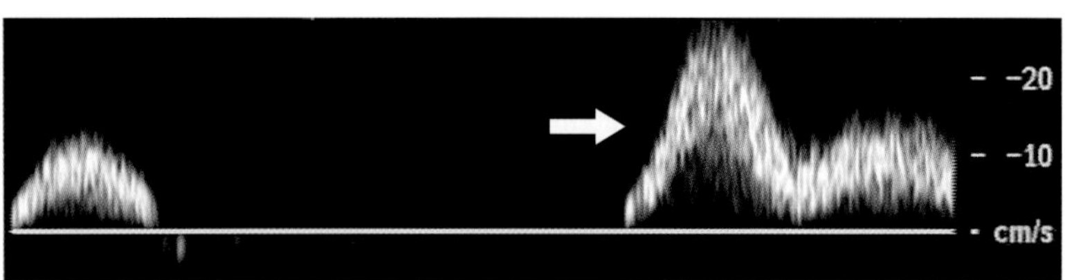

Figure 13.14 • The Valsalva maneuver demonstrates competency of the proximal femoral vein. There is a cessation of normal phasic flow during the Valsalva maneuver followed by a surge of flow during expiration (arrow).

should be a temporary cessation of the normal spontaneous phasic flow pattern in the femoral and common femoral veins. If the SFJ is incompetent, the increase in abdominal pressure will produce significant reflux across the junction (Fig. 13.15). One potential pitfall of using the Valsalva maneuver for the assessment of proximal reflux can occur in patients who have a competent valve in the iliac vein system, which is usually valve-free. In this situation, the proximal valve will protect an incompetent SFJ or proximal superficial femoral vein, and no reflux will be seen. The Valsalva maneuver is not used for the assessment of more distal veins.

Calf compression

To assess the competency of the valves, the flow in the veins toward the heart should be temporarily increased or augmented. The easiest way to produce flow augmentation is to place a hand around the back of the calf and give a prolonged firm squeeze that is then quickly released. It is important to squeeze the belly of the muscle rather than a small portion (Fig. 13.16). In our experience flow augmentation should be sufficiently strong to produce a transient peak flow velocity of >30 cm/s in the main superficial vein trunks so that valve closure should be rapid on the squeeze release. However, this velocity can be difficult to achieve in very small veins. If an inadequate calf squeeze is performed, flow augmentation may be very poor, and this can be a source of conflicting results among different sonographers. For this reason, some units prefer to use a rapid cuff inflator with cuffs around the calf or thigh. The system inflates the cuff to a preset pressure before rapid deflation to provide reproducible compression. The disadvantage of this method is that it can be time-consuming and cumbersome. Manual compression of vein clusters is useful if the varicose veins are located in less common positions, such as the lateral aspect of the calf or thigh. It is also possible to augment flow by asking the patient to dorsiflex and relax the foot a couple of times.

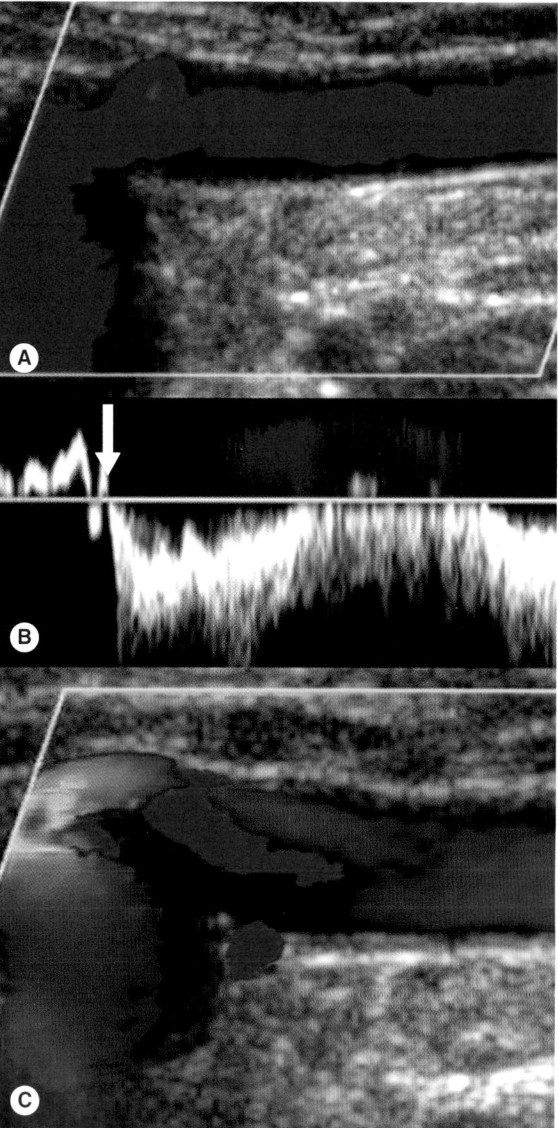

Figure 13.15 • Incompetence of the saphenofemoral junction is demonstrated by color flow imaging and spectral Doppler during a Valsalva maneuver. (A) During inspiration, flow is towards the heart (flow coded blue). (B) The arrow indicates the start of the Valsalva maneuver, with marked reflux demonstrated. (C) Color flow imaging also demonstrates the reflux (flow coded red). Note that the saphenofemoral junction and great saphenous vein are distended during the maneuver.

GRADING OF SUPERFICIAL AND DEEP VENOUS REFLUX

Inconsistent reflux

Ultrasound evaluation of the degree of venous reflux and even the detection of its presence or absence can be poorly reproducible. Many factors change venous tone and hence venous reflux. Limb muscle tone also influences venous flow and reflux. A consistent degree of weight-bearing seems to introduce some reproducibility.

- Reflux is more likely to be recorded later in the day due to hydrostatic effects on the venous system and loss of venous tone
- If the patient feels faint, venous tone changes, increasing the likelihood of reflux in otherwise competent veins
- If the examination room is very cold, the periphery may be vasoconstricted, resulting in reduced filling of the veins which in some cases may lead to reflux being missed or classed as normal
- If the patient is anxious the leg muscles may be tense; it may be difficult to produce an adequate calf squeeze to augment flow. Make sure the patient relaxes the calf muscle
- If the patent is sitting with the mid-thigh on the edge of the examination table, this can have the effect of compressing or cutting into the thigh muscles, making imaging and assessment of the femoral vein difficult, and can also distort the position of the great saphenous vein
- A degree of weight-bearing can be achieved with the legs dependent by placing the foot of the examined leg on a stool
- Weight-bearing can have a variable effect on venous reflux; for example, there are cases when a calf perforator in an edematous leg will show continuous reflux on dependency but this reflux cannot be reproduced with partial or full weight-bearing

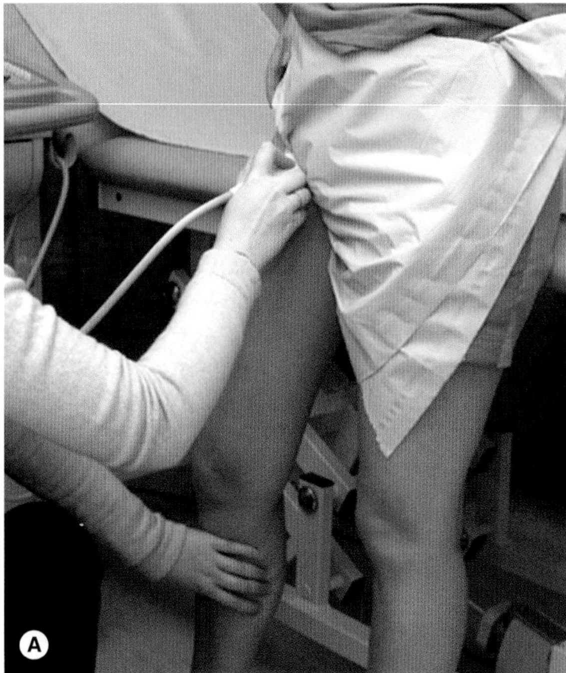

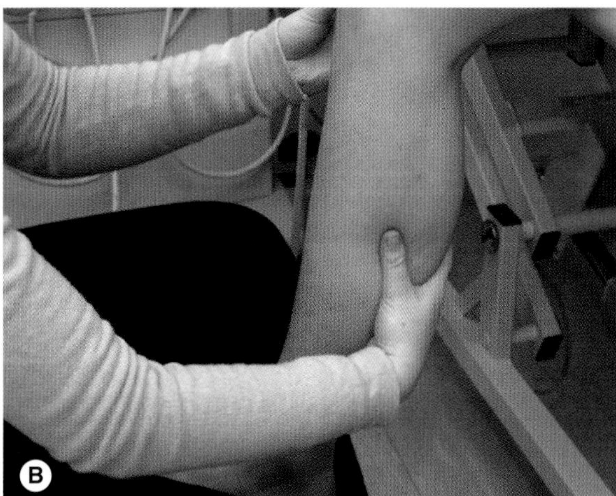

Figure 13.16 • (A) Incorrect placement of the hand around the calf will result in poor augmentation. (B) The belly of the calf muscle should be firmly squeezed, as shown in this example.

Considerable debate surrounds the grading of venous reflux, especially as different patterns of reflux can be observed in the venous system. The following protocol is used by our unit.

With the relevant segment of vein imaged in longitudinal section, the color box is steered to obtain the best angle of insonation to the vein. A calf squeeze is performed and the augmentation of flow demonstrated with color flow imaging. It is often possible to tell from the color flow display if the vein is normal or incompetent. A competent vein will display a burst of flow toward the heart during a calf squeeze, followed by an abrupt cessation of flow during squeeze release, although a very

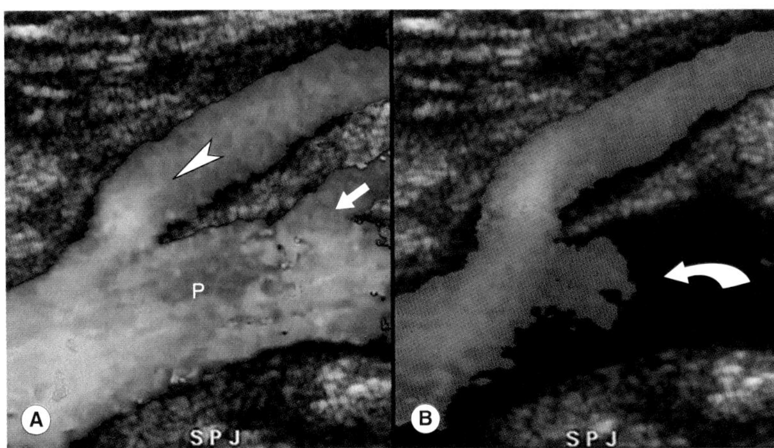

Figure 13.17 • (A) In this color flow image of the saphenopopliteal junction, flow in the small saphenous vein (arrow head) and popliteal vein (P) is toward the heart (coded blue) during distal augmentation. The straight arrow shows the insertion of the gastrocnemius vein. (B) Following squeeze release there is significant retrograde flow (coded red) in the small saphenous vein and popliteal vein above the junction, due to saphenopopliteal junction incompetence. However, no retrograde flow is demonstrated in the popliteal vein below the level of the saphenopopliteal junction, indicating popliteal vein competency at this level (curved arrow).

brief period of retrograde flow may be seen as the valves close. Significant venous reflux will be demonstrated by a sustained period of retrograde flow following calf release (Figs 13.17 and 13.18). However, the grading of venous reflux on the basis of color flow imaging alone can sometimes be misleading. This is because the color flow image may give little impression of the flow volume or may not detect low-volume reflux at all. Spectral Doppler is used to grade the degree and duration of venous reflux (Fig. 13.19). The spectral Doppler sample volume should be large enough to cover the vein lumen, and the angle of insonation should be equal to or less than 60° to obtain a good spectral Doppler trace.

GRADE	REFLUX DURATION
Normal valve function	Rapid valve closure. Reflux duration <0.5 s.
Moderate reflux	Reflux duration of 0.5–<1 s, mild to moderate retrograde flow
Significant reflux	Reflux duration of ≥1 s, large volume of retrograde flow

Table 13.2 Grading of venous reflux

Table 13.2 categorizes the degrees of venous reflux. The same criteria are used for grading venous reflux by calf compression or the Valsalva maneuver. Although the classification of venous reflux can sometimes be subjective and poorly reproducible, many scientific publications have used a reflux duration of >0.5 s to indicate abnormal valve function (Sarin et al. 1994; Evans et al. 1998; Ruckley et al. 2002; Labropoulos et al. 2003). In some cases, the reflux may be so severe that retrograde flow persists for more than 4 s. Finally, it may be possible to misinterpret a competent segment of a large vein as incompetent due to helical motion of flow during augmentation. This is especially true for the popliteal vein just above the knee, as the vein is large at this level, having been joined by a number of veins across and just below the knee.

Some patterns of reflux can be difficult to interpret, and attempts have been made to measure the volume of reflux using ultrasound volume flow measurements. In practice this is too time-consuming to be used routinely, but subjective

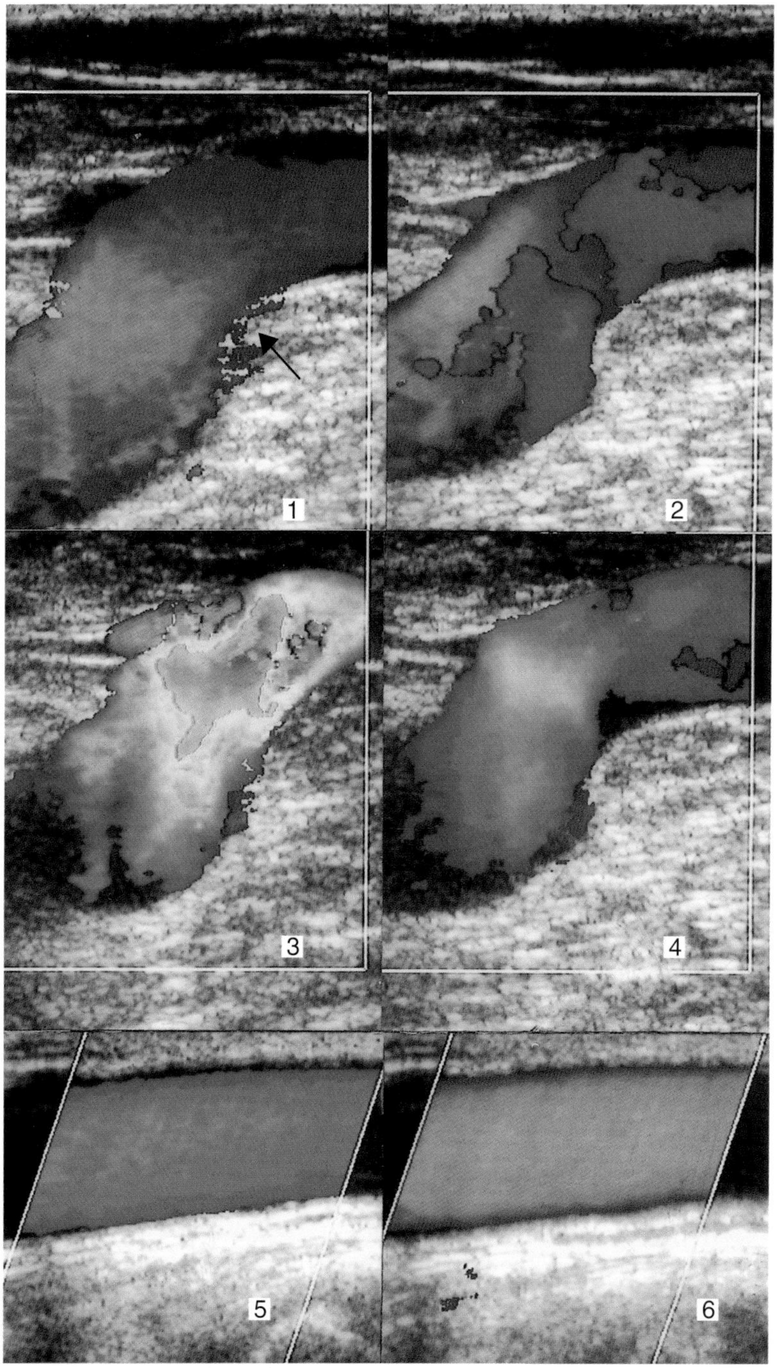

Figure 13.18 • Incompetence of the saphenofemoral junction and great saphenous vein is demonstrated with color flow imaging. Images 1–4 show flow across the junction (arrow) over a 3 s time interval at the end of distal augmentation. In image 1, flow (coded red) is toward the heart just before squeeze release. In images 2 and 3, there is increasing retrograde flow. In image 4, reflux (coded blue) is seen across the junction. Image 5 shows the great saphenous vein with flow toward the heart during augmentation. Image 6 demonstrates marked reflux following squeeze release.

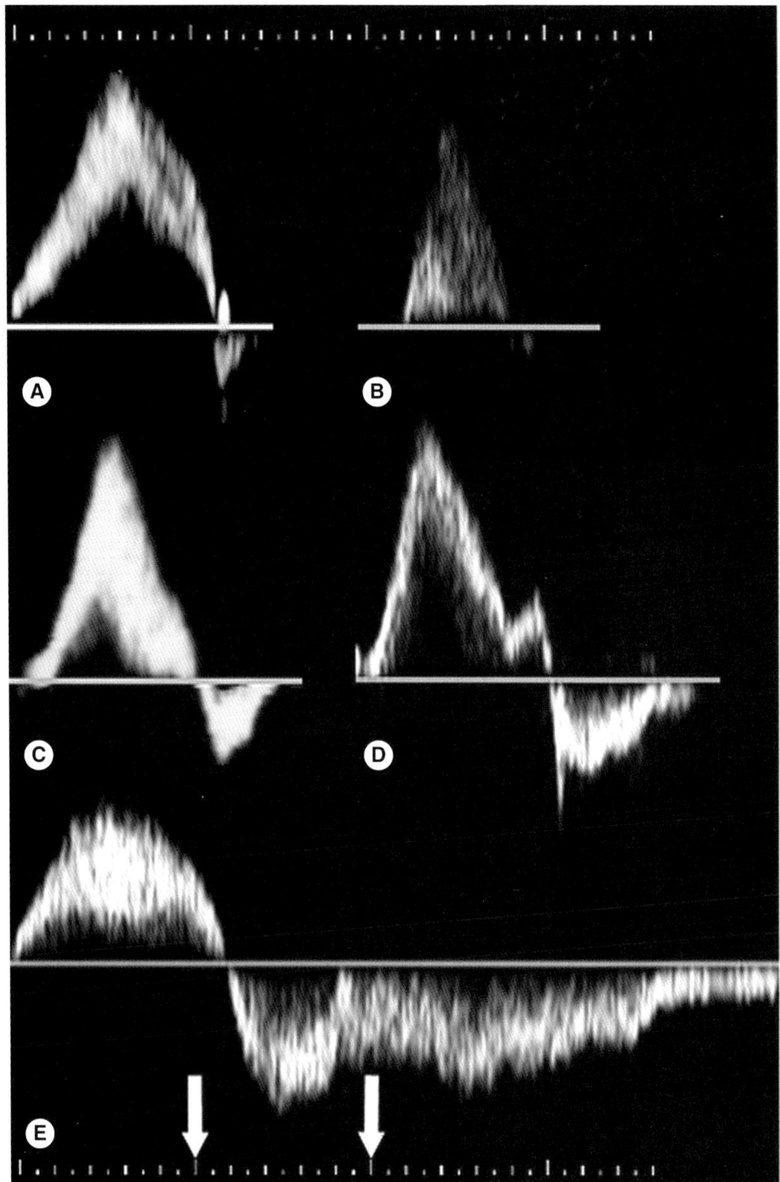

Figure 13.19 • Spectral Doppler is used to assess venous reflux. The scale between the arrows is 1 s. (A) Augmentation of flow in the great saphenous vein following calf compression shows a short duration of normal retrograde flow below the baseline on squeeze release, indicating competent valves. (B) Poor spectral traces can be obtained due to transducer movement during calf augmentation and the measurement should be repeated. (C) Borderline reflux is demonstrated (approximately 0.5 s). (D) Moderate venous reflux of 0.8 s duration. (E) Severe venous reflux >1 s duration.

assessment of the reflux volume can be useful. Trickle or low-velocity reflux can occur due to partially incompetent valves (Fig. 13.20). This can be observed in many veins but is common in the popliteal vein below the knee. It has been speculated that incipient deep venous reflux may occur due to gross superficial varicose veins causing overload of the deep venous system. This may cause some degree of dilation of the deep veins in the lower leg, which impairs normal valve function (Walsh et al. 1994).

Another problem of interpretation can occur when a vein is very large or dilated, as the duration of reflux may be relatively short. However, the volume of reflux can be high due to the large diameter of the vein. In this situation, significant reflux may be suspected if the shape of the spectral Doppler reflux pattern is the same as the augmentation pattern (Fig. 13.21). It may be difficult to augment flow in the veins of patients with gross venous stasis, and very little reflux will occur following distal release. However, the B-mode image often displays aggregation of the blood in the dilated vein as a speckle pattern (Fig. 13.22). Only a small amount of movement in the speckle pattern will be seen during calf compression. The deep venous sinuses in the calf may be dilated and congested with blood, and this appearance can be mistaken for a deep-vein thrombosis (see Ch. 14). In some cases, it may be necessary to complement the duplex scan with other diagnostic tests, such as ambulatory venous pressures or plethysmography.

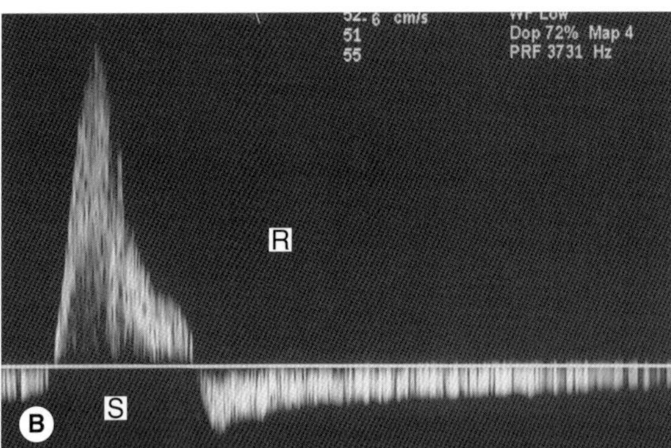

Figure 13.20 • (A) Partial incompetence of a venous valve is demonstrated by an area of retrograde flow (arrow) between the two valve cusps. (B) Spectral Doppler demonstrates trickle or low-velocity reflux (R) in the popliteal vein following distal augmentation (S).

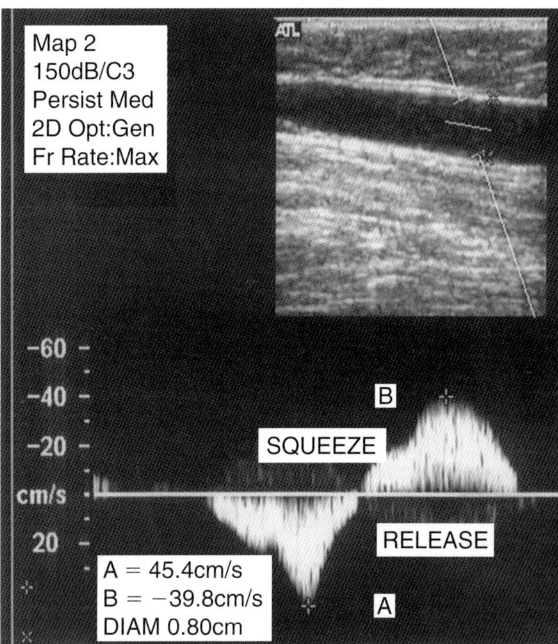

Figure 13.21 • There can be problems in quantifying venous reflux. In this example the great saphenous vein was very large (8 mm diameter), but the duration of reflux (0.9 s) is shorter than that shown in Figure 13.19E. However, the volume of reflux is similar to that demonstrated during augmentation. In this example, the volume of blood flow during reflux is probably very significant due to the size of the vein. It should be noted that volume flow calculations are not routinely used in venous examinations.

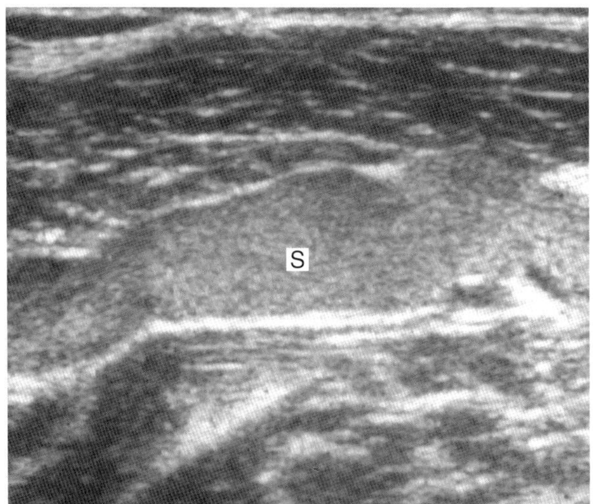

Figure 13.22 • Venous stasis (S) is demonstrated as an echogenic speckle pattern in this B-mode image of a deep calf vein.

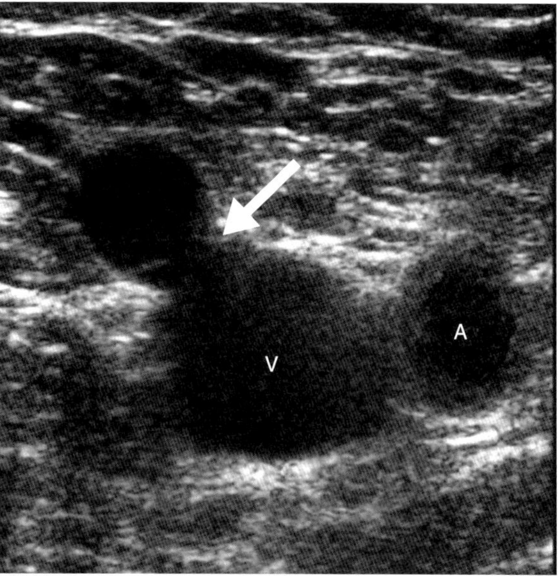

Figure 13.23 • (A) A transverse image of the left common femoral vein demonstrating the position of the saphenofemoral junction (arrow), common femoral vein (V), and common femoral artery (A). This view is sometimes called 'Mickey Mouse,' for obvious reasons. This junction is reasonably large and would need investigating for incompetence.

SCANNING PROTOCOL FOR THE LOWER-LIMB VENOUS SYSTEM

Advice

It is often quicker to image the varicose veins distally and follow them back to their supply.

A venous preset should be selected on the duplex scanner, which should typically set the pulse repetition frequency at 1000 Hz. The color wall filter should also be set at a low level. A high-frequency transducer is normally used for scanning superficial varicose veins, although a mid-frequency transducer may be needed for large legs. A mid-frequency transducer is usually required for imaging the deep veins and junctions. A combination of B-mode, color flow imaging, and spectral Doppler is used throughout the examination. The assessment of venous reflux is performed with the transducer in a longitudinal plane to the vein but initial identification of reflux is often better performed in transverse with cephalad transducer angulation. Also, the assessment of perforator competency may require the probe to be oriented into other imaging planes to follow its course. It is necessary to perform an examination of the femoral and popliteal veins during any vein assessment to assess the competency, as the superficial veins can act as collateral pathways if the deep veins are obstructed, and surgery of the superficial veins would be contraindicated and potentially damaging.

Assessment of the GSV and deep veins of the thigh and knee

1. The SFJ is located by first identifying the common femoral vein in transverse section just below the level of the inguinal ligament. The anatomy in this region is demonstrated in Figure 9.8. The common femoral vein lies medial to the common femoral artery and is normally larger than the artery. The SFJ will be seen on the anteriomedial side of the common femoral vein (Fig. 13.23). It is usual to see other tributaries joining the SFJ. Remember that these tributaries may be the main

supply to the varicose veins, especially the AASV.

2 The transducer should then be rotated so that the common femoral vein and SFJ can be seen in longitudinal section (Figs 13.11B and 13.24). The competency of the common femoral vein, SFJ, and proximal GSV can be assessed using distal compression and the Valsalva maneuver. The origin of the femoral vein, which lies below the level of the SFJ, should also be assessed for competency. Large visible branches dividing from the SFJ, especially the AASV, can also be checked for competency.

3 The GSV is examined in transverse section along the medial thigh to the knee. In transverse section, it is often possible to see the GSV running directly into varicose areas. Large perforators and tributaries are relatively easy to identify. Large thigh perforators should be assessed for competency. The GSV is then followed in longitudinal section from the SFJ to the knee and assessed for competency at frequent intervals. This is because the SFJ and proximal GSV may be competent, but there may be segmental reflux in the upper, mid-, or lower thigh, beyond incompetent valve sites, perforators, or branches. It is even possible for the main trunk of the GSV to be competent, with isolated incompetence of side tributaries that supply superficial varicose areas in the thigh or calf. Another common finding is incompetence of the proximal GSV to the level of an incompetent superficial thigh tributary that exits the saphenous compartment. Beyond the incompetent tributary, the GSV can be competent, very small, hypoplastic or absent (Fig. 13.6). It is also not infrequent to find a superficial tributary re-entering the saphenous compartment lower down in the leg and for the GSV to become incompetent again beyond this point. The size of the GSV is often seen to increase where the tributary joins. The GSV or a large tributary can also be incompetent proximally, flowing into a competent perforator in the mid-thigh, becoming competent below the perforator. There can be numerous variations to the patterns described above, especially in the thigh and knee region.

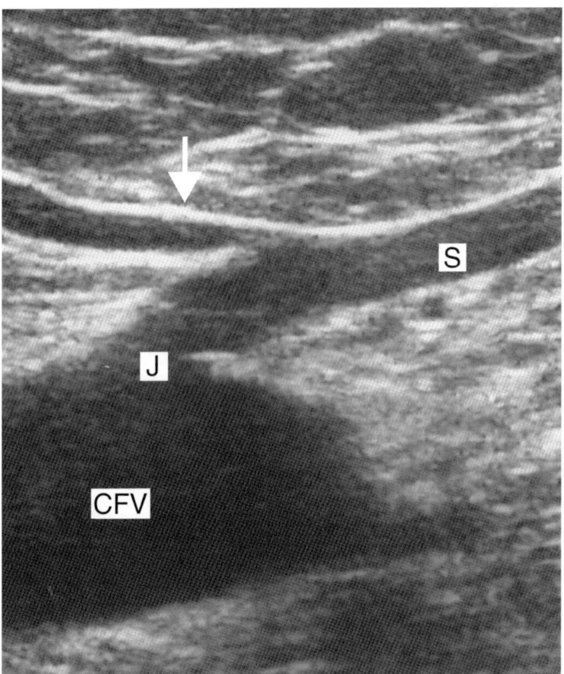

Figure 13.24 • A longitudinal image of the distal common femoral vein (CFV), saphenofemoral junction (J), and proximal great saphenous vein (S). A superior tributary is seen draining to the great saphenous vein, just proximal to the junction (arrow). It is often not possible to image the femoral vein distal to the saphenofemoral junction in the same plane.

4 The femoral vein and proximal popliteal vein above the knee should be assessed for patency and competency. They are imaged from a medial thigh position in longitudinal section. The femoral and popliteal veins lie deep to their respective arteries when imaged from this position.

5 The GSV is then followed in transverse section across the knee along the medial aspect of the calf to ankle. Assessment of the superficial foot veins, comprising the dorsal arch and medial and lateral marginal veins, is not normally necessary. These veins are the anatomic origins of the GSV and SSV. It is common to see large tributaries dividing from the main trunk of

the GSV in the calf. Posteromedial varicose tributaries of the GSV in the upper calf sometimes interconnect to the SSV system in the posterior calf, causing SSV incompetence below this level (Fig. 13.25). The GSV and its major tributaries are then assessed in a longitudinal section using distal compression to augment flow. However, the varicose veins may be so obvious in the calf that little time needs to be spent on assessing the GSV at this level if it is the supply to the varicose areas. The GSV can also supply varicose areas on the lateral aspect of the calf, via incompetent tributaries that run over the front of the shin. There is considerable debate about the need to examine all calf perforators by duplex, and whether this is done may depend upon local protocols. In many cases perforators connect to side branches of the GSV and not to the main trunk.

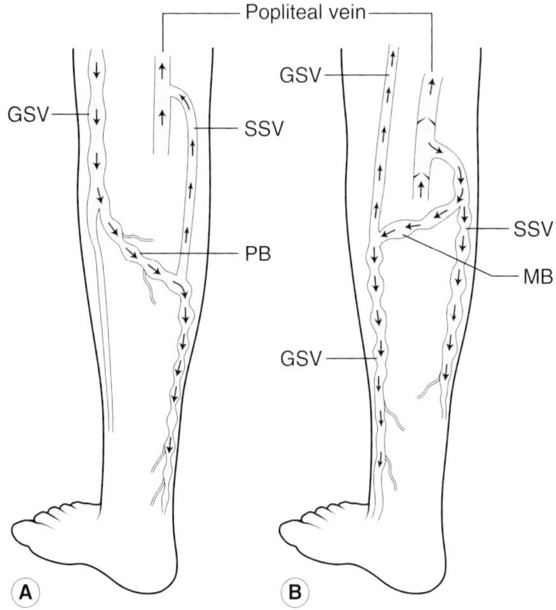

Figure 13.25 • (A) Posterior varicose branches (PB) of the great saphenous vein may interconnect to the small saphenous vein (SSV) distribution in the posterior calf, causing SSV incompetence below the point of communication. ↑, competent veins; ↓, incompetent veins. (B) Medial varicose branches (MB) of the SSV can interconnect to the great saphenous vein (GSV) in the calf, leading to segmental GSV incompetence.

6 The popliteal vein above and below the knee is examined from the popliteal fossa and assessed for patency and competency. The popliteal vein lies superficial to the popliteal artery when imaged from the popliteal fossa. Some clinicians request an assessment of the gastrocnemius veins. The investigation then continues with an assessment of the SSV.

Assessment of the SSV

Preoperative marking of the position of the saphenopopliteal junction

The position of the saphenopopliteal junction can be marked preoperatively with the aid of duplex scanning, because of its highly variable position. Some surgeons ask for a mark to be made on the skin corresponding to the position of the junction. However, others prefer a mark over the small saphenous vein just distal to the junction, so that the vein can be identified and followed back to the junction. Alternatively, a cross can be placed over the junction with a line drawn indicating the path of the small saphenous vein to the point where it becomes superficial. It is important for the surgeon and sonographer to agree on a system of marking to avoid any misunderstandings.

1 The SSV is initially easier to locate just below the popliteal fossa in transverse section, where it will be seen lying within the superficial saphenous compartment (Figs 13.4B and 13.26). It is sometimes very small and easy to miss. The SSV is followed proximally into the popliteal fossa in transverse section, where it will be seen to perforate the muscular fascia and run deep to join the popliteal vein at the saphenopopliteal junction. The proximal SSV can curve medially or laterally toward the saphenopopliteal junction (Fig. 13.27). The actual junction can be located on the anterior, medial, lateral, or, occasionally, posterior aspect of the popliteal

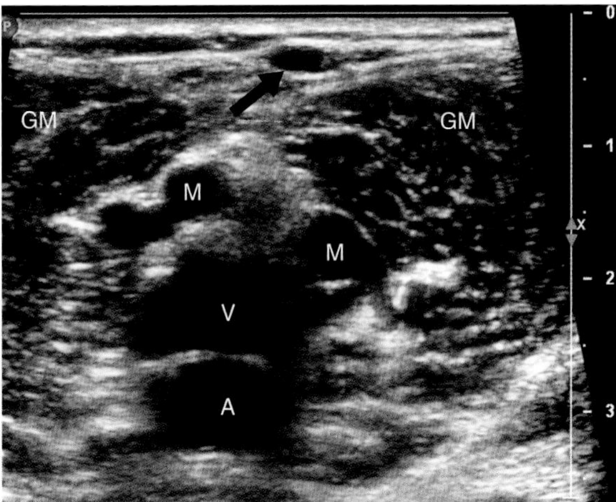

Figure 13.26 • A transverse B-mode image just below the popliteal fossa shows the position of the small saphenous vein (arrow) lying in the superficial, saphenous compartment, with the gastrocnemius muscles (GM) visible. The popliteal vein (V) and muscular veins (M) are seen below the fascia. The popliteal vein lies superficial to the popliteal artery (A) when imaged from this position.

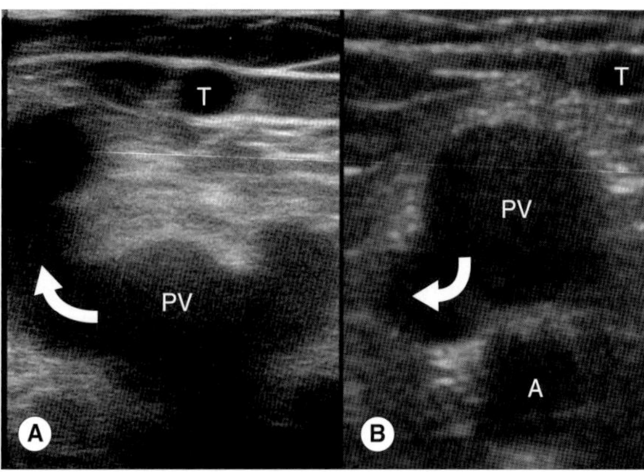

Figure 13.27 • Two transverse images of the right popliteal fossa showing abnormally large saphenopopliteal junctions (arrows). (A) The junction is seen at the 9 o'clock position relative to the popliteal vein (PV). A thigh extension vein (T) is seen in this image. (B) The junction is located in a slightly different position. The popliteal artery (A) is seen in this image. The saphenopopliteal junction can be located in a range of positions with respect to the popliteal vein, although it is more commonly located on the lateral side.

vein when viewed from the popliteal fossa. In some situations, the junction and proximal SSV can be extremely tortuous, with the vein doubling back on itself in a S-shape longitudinally, while following a tortuous path in either the medial or lateral direction. This leads to a very confusing image in which it is even possible to see different sections of the proximal SSV in the same scan plane. Slow, careful movement of the probe should be used to track the vein back to the popliteal vein. It is also possible to mistake tributaries of the gastrocnemius vein for the SSV if they run superficially within the gastrocnemius muscle. Care should be used when identifying the anatomy in this area and it is important to be able to identify the saphenous compartment for correct identification of the SSV. Finally, a large perforator from the popliteal vein, separate from the SSV, can sometimes be found in the popliteal fossa, supplying superficial varicose areas (Fig. 13.28). It is more common for this perforator to be located on the lateral aspect of the popliteal fossa or lower thigh. The varicose veins supplied by the perforator can be completely independent of the SSV, which may be normal throughout its length.

2 The saphenopopliteal junction and proximal SSV are then imaged in longitudinal section (Fig. 13.29). In some cases, the junction is tortuous, and rotation of the probe is required to allow the junction to be visualized. The saphenopopliteal junction and proximal SSV should then be assessed for reflux with a strong calf squeeze. If not already performed previously, the competency of the above- and below-knee popliteal vein should be assessed.

3 As described previously, there is considerable anatomical variation in the position of the saphenopopliteal junction (Figs 13.8 and 13.30). In some cases, it may be

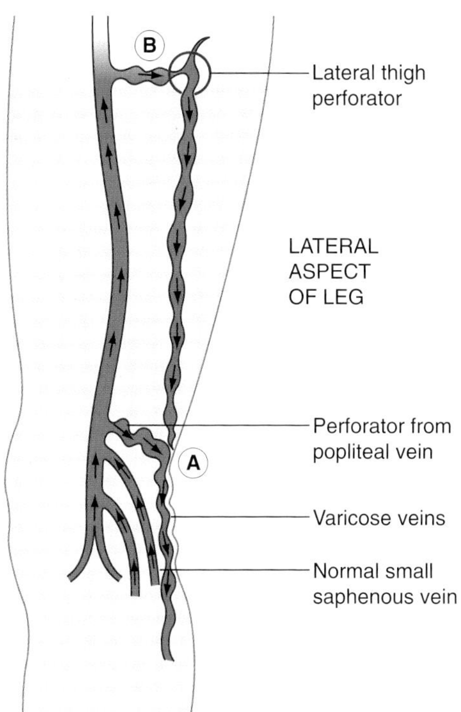

Figure 13.28 • The saphenopopliteal junction and small saphenous vein may be competent but an incompetent perforator dividing from the popliteal vein can supply varicosities in the popliteal fossa and calf, as shown in this diagram (A). Varicose areas on the lateral thigh and calf can also be supplied via upper lateral thigh perforators (B). It is often difficult to trace the perforator to its connection to the deep vein.

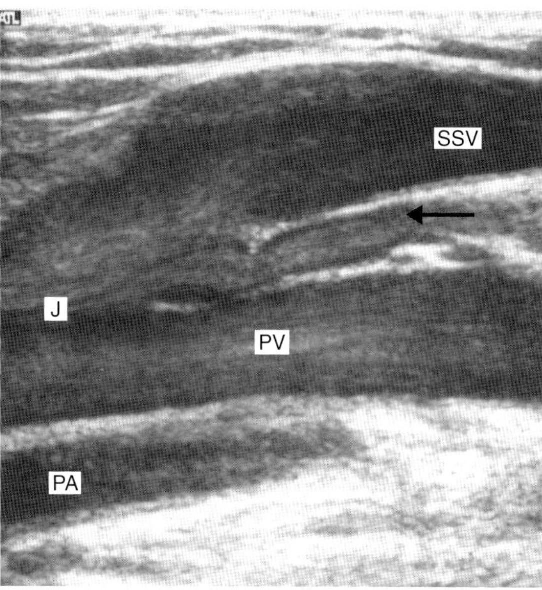

Figure 13.29 • A longitudinal image of the popliteal fossa demonstrating a dilated saphenopopliteal junction and proximal small saphenous vein (SSV). There is a small deep vein (arrow) joining the SSV at the level of the junction (J) to the popliteal vein (PV). The popliteal artery (PA) lies below the vein. It is not always possible to see the junction in this plane or this clearly, especially if it lies to the medial or lateral side of the popliteal vein.

impossible to identify, owing to the height of the junction in the posterior thigh. The TE, if present, can be the source of SSV incompetence. In this situation, it is possible to follow the TE, which will be seen to run as a continuation of the SSV, in transverse section up the posterior thigh to its origin, which may be from a number of sources, as shown in Figure 13.8. The Giacomini vein tends to run in a layer of fascia as it courses towards the GSV, which can aid its identification. It is possible to misidentify very superficial posterior thigh branches of the GSV as the Giacomini vein.

4 In transverse section, the SSV is followed distally from the popliteal fossa along the posterior aspect of the calf, to the posterolateral aspect of the ankle. The SSV is then assessed for reflux along its length in longitudinal section. If the vein is small, it is difficult to demonstrate flow during compression. Large perforators can be assessed for competency. Varicose tributaries from the GSV can interconnect to the SSV system. Conversely, medial varicose tributaries of the SSV may also interconnect to the GSV system (Fig. 13.25B). The SSV can also supply varicose areas on the lateral and anterior aspects of the calf via branches. Varicose tributaries of the lateral thigh system can also join the SSV at a variable level, with the SSV being competent proximal to this point.

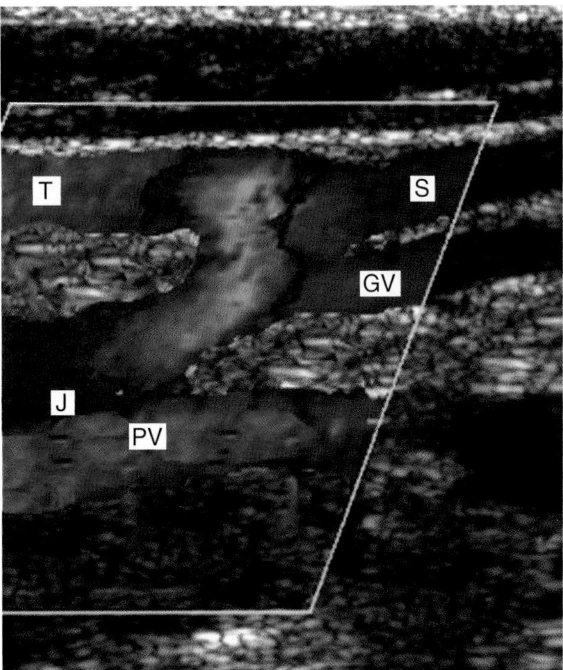

Figure 13.30 • An anatomical variation involving the proximal small saphenous vein (SSV). In this image the SSV (S) continues to run up the posterior thigh as the thigh extension (T). A gastrocnemius vein (GV) also drains to the SSV just proximal to the saphenopopliteal junction (J) forming a common trunk. The popliteal vein (PV) is demonstrated in this image.

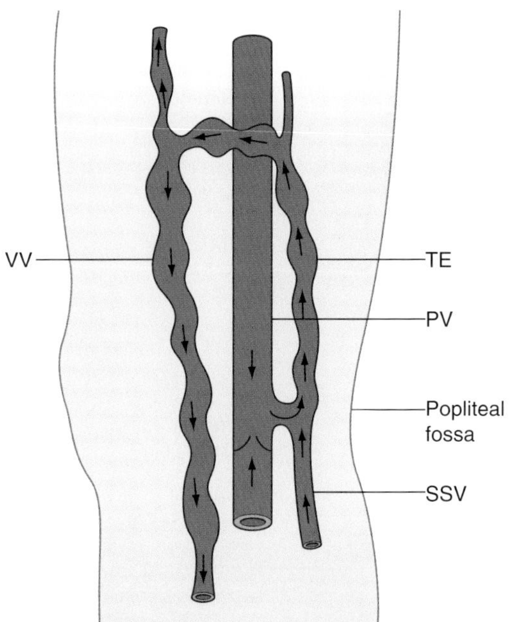

Figure 13.31 • Paradoxical reflux can occur in the thigh extension (TE) vein of the small saphenous vein (SSV) due to incompetence of the saphenopopliteal junction leading to a siphon effect, causing blood to flow up the TE which feeds into the varicose veins (VV).

Concluding the scan

Some varicose veins may lie in more unusual distributions, such as the anterior aspect of the calf or lateral aspect of the thigh. In these situations, it is important to follow the varicose areas proximally in transverse section to identify the supply. The supply is frequently from varicose branches of the GSV or SSV, depending on the location of the varicose areas. One such example is incompetence of the AASV from the SFJ. This vein often supplies varicose areas on the anterior aspect of the thigh and lateral calf. The main proximal trunk of the GSV can be competent or incompetent in this situation. Varicose veins running along the lateral aspect of the thigh and calf can be related to isolated perforators located on the lateral or posterolateral aspect of the upper thigh and buttock (Fig. 13.28). Varicose veins in the lower thigh and calf can be supplied by the TE. In this unusual situation, blood flows in a loop, across an incompetent saphenopopliteal junction and up the TE vein, which then feeds the superficial varicosities running down the leg. This paradoxical situation is similar to a siphon effect, but flow will eventually make its way down into the calf via the incompetent veins, in the correct gravitational direction (Georgiev et al. 2003) (Fig. 13.31). The main trunk of the SSV can be competent or incompetent in this situation. In some patients, it may be impossible to define clearly the source of the varicose veins, especially if they are very small, are diffusely distributed, and generally run into very small superficial tributaries.

Vulval varicosities and pelvic incompetence

Vulval varicosities can develop during pregnancy and most regress after birth. However, persistent vulval varicosities are due to incompetence of the pelvic veins, including the ovarian or internal iliac veins. Vulval varicosities can supply varicose veins in the leg and this source is sometimes overlooked or missed by clinicians. These veins may either render the GSV incompetent or remain isolated from it. The sonographer should always be suspicious of veins that are running towards the inner aspect of the groin, especially if they run behind the adductor longus tendon, which is normally easy to feel. The detailed investigation of ovarian veins requires transvaginal ultrasound scanning and the description is outside the scope of this book. Ovarian and pelvic veins can be treated effectively by coil embolization.

B-mode appearance of varicose veins and perforators

Varicose veins are easy to identify on the B-mode image. They appear as single or multiple dilated tortuous vessels that vary randomly in diameter as the probe is swept across the varicose area (Fig. 13.32). They are superficial and may be located in the thigh as well as the calf. The main trunk supplying varicose areas, such as the GSV in the thigh, may be dilated but often has a reasonably even caliber and is frequently not visible on the skin surface. Occasionally a large localized dilation can be seen in the main trunk, called a varix (Fig. 13.32B). The easiest way of locating perforators is to run the transducer steadily along the trunk of the superficial vein in transverse section. A break in the fascia will be seen on the B-mode image as the perforator runs between the subcutaneous and subfascial areas (Fig. 13.33).

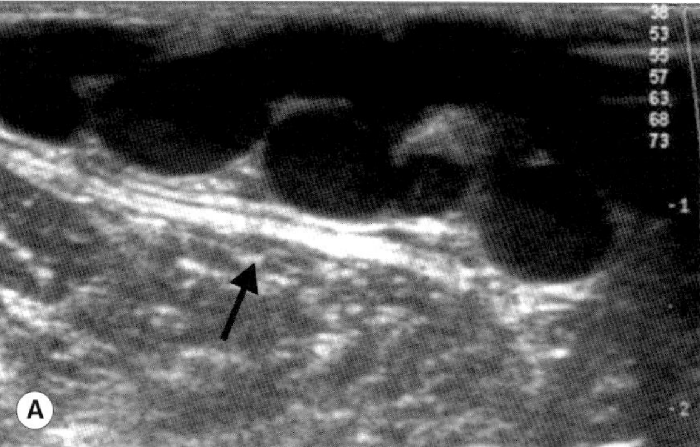

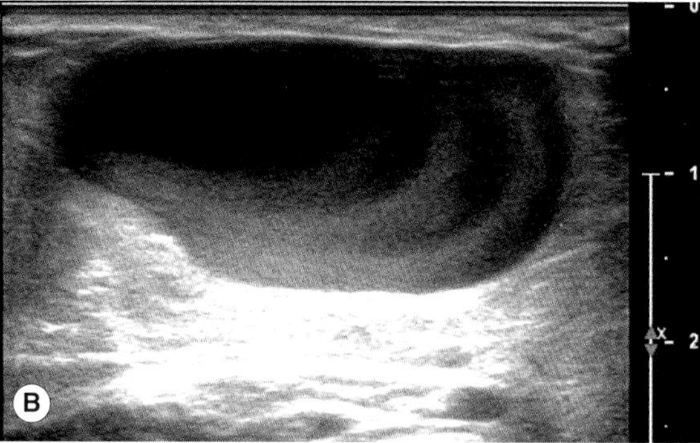

Figure 13.32 • (A) A transverse image of tortuous dilated varicose veins. The muscular fascia is indicated by the arrow. (B) A large varix involving the great saphenous vein.

INVESTIGATION OF RECURRENT VARICOSE VEINS

Some patients develop recurrent varicose veins over a variable time period following surgery. Recurrent varicose veins are veins which have become varicose after the original treatment (Browse et al. 1999). The scanning technique for the investigation of recurrent varicose veins is very similar to that used for the investigation of primary varicose veins. However, it is important to keep an open mind as to the source of the recurrent veins, as their supply can be unpredictable. It is often easier to begin the examination at the level of the varicose areas in transverse section and work proximally to the point of supply. The use of color flow imaging during calf augmentation can allow smaller varicose veins to be followed proximally if the B-mode imaging is poor. Some of the main causes of recurrent varicose veins are summarized below.

Possible causes of GSV recurrences

Incomplete ligation of the saphenofemoral junction

Normally the junction should be ligated and any tributaries divided (Fig. 13.34A). However, due to misidentification or inadequate dissection, it is possible to ligate only a tributary during surgery, rather than the main junction. The level of the SFJ

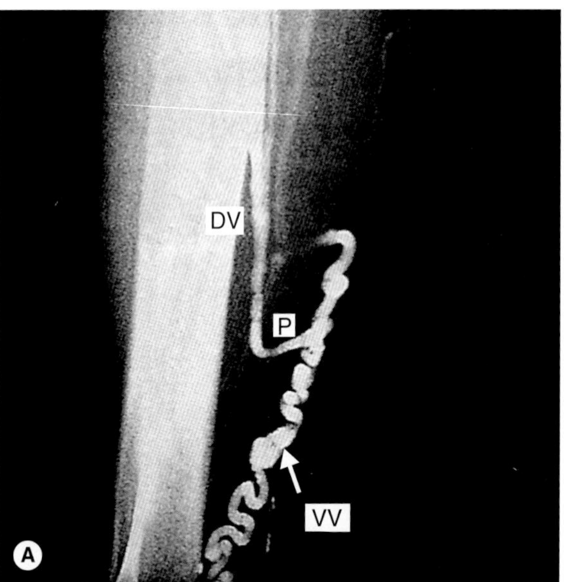

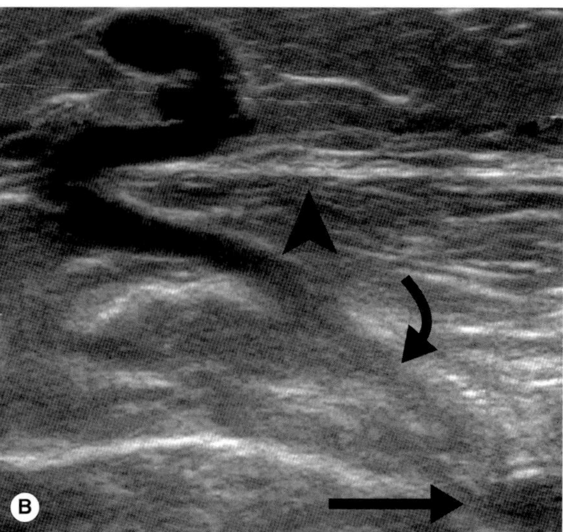

Figure 13.33 • (A) A venogram demonstrating a perforator (P) running between the deep veins (DV) and varicose veins (VV). (B) A B-mode image demonstrating a large perforator. The fascia is demonstrated by the arrowhead, and there is a clear break in the fascia as the perforator runs between the deep and superficial compartments. It may be difficult to display the entire path of a perforator clearly in a single image, as evidenced in this example (curved arrow). The position of the femoral vein is shown by the straight arrow.

should be examined in transverse section, where it is easy to identify a large patent junction. Sometimes the scan demonstrates that the main trunk of the GSV has been ligated just distal to the SFJ but a tributary has been left intact. This tributary then supplies the varicose veins or intact GSV trunk, if the GSV has not been stripped. This is often the case when the AASV is found to be intact at the level of the SFJ. It frequently supplies varicose areas in the anterior and medial aspects of the thigh, which in turn run into the calf (Fig. 13.35). Occasionally, there may be a very small recurrent junction that can be difficult to identify without the aid of color flow imaging (Fig. 13.34B).

Incompetent tributaries

In some cases, the SFJ has been ligated, but small tributaries from the inner aspect of the groin or from the lower abdominal wall supply varicose areas in the GSV distribution or the main GSV trunk, if it has not been stripped. These tributaries are often supplied from pudendal, perineal, or superficial epigastric veins. Typically, the scan will demonstrate varicose veins, or an intact trunk if this has not been stripped in the upper thigh, breaking up into small tributaries before disappearing toward the inner aspect of the groin. These tributaries are usually seen as a fine, diffuse web of veins on the color flow image. Sometimes these tributaries may run close to the femoral vein, but no direct connection will be identified (Fig. 13.34C). It is also possible for recurrent varicose veins to be supplied from veins running from the lower abdominal wall.

Neovascularization

It has been suggested that neovascularization or regrowth can occur between the femoral vein and superficial varicose veins at the groin following ligation of the SFJ (Jones et al. 1996). These small veins then supply the GSV, if it had not been stripped, or proximal recurrent varicose veins. Duplex scanning will reveal a diffuse web of small tortuous veins in the groin, with a small connection to the femoral vein that may be impossible to follow without the aid of color flow imaging.

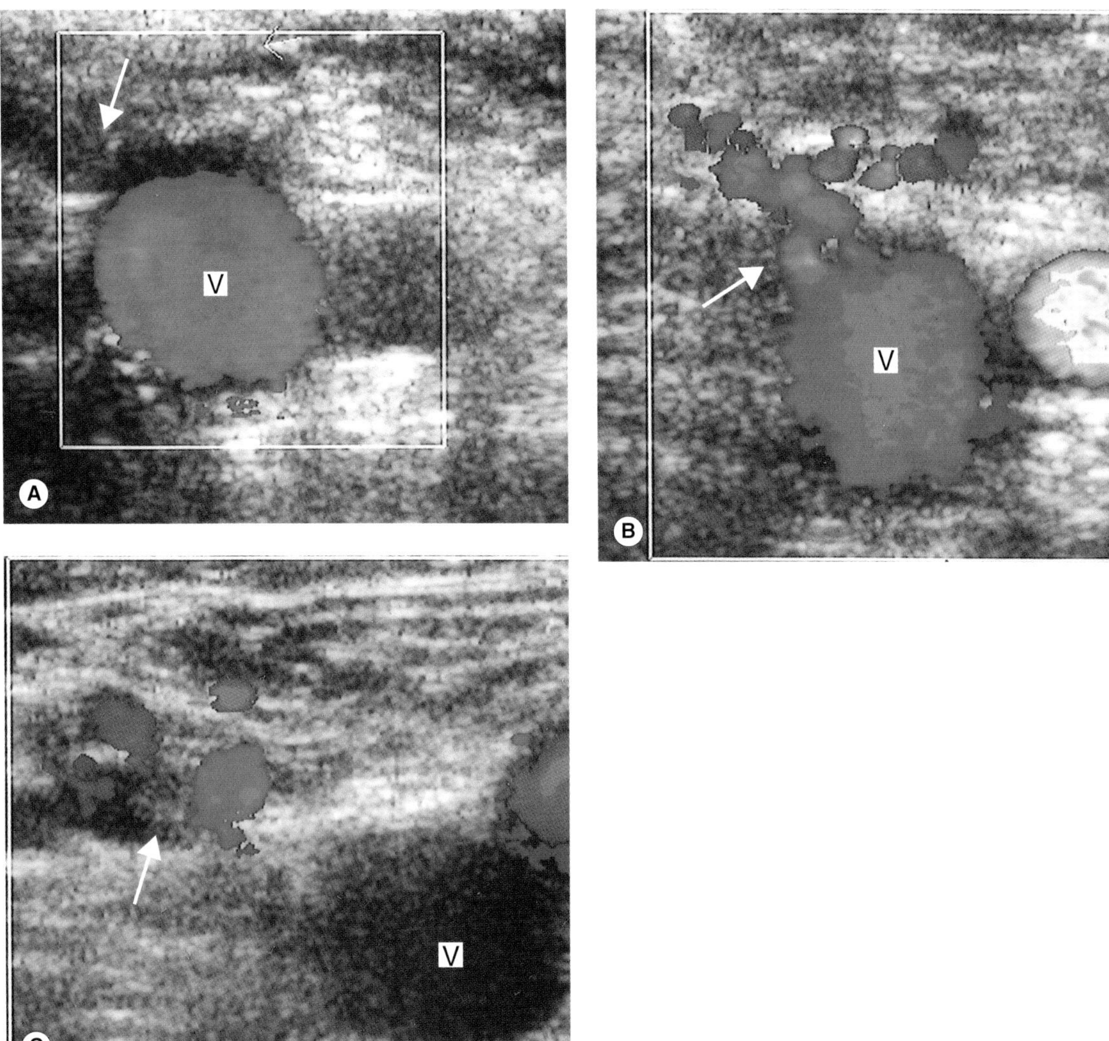

Figure 13.34 • Three examples of ultrasound findings at the level of the saphenofemoral junction following surgery. The femoral vein (V) is seen in all three images. (A) The saphenofemoral junction (arrow) has been completely ligated by surgery. (B) A small recurrent junction (arrow) is seen to supply a diffuse network of small veins. (C) The saphenofemoral junction has been ligated but a diffuse web of small veins is seen adjacent to the vein (arrow).

Thigh or calf perforators

Recurrent varicose veins can be supplied by thigh or calf perforators (Fig. 13.33). Large thigh perforators are relatively easy to identify by following the varicose trunk up the medial thigh in transverse section, where it will be seen to connect directly, or via side branches, to the perforator. Perforators to the deep veins can have very tortuous courses. If a mid-thigh perforator is the main supply to the varicose areas, there may be only small, or no, varicose veins seen above the level of the perforator. Duplex scanning can be used to mark the location of perforators preoperatively.

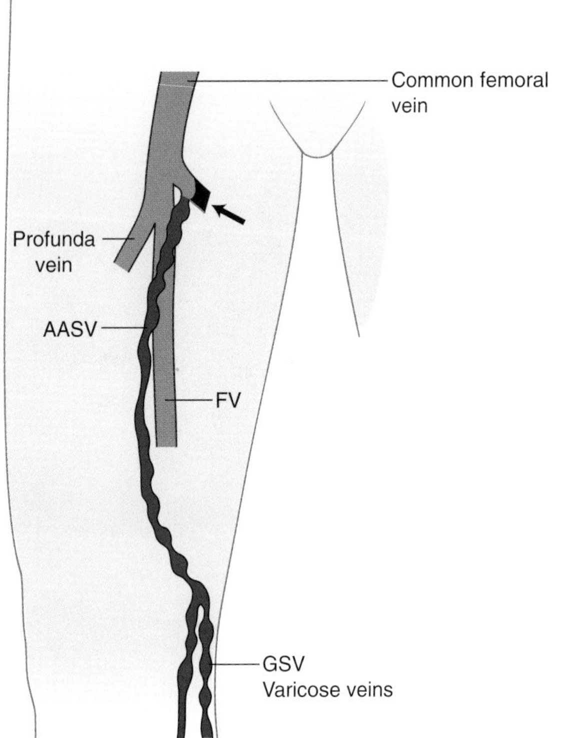

Figure 13.35 • Incomplete ligation of the saphenofemoral junction can be the cause of recurrent varicose veins. In this example the anterior accessory saphenous vein (AASV) has been left intact following incomplete ligation of the junction (arrow). The AASV now supplies the varicose areas shown on the diagram. FV, femoral vein; GSV, great saphenous vein.

Incomplete stripping of the GSV trunk in the thigh

Sometimes the SFJ has been ligated, but the vein stripper has been passed down a tributary of the GSV, leaving the majority of the main trunk intact. The image will demonstrate the presence of an incompetent GSV trunk that breaks into small tributaries toward the groin with a variable supply, as described in some of the examples above.

Incompetence of the SSV

Varicose veins in the GSV distribution of the calf can occur due to incompetence of the SSV. In this situation, posteromedial varicose branches of the SSV interconnect to the GSV distribution (Fig. 13.25B).

Nonidentifiable source

In some instance small diffuse tortuous varicose veins may be present superficially in the GSV distribution and no obvious major source can be located. These veins can be avulsed or treated with sclerotherapy.

Possible causes of SSV recurrences

Incomplete ligation of the saphenopopliteal junction

Recurrence can occur if there has been incomplete ligation or misidentification of the saphenopopliteal junction during surgery. With the transducer in transverse section, the SSV can be followed proximally, where it will be possible to see the saphenopopliteal junction clearly.

Incompetent thigh extension vein or Giacomini vein

In some circumstances a large incompetent TE vein may run directly into the SSV, or varicose areas, at the popliteal fossa. Starting in a transverse section just below the popliteal fossa, the SSV is identified and followed proximally. The saphenopopliteal junction should not be seen if it has been correctly ligated. However, the SSV continues to course up the posterior thigh as the TE. The TE vein can have a variable supply, as described previously.

Incompetent perforators

These perforators may arise from variable positions and can be found above the popliteal fossa, at the popliteal fossa, or arising from the gastrocnemius and soleal veins. Perforators arising in the region of the popliteal fossa can follow very tortuous routes. Perforators supplying varicose areas in the SSV distribution are easiest to identify in transverse section.

GSV incompetence

Varicose veins in the SSV distribution can occur due to GSV incompetence. Incompetent posterior veins in the GSV distribution, which are not prominent on the skin surface, may run into the SSV system in the upper posterior calf, where the veins become more prominent. The surgeon performing the original surgery may have assumed that these varicose veins were related to saphenopopliteal junction incompetence and ligated the junction, but in fact the SSV was competent above the point of communication between the GSV and the SSV. Therefore, ligation of the saphenopopliteal junction will not have controlled the varicose veins (Fig. 13.25A).

Diffuse varicosities in the popliteal fossa

Diffuse varicosities distinct from the saphenopopliteal junction or SSV may resupply the SSV. In this situation, although the saphenopopliteal junction has been ligated, the SSV trunk is supplied by numerous small superficial tributaries that are difficult to follow to any major source.

ASSESSMENT OF PATIENTS WITH SKIN CHANGES AND VENOUS ULCERATION

Many patients with venous ulcers have never had varicose vein surgery, whereas others may have had a number of previous operations. However, the basic technique for assessing patients with venous ulceration is similar to the technique for the assessment of varicose veins. Many patients are elderly and are unable to stand during the examination, but the leg should be in a dependent position to assess for reflux. This is best achieved by hanging the leg over the side of the examination table with the feet resting on a stool. It is necessary to remove any pressure or compression dressings, as these may reduce venous reflux, leading to false results. Patients with venous ulceration are more likely to have deep venous incompetence or obstruction than patients with simple varicose veins. Therefore, it is important to assess the deep veins carefully. It is often easier to start the scan by examining the popliteal vein from the popliteal fossa, as many surgeons will not perform superficial surgery if there is gross reflux in the popliteal vein above and below the knee, and a less detailed scan of the superficial vein system may be required.

There are a number of problems associated with the assessment of patients with venous ulcers. It can be difficult to image the deep veins in obese patients with large legs. In this situation, it may be worth trying a low-frequency abdominal transducer to image the deep veins. Sometimes the calf is too ulcerated or sore to perform calf compression for the assessment of reflux. In such cases, try squeezing the upper portion of the calf, where there may be less ulceration or skin change. If in doubt, warn the patient that the test could be uncomfortable, as many patients are willing to cooperate but may be distressed if no prior warning of discomfort is given. In rare cases, some analgesia may be required. It can be difficult to assess the competency of veins in patients with continuous high-volume flow (hyperemic flow) in the superficial and deep veins due to infection. The high-volume flow toward the heart can lead to a reduction in reflux duration (Fig. 13.36). Under

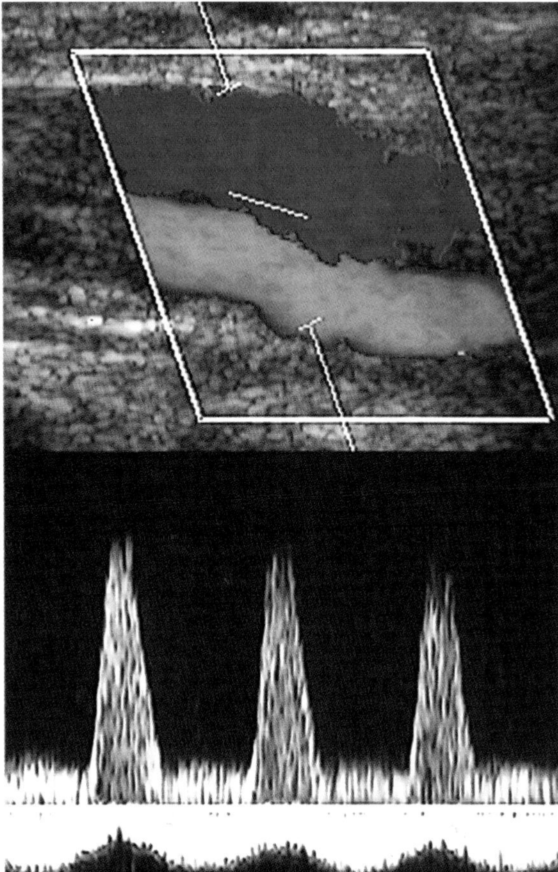

Figure 13.36 • An example of hyperemic flow patterns in the superficial femoral artery and femoral vein due to infection in the lower leg. The arterial signal, above the baseline, demonstrates high-volume flow throughout the cardiac cycle. There is continuous high-volume flow in the vein, shown below the baseline.

these circumstances it is very difficult to examine the function of the veins, but it may be an indication that the leg is infected. Appropriate action, such as antibiotic therapy and leg elevation, may need to be taken to reduce the infection or cellulitis. The leg can be reassessed when the hyperemia subsides. In contrast, it can be difficult to generate flow or reflux in some immobile patients with edema.

ENDOVENOUS ABLATION OF VARICOSE VEINS

EVLT and RFA of varicose veins are minimally invasive catheter-based techniques that can avoid the need for open surgery and vein stripping (Fig. 13.37). Both systems use heat to destroy the vein but different methods are used to generate the heat. The treatment procedure is similar for EVLT and RFA, with the tip of the catheter positioned just below the relevant junction, usually the SFJ or saphenopopliteal junction. The injection of large amounts of diluted local anesthetic solution (tumescent anesthesia), to surround the length of the vein, protects perivenous tissue from heat damage by acting as a heat sink once heating is activated. The tumescence also reduces the vein diameter by compression, removing blood and ensuring better contact between the vein wall and catheter and more efficient transfer of energy or heat. The catheter is then withdrawn at a predetermined rate to destroy the vein. Specialized stylet-type catheters are also available to treat perforators.

Technology

Introduction

Medical devices and accessories are undergoing constant development and refinement and for this reason we are not providing detailed specification of catheters or accessories, as this is beyond the remit of this book. For comprehensive information

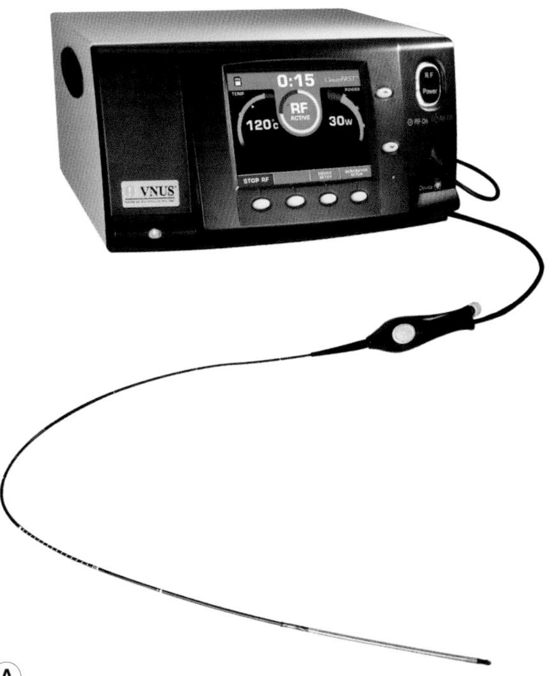

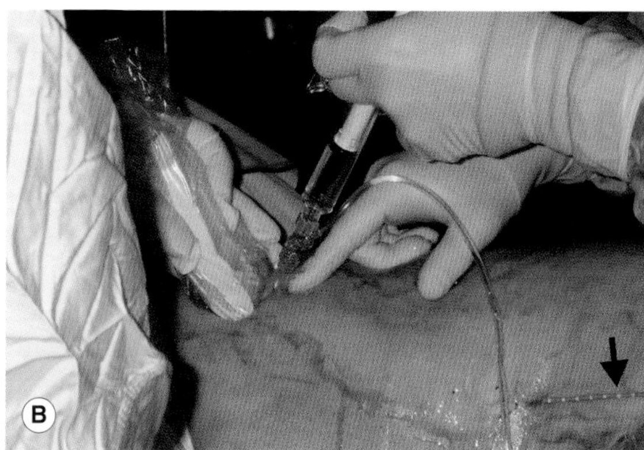

Figure 13.37 • Examples of endovenous technology and treatment. (A) A VNUS ClosureFAST radiofrequency catheter and VNUS RFG Plus radiofrequency (courtesy of VNUS Medical Technologies). (B) Injection of tumescence under ultrasound guidance. The sheath and its markings are clearly shown in this image (arrow).

concerning equipment, accessories, and device-specific protocols (catheter pullback speeds, etc.) the reader should contact the appropriate manufacturer.

Radiofrequency ablation

A radiofrequency generator delivers high-frequency alternating electromagnetic energy (radiofrequency) to the electrodes located at the end of the catheter. There is a central electrode surrounded by an outer group of collapsible electrodes or tufts that make contact with the vein wall. The radio waves do not conduct the heat but it is the resistance to these waves in the surrounding tissue, causing excitement of the molecules in the tissue, that causes resistive heating. The injection of tumescence anesthesia to collapse the vein ensures good contact between the vein wall and outer electrodes. The vein is typically heated to 85 °C and a thermocouple in the tip allows for accurate monitoring and automatic maintenance of this temperature. The heat induces venous spasm and collagen shrinkage, damaging the vein wall, leading to occlusion. Catheter pullback speeds are relatively slow compared with laser, which heats the vein to a much higher temperature. However, a new RFA catheter has been introduced that has an active element length of 7 cm, allowing for rapid treatment of sequential segments, and it is possible that this will supersede the original design (Dietzek 2007).

Endovenous laser therapy

Laser (light amplification by stimulated emission of radiation) creates high-energy bundled light that is monochromatic (all one wavelength) and releases direct thermal energy that heats both the blood and adjacent vein wall, causing destruction of the cells in the vein wall (van den Bos et al. 2008). The tip reaches temperatures in the region of 800 °C. The use of tumescence to compress the vein increases the contact surface area. The term fluence refers to the total amount of energy applied per unit area and is measured in J/cm^2. The laser energy delivered to the vein depends, amongst other factors, on the output setting of the device and the pullback speed of the catheter. The quicker the pullback speed, the less energy is delivered to the surface area of the vein. The energy produced by the laser is sufficient to vaporize the blood, creating bubbles that can be seen on the ultrasound image.

Ultrasound equipment

Almost all modern ultrasound scanners used for imaging peripheral venous disease should be suitable for guiding endovenous procedures. This also includes most portable scanners, providing they have a large enough screen. Typically, flat linear array transducers with a frequency in the range of 5–12 MHz are suitable for guidance, providing good images of wires and catheters. High-frequency probes can provide excellent resolution of the main superficial venous trunks but may provide suboptimal images of the SFJ or saphenopopliteal junction in larger patients and in certain cases could lead to problems in the precise positioning of the catheter tip relative to a junction. To ensure sterility of the procedure, the transducer can be placed in a sterile probe cover containing ultrasound gel with a sterile sleeve covering the transducer cable.

The procedure

A video showing key ultrasound images of the procedure is included on the DVD. A pretreatment scan should have been performed to ensure the veins are suitable for endovenous treatment. In most cases, the main trunk of the GSV or SSV is treated but it is possible to treat other veins providing they fulfill treatment criteria (Table 13.3). The following detailed description is for EVLT treatment of the GSV.

The patient should be in a supine position on the treatment table. Prior to vein puncture, the GSV should be scanned to identify the optimum site for catheter access. Ideally for the GSV, this is around the knee level where the vein is usually superficial and nerve injury is less likely to occur. It is also useful to image the SFJ to ensure that good images of the junction can be obtained. This also allows the operator to optimize the gray-scale image controls for guiding the procedure. As the procedure is commenced, the operating table is tilted in a foot-down position to distend the vein for easier identification and puncture of the vein. For patients undergoing a local anesthetic procedure, some local anesthetic can be injected into the skin at the

The main inclusion and exclusion criteria can include the following, although these may change with technological development:
INCLUSION CRITERIA
• Primary or recurrent truncal varicosities without significant tortuousity • Veins >2 mm in diameter but preferably > 3 mm • Treatable length of at least 10–12 cm
EXCLUSION CRITERIA
• Very small veins <2 mm diameter • Tortuous veins • Grossly dilated veins • Veins containing acute thrombophlebitis • Chronic scarring due to previous thrombophlebitis • Patients with acute deep-vein thrombosis

Table 13.3

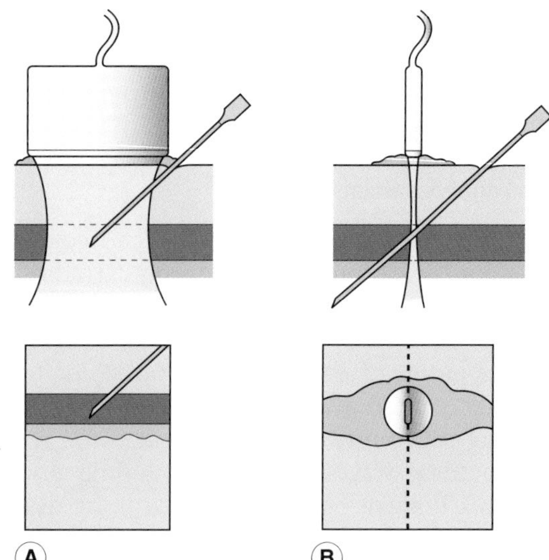

Figure 13.38 • Schematic diagrams of venous cannulation which can be performed in the longitudinal (A) and transverse imaging planes (B). The disadvantage of the transverse plane is that the needle tip may be out of plane and lie deeper than suspected from the image, as shown by the dashed parts of the line.

region of the puncture site. The vein is then cannulated under ultrasound guidance. This can be performed using transverse or longitudinal imaging of the vein, as shown in Figure 13.38, and depends on personal preference. The advantage of longitudinal imaging is that the tip and shaft of the cannula can be seen within the image once the cannula is in alignment with the vein. Using transverse imaging, it is possible that the cannula may be inserted too deep, with the tip lying below the vein, but the ultrasound image may show an oblique image of a short section of the shaft close to the vein, giving the false impression that this represents the tip (Fig. 13.38). However, the transverse plane is sometimes easier to use if the vein is lying in a very superficial position.

When the needle tip makes contact with the vein, it will cause an indentation of the vein wall and at this point slightly more pressure is applied to the needle to pierce the wall.

Once the vein has been cannulated, a guide wire is then passed into the vein. The wire is advanced so that it runs across the SFJ. The passage of the guide wire is followed by ultrasound. It is not uncommon for the wire to loop or snag, especially in dilated or tortuous areas of the vein. Local external compression or 'stretching' of the vein with fingers will usually solve this problem and facilitate passage of the guide wire. The introducing cannula is then removed and a flexible sheath passed over the guide wire and advanced across or to the level of the SFJ. The sheath has markings every centimeter to enable accurate pullback speed when the laser is activated (Fig 13.37B). Some sheaths have a pre-dilator with a sharp tip to increase rigidity and improve venous access. Manufacturers have also produced sheath tips that are loaded with tungsten or ceramic material to make imaging easier.

The guide wire and pre-dilator are then removed. The sheath should be in a position so that it is approximately 2–4 cm distal to the junction as seen on a longitudinal ultrasound image. The laser fiber is then inserted into the sheath. The laser fiber has a locking device so that it can be inserted to the correct length and will be seen to project 2 cm beyond the sheath tip (Fig. 13.39C). It is absolutely essential to confirm that the laser tip extends beyond the end of the sheath, otherwise the end of the sheath will be transected once the laser is

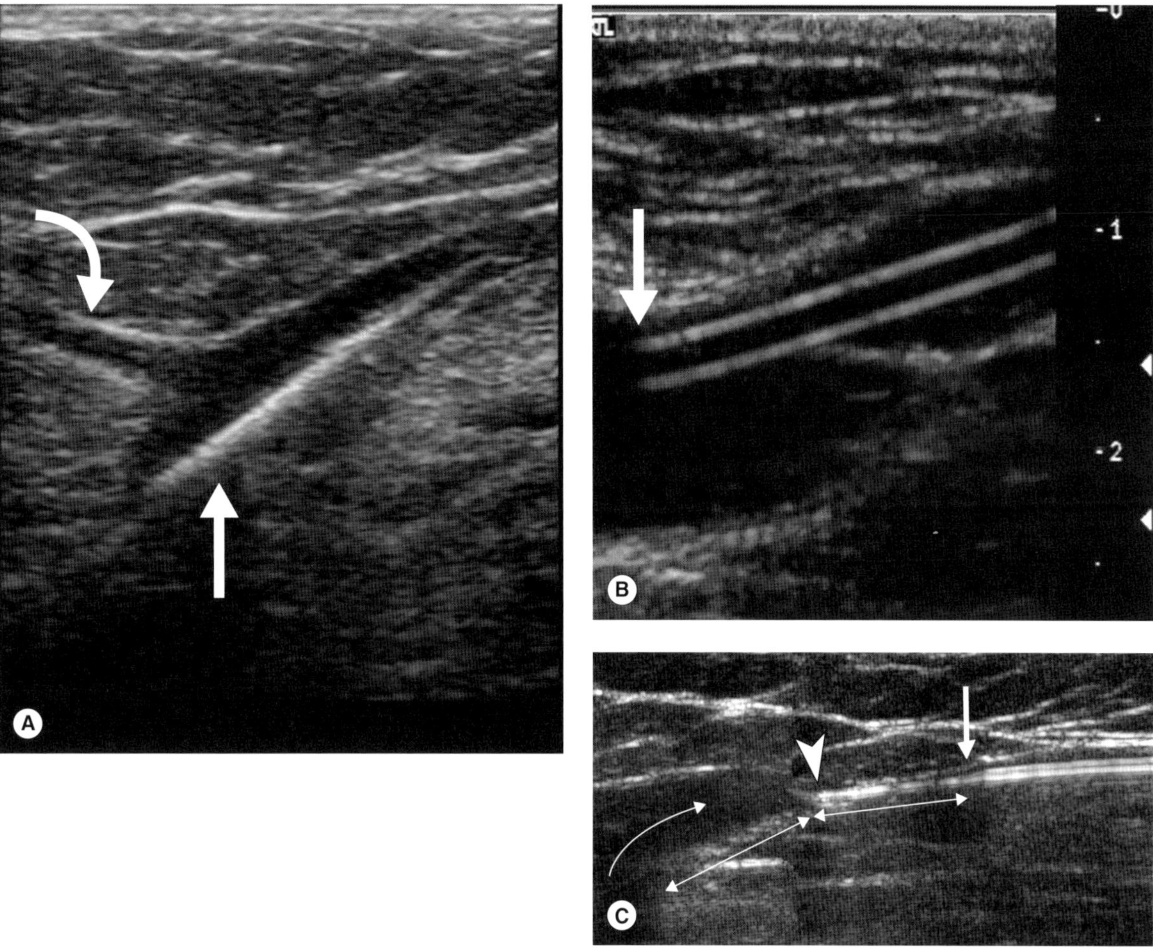

Figure 13.39 • Examples of endovenous wires and catheters. (A) A guide wire is seen within the great saphenous vein (GSV) and across the saphenofemoral junction (SFJ: straight arrow). Note the superficial epigastric vein (curved arrow). The laser or radiofrequency catheter tip should be placed distal to this tributary (see text). (B) The sheath tip is clearly seen (arrow). (C) A laser catheter has been positioned below the SFJ. The tip (arrowhead) can be seen protruding 2 cm beyond the sheath. The small step indicating the end of the sheath is visible (straight arrow). The curved arrow runs through the center of the GSV from the SFJ towards the laser tip. The double-headed lines indicate 2 cm distance.

activated and will remain in the patient. The laser tip also has a red guide light that should be visible through the skin in nonobese patients.

The next important stage is to position the laser tip so that it lies 2 cm from the SFJ, as seen on longitudinal imaging, by gently withdrawing or advancing the sheath. It is advantageous to do this before the injection of tumescence, as imaging of the junction can be more difficult once the tumescence has infiltrated the tissues in this area. Some clinicians place the tip slightly closer to the junction or just distal to the junction of the superficial epigastric vein, which is normally the first tributary of the SFJ (Fig. 13.39A). Theoretically this preserves flow at the junction and prevents thrombus extending from the GSV across the junction.

The operating table is now placed into a head-down (Trendelenburg) position to empty the vein

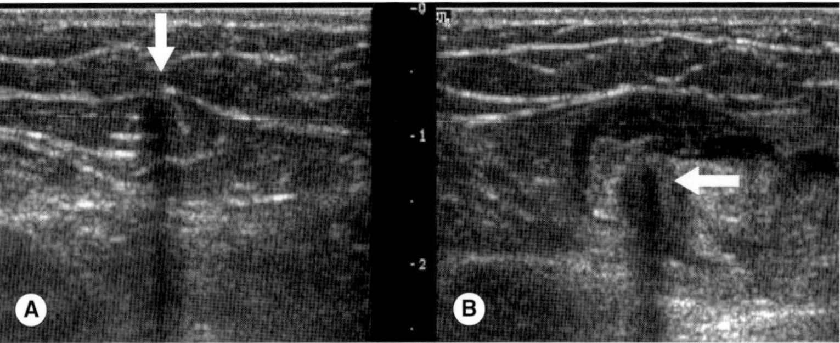

Figure 13.40 • (A) An image of the great saphenous vein before injection of tumescence. The position of the great saphenous vein is seen below the arrow. An acoustic shadow is seen in the image due to the laser catheter within the vein. (B) Injection of tumescence fluid has dilated the saphenous compartment. The vein position is shown by the arrow.

of blood, providing better contact between the laser tip and vein wall and allowing more efficient transfer of heat to damage the vein wall. The next phase of the procedure involves the injection of tumescence, normally saline containing local anesthetic, in the perivenous space along the length of the vein (Fig. 13.40). The tumescence has four main functions. Firstly, it provides cooling and offers some perivascular tissue protection against heating or burns. Secondly, it provides pain relief. Thirdly, the vein tends to collapse, removing blood and improving surface contact between the laser and vein wall. Finally, injection of the tumescence will 'sink' the position of superficial veins relative to the skin surface, to ensure that there is at least 1 cm between the vein and the skin surface to avoid skin burns. Superficial veins which often sit above the saphenous compartment may require a substantial amount of tumescence to achieve this. The tumescence is delivered by a series of punctures along the length of the vein under transverse ultrasound imaging (Fig 13.37B).

The GSV usually lies in the saphenous compartment, which has a layer of fascia superficial to the vein and it is important to penetrate this layer of fascia with the needle tip so that the anesthetic fluid enters the saphenous compartment. Starting distally, the needle tip is advanced so that the tip is adjacent to the vein and then the solution is injected so that there is obvious splaying of the perivenous tissues, indicating that the vein is surrounded by a cuff of fluid. The tumescnce will tend to diffuse more with veins that lie superficial to the saphenous compartment. The syringe can be discharged a number of times using the same puncture so that fluid tracks along the perivenous space around the vein to avoid too many injections, especially if the procedure is being performed under local anesthetic. Once the vein is surrounded by tumescence the position of the laser tip can be rechecked to ensure it has not become accidentally displaced.

Finally, the laser is activated and the catheter withdrawn at an appropriate speed to destroy the vein. Ultrasound can be used to follow the catheter pullback, although this is not usually necessary. The energy supplied to the laser tip also heats the surrounding blood and this can be clearly seen as echogenic areas. It is very common to see streaming of echogenic reflections moving proximally towards the common femoral vein. This probably represents steam bubbles and may appear disconcerting when first seen. The length of the vein is treated down to a few centimeters above the puncture site and finally the sheath and laser are withdrawn. Ultrasound can then be used to ensure the patency of the common femoral vein. Finally, some compression bandaging is applied to the leg, normally for a number of days.

The main complications of the procedure are shown in Table 13.4. The most serious procedural complication involves misidentification of

PROCEDURAL	COMMENT
Inability to cannulate vein	May be due to spasm or inexperience. If spasm occurs, the vein may need to be punctured above the original puncture site
Vein spasm	Can make passage of the sheath difficult
Incorrect placement of catheter tip	Rare and can be avoided by following protocols
POST-PROCEDURE	
Excessive pain	Usually resolves with analgesia
Skin burns	Rare
Recanalization of vein	
Deep-vein thrombosis	
Thrombophlebitis	

Table 13.4 Complications associated with endovenous ablation

anatomy leading to the placement of the tip in the wrong position or even a deep vein. In addition the treatment tip must always extend beyond the sheath tip.

The treatment of the SSV is the same as the procedure described above but the anatomy is far more variable and care should be used in the positioning of the tip of the catheter. There is some evidence that deep-vein thrombosis is more likely to be associated with the treatment of a SSV that drains directly to the saphenopopliteal junction with no other tributaries, unlike the saphenofemoral junction where flow in the superficial inferior epigastric vein or other tributaries can maintain patency of the SFJ (Fig. 13.41). It has also been suggested that greater volumes of tumescence may be required during ablation of the SSV to prevent any thermal injury to the sural nerve, which is in close proximity to the vein. It is also possible to treat incompetence of the Giacomini vein with endovenous techniques.

Radiofrequency treatment

The ultrasound guidance follows a similar pattern to that described for EVLT but a shorter introducer sheath is used. The primary difference is the appearance of the RFA catheter tip. However, a new radiofrequency catheter that does not include a tuft of outer electrodes has recently been introduced, which is shown in Figure 13.37A.

Follow-up

Data on the effectiveness of endovenous ablation suggest good outcomes with low recanalization rates and high patient satisfaction. A randomized trial comparing EVLT with surgery has indicated comparable results but an earlier return to normal activity following EVLT (Darwood et al. 2008). Ultrasound is the ideal modality for follow-up to assess outcomes and complications (Fig. 13.41). Potential complications are show in Table 13.4.

FOAM SCLEROTHERAPY

The foam is formed by mixing liquid sclerosant with air using two syringes linked by a three-way

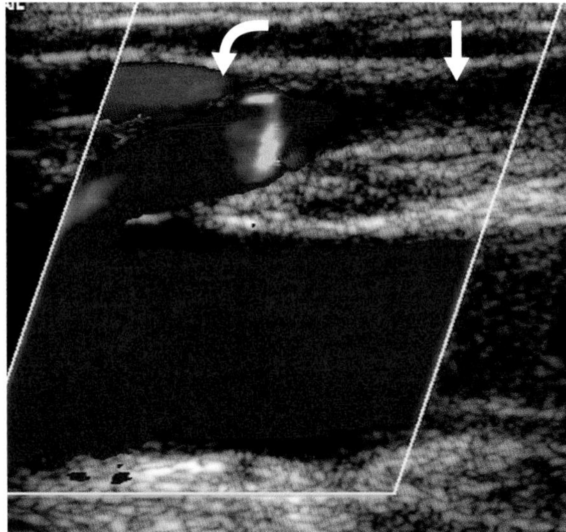

Figure 13.41 • The appearance of the saphenofemoral junction after successful endovenous treatment. The great saphenous vein is occluded (arrow). The saphenofemoral junction remains patent due to flow entering from a preserved superficial epigastric tributary (curved arrow).

tap. Foam sclerotherapy can be used to treat varicose veins and the main trunks of the GSV and SSV. The injection of foam displaces the blood and causes damage to the endothelium of the vein wall and subsequent fibrosis and occlusion. Ultrasound can be used to guide the cannulation and injection of the foam into the appropriate superficial veins. Many surgeons elevate the leg before injecting the foam to empty the vein. The progress of the foam can be monitored with ultrasound during the injection. The foam can be milked along the vein with the aid of the transducer. Ultrasound compression of the saphenofemoral or saphenopopliteal junction is often used to prevent the foam entering the deep system. In practice, it is not infrequent to see some foam that has entered the deep venous system via perforators, but this will be rapidly diluted.

OTHER DISORDERS OF THE VENOUS SYSTEM

Superficial thrombphlebitis

Superficial thrombophlebitis is an inflammatory process that involves the superficial veins (see Ch. 14). The superficial vein may become partially or fully thrombosed. Typically, the area around the phlebitis is reddened, tender, and hot, and the superficial vein may be swollen and hard. Phlebitis is normally treated with analgesia and anti-inflammatory drugs, but superficial vein stripping or saphenofemoral or saphenopopliteal junction ligation may be required.

Klippel–Trenaunay syndrome (KTS)

KTS is a congenital condition and consists of a range of abnormalities that can involve the skin capillaries, often causing nevi (birthmarks or port-wine stains), bone and soft-tissue hypertrophy (excessive limb growth) and venous varicosities. Each case of KTS is unique, and often only one limb is affected, but other areas of the body may also be involved. Abnormalities of the venous system range in severity (Browse et al. 1999). Visible varicose veins vary from very minor to severe and can be widely distributed throughout the leg. Varicosities are commonly seen on the lateral aspect of the thigh and calf. In some cases of KTS, the deep veins may be abnormal. Abnormalities can include absence of parts of the deep venous system, unusually small deep veins, or large, dilated deep veins with nonfunctioning valves. It is therefore very important to scan the deep venous system in all patients with KTS to detect any deep venous abnormalities, before treating any large superficial varicosities by surgery (Eifert et al. 2000).

Venous hemangioma

Venous malformations can occur anywhere in the body and consist of an abnormal network of veins. Venous hemangiomas vary in size and can be very extensive. They can occur in the superficial tissues, muscles, or organs. They can cause pain and swelling and may be disfiguring when they are superficial. Duplex scanning can be useful for imaging venous malformations to exclude evidence of arteriovenous fistulas, but it can be difficult to define the full extent of the lesion, especially if it is deep or involves joints. When imaging very superficial lesions, it is important not to apply too much pressure with the transducer, as this may occlude the veins. Other imaging techniques, such as magnetic resonance imaging, are often used to investigate the extent of the malformation, especially if it is diffusely distributed in muscles.

REPORTING

Duplex assessment of varicose veins is a dynamic technique, and it can be difficult to demonstrate this quality on hard copy, although recordings of reflux patterns, as seen on the spectral Doppler display, may be useful. It is therefore easier to provide a functional map of the venous system, as shown in Figure 13.42. The superficial veins can be drawn on to the diagram, and black arrows pointing toward the heart indicate normal competent veins. Red arrows pointing toward the feet indicate venous reflux. This diagram can be accompanied by a brief report outlining any limitations of the scan. This type of report is easy for the surgeon to interpret in a busy outpatient clinic and is also useful to show to the patient, as it provides a clear explanation of the problem.

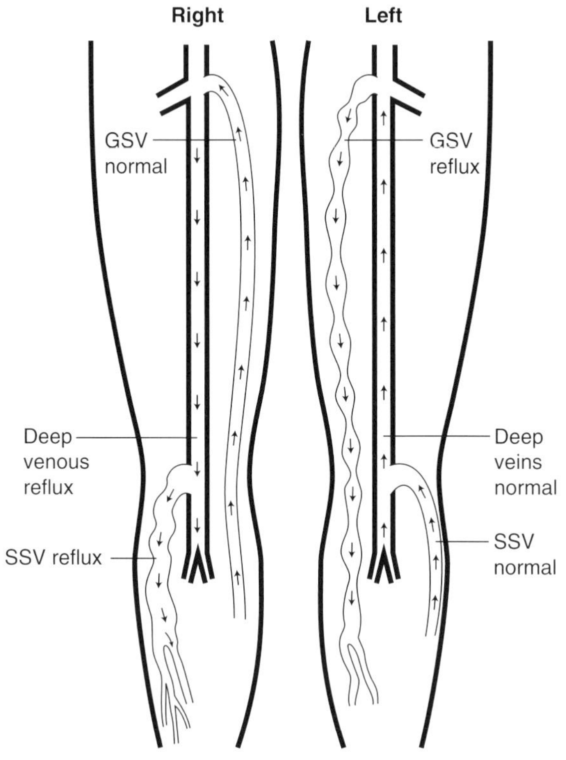

Figure 13.42 • The use of diagrams makes it easier for the clinician to interpret the findings of a venous duplex examination (see text). GSV, Great saphenous vein; SSV, small saphenous vein.

References

Abu-Own A, Scurr J H, Coleridge Smith P D 1994 Saphenous vein reflux without incompetence at the saphenofemoral junction. British Journal of Surgery 81: 1452–1454

Browse N, Burnand K G, Irvine A T et al. 1999 Diseases of the veins, 2nd edn. Arnold, London, pp 191–248

Caggiati A, Bergan J J, Gloviczki P et al. 2002 Nomenclature of the veins of the lower limbs: an international interdisciplinary consensus statement. Journal of Vascular Surgery 36: 416–422

Caggiati A, Rippa Bonati M, Pieri A et al. 2004 1603–2003: four centuries of valves. European Journal of Vascular and Endovascular Surgery 28: 439–441

Callam M J 1994 Epidemiology of varicose veins. British Journal of Surgery 81: 167–173

Cavezzi A, Labropoulos N, Partsch S et al. 2006 Duplex ultrasound investigation of the veins in chronic venous disease of the lower limbs – UIP consensus document. Part II. Anatomy. European Journal of Vascular and Endovascular Surgery 31: 288–299

Coleridge-Smith P, Labropoulos H, Partsch H et al. 2006 Duplex ultrasound investigation of the venous disease of the lower limbs – UIP consensus document. Part I. Basic principles. European Journal of Vascular and Endovascular Surgery 31: 83–92

Darwood R, Theivacumar N, Dellagrammaticas D et al. 2008 Randomized clinical trial comparing endovenous laser ablation with surgery for the treatment of primary great saphenous veins. British Journal of Surgery 95: 294–301

Dietzek A 2007 Endovenous radiofrequency ablation for the treatment of varicose veins. Vascular 15: 255–261

Eifert S, Villavicencio J L, Kao T C et al. 2000 Prevalence of deep venous anomalies in congenital vascular malformations of venous predominance. Journal of Vascular Surgery 31: 462–471

Eklöf B, Rutherford R, Bergan J et al. 2004 Revision of the CEAP classification for chronic venous disorders: consensus statement. Journal of Vascular Surgery 40: 1248–1252

Evans C J, Allan P L, Lee A J et al. 1998 Prevalence of venous reflux in the general population on duplex scanning: the Edinburgh Vein Study. Journal of Vascular Surgery 28: 767–776

Evans C J, Fowkes F G, Ruckley C V et al. 1999 Prevalence of varicose veins and chronic venous insufficiency in men and women in the general population: Edinburgh Vein Study. Journal of Epidemiology and Community Health 53: 149–153

Georgiev M, Myers K A, Belcaro G 2003 The thigh extension of the lesser saphenous vein: from Giacomini's observations to ultrasound scan imaging. Journal of Vascular Surgery 37: 558–563

Jones L, Braithwaite B D, Selwyn D et al. 1996 Neovascularisation is the principal cause of varicose vein recurrence: results of a randomised trial of stripping the long saphenous vein. European Journal of Vascular and Endovascular Surgery 12: 442–445

Labropoulos N, Tiongson J, Pryor L et al. 2003 Definition of venous reflux in lower extremity veins. Journal of Vascular Surgery 38: 793–798

Lambourne L A, Moffatt C J, Jones A C et al. 1996 Clinical audit and effective change in leg ulcer services. Journal of Wound Care 5: 348–351

Magnusson M B, Nelzen O, Risberg B et al. 2001 A colour Doppler ultrasound study of venous reflux in patients with chronic leg ulcers. European Journal of Vascular and Endovascular Surgery 21: 353–360

Ruckley C V, Evans C J, Allan P L et al. 2002 Chronic venous insufficiency: clinical and duplex correlations. The Edinburgh Vein Study of venous disorders in the general population. Journal of Vascular Surgery 36: 520–525

Sarin S, Sommerville K, Farrah J et al. 1994 Duplex ultrasonography for assessment of venous valvular function of the lower limb. British Journal of Surgery 81: 1591–1595

Scriven J M, Hartshorne T, Bell P R et al. 1997 Single-visit venous ulcer assessment clinic: the first year. British Journal of Surgery 84: 334–336

Stuart W P, Adam D J, Allan P L et al. 2000 The relationship between the number, competence, and diameter of medial calf perforating veins and the clinical status in healthy subjects and patients with lower-limb venous disease. Journal of Vascular Surgery 32: 138–143

Van den Bos R, Kockaert M, Neumann H et al. 2008 Technical review of endovenous laser therapy for varicose veins. European Journal of Vascular and Endovascular Surgery 35: 88–95

Walsh J C, Bergan J J, Beeman S et al. 1994 Femoral venous reflux abolished by greater saphenous vein stripping. Annals of Vascular Surgery 8: 566–570

Further reading

Bellard G, Nicolaides A N, Veller M 1995 Venous disorders. W B Saunders, London

Browse N, Burnand K G, Irvine A T et al. 1999 Diseases of the veins, 2nd edn. Arnold, London

Greenhalgh R M (ed.) 1995 Vascular imaging for surgeons. W B Saunders, London

Duplex assessment of deep venous thrombosis and upper-limb venous disorders

14

Tim Hartshorne and David Goss

CONTENTS

INTRODUCTION

Deep venous thrombosis (DVT) is a common disorder that can lead to fatal pulmonary embolism (PE); the combined condition is described as venous thromboembolism (VTE). Duplex scanning is considered to be the method of choice for the imaging of DVT, with other imaging techniques reserved for technically incomplete or difficult duplex examinations. Duplex scanning can be used for serial investigations to monitor the progression and outcome of thrombosis. In addition, duplex scanning can be useful for assessing the long-term damage to veins and valve function as a result of chronic postthrombotic syndrome (Haenen et al. 2002). This can lead to the development of lower-limb venous hypertension and possible leg ulceration. This chapter provides a description of duplex scanning techniques for the diagnosis of DVT and also considers other pathologic conditions that may mimic the symptoms of venous thrombosis.

EPIDEMIOLOGY AND PATHOLOGY OF DVT

DVT usually affects the lower-limb veins, but it can also occur in the upper limbs, especially in conjunction with catheter access or malignancy. The published data on the epidemiology of DVT and PE demonstrate some variability, and reported rates of DVT and thromboembolism appear to be partly dependent upon methods of data collection (autopsy records, discharge diagnoses, and so forth) and the patient population studied. A systematic review by Fowkes et al. (2003) indicated an incidence of DVT in the whole general population of approximately 5 per 10 000 per annum. However, the incidence was highly dependent upon age and increased from 2–3 per 10 000 person years at age 30–49 years to 20 per 10 000 person years at age 70–79 years. Around 40% cases of DVT were found to be idiopathic (of unknown cause). The annual rate of PE is somewhere in the region of 6 cases per 10 000 in the general population (Nicolaides et al. 1994). A review by White (2003) indicated that death occurs in approximately 6% of DVT cases and 12% of PE cases within 1 month of diagnosis. Open or healed venous ulceration occurs in around 1% of the general adult population, with a proportion attributed to postthrombotic syndrome (Fowkes et al. 2001). The early detection and treatment of DVT can therefore reduce the subsequent risk of mortality or long-term morbidity.

Virchow (1846) described the association between thrombosis in the legs and emboli in the lung. The factors predisposing to thrombosis are described by his famous triad of coagulability of the blood, damage to the vein wall or endothelium, and venous stasis. Venous thrombi are believed to originate in valve cusp pockets (Fig. 14.1) or in the deep venous muscular sinuses, such as the soleal veins. DVT most commonly occurs in the calf veins and can propagate to the proximal veins. In the lower limb the popliteal vein is usually described as a proximal vein. It is not necessary for all the calf veins to be affected in order for proximal propagation to occur. It is believed that approximately 10–20% of calf vein thrombi propagate to the deep veins across and above the knee (Khaw 2002; Labropoulos et al. 2002). This is thought to be associated with an increased risk of PE. Isolated thrombosis of the proximal veins, such as the femoral or iliac veins, is less common and can be due to trauma, surgery, pregnancy, or malignancy. Proximal and distal propagation of thrombus can occur in this situation. Venous stasis can also lead to DVT, and this is why patients undergoing periods of bed rest or immobility are at greater risk of developing thrombosis. In fact hospitalized patients with medical illnesses have a similar risk of VTE as those undergoing major general surgery (Anderson & Spencer 2003).

There is evidence to suggest that long-haul air travel is associated with an increased risk; this risk may be low but, as with VTE generally, additional factors increase the risk. The main risk factors associated with the development of venous thrombosis are shown in Box 14.1. In the early stages of a DVT, it is possible for a large proportion of the clot to be nonadherent to the vein wall. This is termed a free-floating thrombus. In this situation there is a

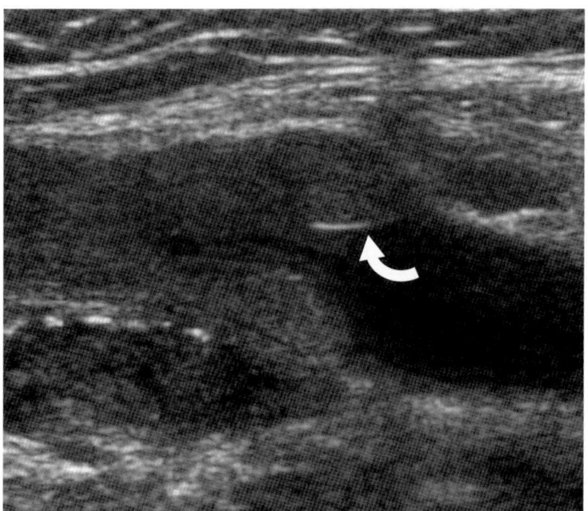

Figure 14.1 • A longitudinal B-mode image of a deep vein. Note the venous stasis above the valve sites. The anterior valve cup is visible in this image (curved arrow).

BOX 14.1 Risk factors for the development of deep venous thrombosis

- Coagulation disorders
- Immobilization
- Surgery and trauma
- Malignancy
- Septicemia
- Oral contraceptives
- Increasing age
- Stroke
- Heart failure
- Previous history of deep vein thrombosis
- Long-haul air travel
- Other long distance travel (such as coach)
- Pregnancy
- Other leg pathology

risk of detachment, leading to PE. As thrombus becomes older (7–10 days), it becomes more organized and adherent to the vein wall.

Signs, symptoms, and treatment of DVT

The symptoms of PE include the following:

- Acute dyspnea (sudden breathlessness)
- Pleuritic chest pain
- Hemoptysis (coughing up blood)
- Right-sided heart failure or cardiovascular collapse.

The clinical diagnosis of DVT is unreliable and inaccurate in up to 50% of cases (Cranley et al. 1976; Beyer & Schellong 2005). However, typical symptoms include the development of acute calf pain associated with localized tenderness, heat, and swelling. The superficial veins may also be dilated. If the thrombosis involves the proximal veins, there may be significant swelling of the calf. Unfortunately, other conditions, such as cellulitis and edema, can mimic the symptoms of DVT. In some cases of DVT the patient may be asymptomatic, especially if the thrombus is small or distal. In extreme cases of DVT the outflow of the limb is so severely reduced that the arterial inflow may become obstructed, leading to venous gangrene. This condition is called phlegmasia cerulea dolens. The foot may appear blackened and the limb swollen and blue, even when elevated.

PE occurs when a segment of thrombus breaks loose, travels through the right side of the heart, and lodges in branches of the pulmonary artery. This leads to a perfusion defect in the arterial bed of the lungs.

Computed tomographic pulmonary angiography (CTPA) is the recommended initial imaging method in suspected PE, superseding the isotope ventilation/perfusion (*VQ*) scan.

The high risk of VTE amongst both medical and surgical hospital inpatients has resulted in guidelines from various national and professional bodies as to the best preventive measures (Cayley 2007; National Institute for Clinical Excellence 2007). The prophylaxis of DVT includes the use of mechanical prevention in the form of graduated compression stockings and pneumatic compression devices which increase venous return and therefore reduce the risk of venous stasis. Patients at higher risk may be given low-molecular-weight heparin, which carries a lower risk of bleeding than unfractionated heparin.

In the presence of DVT, the aim of treatment is to prevent thrombus extension and pulmonary embolus and in the longer term to reduce the likelihood of recurrent DVT and postthrombotic syndrome. Treatment is usually with anticoagulation drugs. The initial treatment is with low-molecular-weight heparin, which is converted to long-term therapy with oral anticoagulants, such as warfarin. Occasionally, devices called vena caval filters are positioned in the vena cava when there is a high risk of embolization to the lungs. Surgery is rarely performed to remove thrombus from the femoral and iliac veins.

The investigation and treatment of isolated calf vein thrombosis remain a contentious issue (Lohr et al. 1991; Meissner et al. 1997; Kearon 2003). It is beyond the scope of this book to consider the debate in any detail, but sonographers should be aware of the controversies surrounding this area; most DVTs start in the calf and most resolve but proximal progression does occur. Other issues in the calf are the extra time to extend the scan from distal popliteal to calf veins, the ability to visualize calf veins adequately, and accuracy of detecting DVT in the calf.

Investigations for diagnosing DVT

Traditionally, X-ray venography was the main test used for the diagnosis of DVT. It involves an injection of a contrast agent into the venous system via a dorsal foot vein. In some cases it proves impossible to cannulate a foot vein, and in some situations patent deep calf veins do not fill with contrast agent (Bjorgell et al. 2000). Currently, duplex scanning is the preferred method of imaging DVT. It is often combined with pre-imaging tests in a defined management pathway or protocol. These pathways have been developed because of financial pressures and a desire to provide a coherent and efficient service. The protocols may be complex and are usually expressed in a diagnostic/treatment algorithm (Fig. 14.2). Algorithms differ in detail (Sampson et al. 2005), with DVT ruled out on low

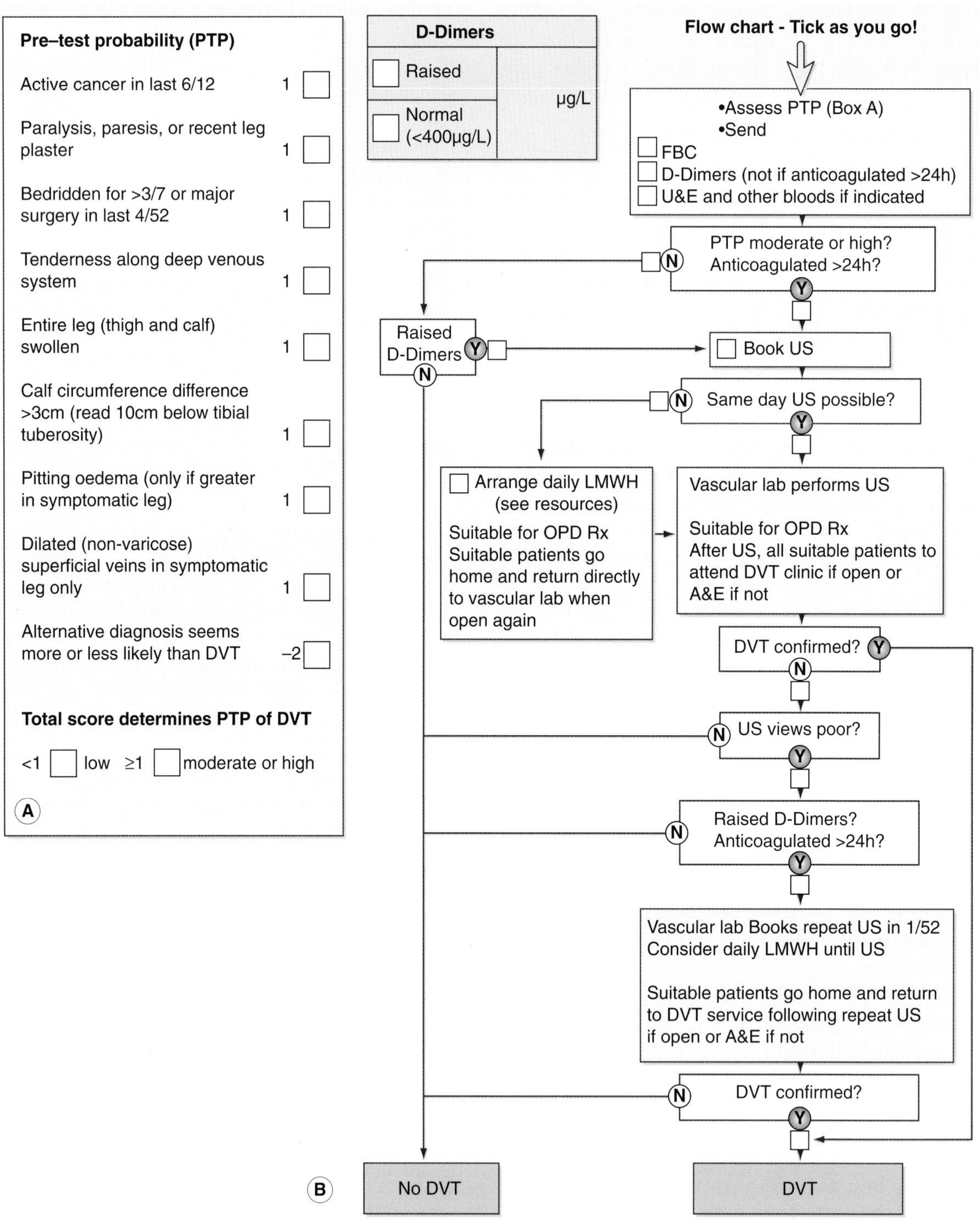

Figure 14.2 • An example of a screening protocol for deep venous thrombosis (DVT). (A) Pretest probability score (Wells score). (B) A flow chart for investigations (courtesy of Kings College Hospital, London). FBC, full blood count; U&E, urine and electrolytes; US, ultrasound; LMWH, low-molecular-weight heparin; OPD, outpatients department; A&E, accident and emergency.

clinical risk and negative D-dimer but sometimes still requiring ultrasound.

Most, but not all, positive diagnosis is by ultrasound. The process normally begins with a clinical assessment, including a risk probability score derived from a set of standard questions. The lower the score, the lower the probability of DVT. An example is given in Figure 14.2, which is based on the Wells score (Wells 2007). The next stage usually involves a biochemical assay to measure D-dimer levels in the blood. D-dimers are products that are formed by the interaction of fibrin, contained in thrombus, and plasmin. Increased levels of D-dimer are associated with the presence of DVT. Unfortunately, increased levels of D-dimer are also found in other conditions, such as malignancy, infection, and trauma. Therefore, the D-dimer test has a high sensitivity but low specificity for the presence of DVT. Despite low specificity, negative predictive values as high as 98% have been reported (Bradley et al. 2000). A negative predictive value indicates the probability that patients will not have the disease in those who have a negative test outcome. (It has been suggested that a combination of a low risk probability score and negative D-dimer test may be useful pre-selection tools to avoid unnecessary duplex examinations; Aschwanden et al. 1999; Orbell et al. 2008.).

Most ultrasound examinations use compression of the vein to confirm patency. This normally involves full examination of the deep veins from the groin to the calf. However, there is evidence that a limited compression test involving two- or three-point compression at the common femoral vein, popliteal vein, and distal popliteal vein (third point) is a method of excluding DVT, in that the cohorts of patients with negative scans and no treatment have low rates of VTE complication at follow-up (Cogo et al. 1998; Khaw 2002). Where the distal veins were not scanned and when clinical suspicion remains or where there are incomplete views of the calf veins, a repeat ultrasound at 1 week may be used to detect progression to distal popliteal vein level.

Magnetic resonance imaging and CT scanning are used for imaging the iliac veins and vena cava when other imaging tests are inadequate or impossible.

PRACTICAL CONSIDERATIONS FOR DUPLEX ASSESSMENT OF DVT

Objectives of the scan

- Exclude or confirm the presence of a deep venous thrombosis
- To identify the location of the thrombus, which veins are involved, and its proximal extent, as this will influence subsequent treatment
- Identify other conditions that may mimic deep venous thrombosis, such as thrombophlebitis

Advice

It is important not to overextend the knee when examining the popliteal vein, as this can lead to collapse or occlusion of the vein.

The main diagnostic criterion used to exclude DVT is complete collapse of the vein under transducer pressure. Color flow imaging and spectral Doppler can also be used during the assessment. Color flow imaging may aid vein identification and improve diagnostic confidence. About 20 minutes should be allocated for a full scan of one leg from the groin distally, including the calf veins.

The legs should be accessible and the patient made as comfortable as possible. In very rare situations, the patient may require some sedation or analgesia before the examination if the limb is extremely painful. It is helpful to ask the patient to point to any areas of discomfort or tenderness, especially in the calf, as this can often be located over the site of the thrombosis. This region should be carefully examined by duplex scanning.

The examination room should be at a comfortable ambient temperature to prevent vasoconstriction (>20 °C). Wherever possible, the legs should be examined in a dependent position in order to fill and distend the veins. Ideally, the patient should be examined with the legs tilted downward from the head by at least 30° (reverse Trendelenburg position). Alternatively, the patient can be examined in a standing position, with the leg to be examined minimally weight-bearing and the patient holding a hand rail or equivalent for support. The calf veins and popliteal fossa are easier to scan with the legs extended, hanging over the side of the examination table, and the feet resting on a stool. Wherever possible, immobile or sick patients should be tilted into a reverse Trendelenburg position, although there may be situations in which the patient cannot be moved, such as in the intensive care unit.

DEEP-VEIN EXAMINATION FOR ACUTE DVT

A mid-frequency, flat linear array transducer should be used for examining the femoral, popliteal, and calf veins. The iliac veins are examined using a low-frequency curved linear array transducer. The scanner should be configured for a venous examination. The color pulse repetition frequency should be low, typically 1000 Hz, to detect low-velocity flow. The color wall filter should also be set at a low level, and the spectral Doppler sample volume should be increased in size to cover the vessel, so that flow is sampled across the lumen.

Ultrasound compression is the main method of confirming vein patency. If direct transducer pressure is applied over a vein it will collapse, as the blood pressure in the deep veins is low, unlike the pressure in the adjacent artery, and the walls will be seen to meet (coapt). The adjacent artery should demonstrate little or no distortion. In contrast, if there is thrombus in the vein it will not collapse. This technique is demonstrated in Figures 14.3 and 14.4. It should be noted that fresh thrombus, which is soft, can partially deform. Compression should be applied at frequent intervals along the length of a vein to confirm patency. Partial collapse of the vein suggests the presence of nonoccluding thrombus. In this situation, the adjacent artery may be seen to deform as the probe pressure is increased to confirm partial obstruction in the vein. Transducer compression should be applied in the transverse imaging plane rather than the longitudinal plane. This is because it is easy to slip to one side of the vein as pressure is applied in the longitudinal plane, and this may mimic compression of the vein when observed on the B-mode image. In some areas the veins lie too deep for compression to be used, such as in the pelvis and sometimes at the adductor canal or calf. Color flow imaging is useful for demonstrating patency in this situation. In order to display flow when using color flow imaging in the transverse plane, some tilting of the transducer is often necessary to obtain a Doppler angle to the vein.

The following guidelines can be used in any sequence, depending upon the areas that require

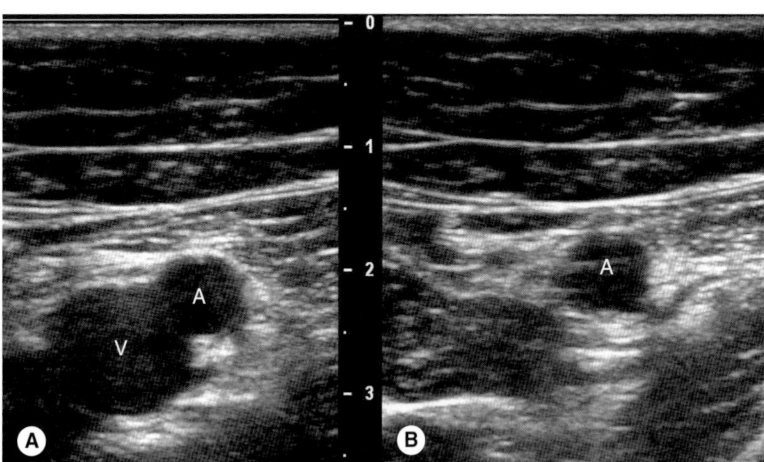

Figure 14.3 • (A) A transverse image of the left femoral vein (V) and superficial femoral artery (A). (B) Patency of the femoral vein is demonstrated by complete collapse of the vein during transducer pressure.

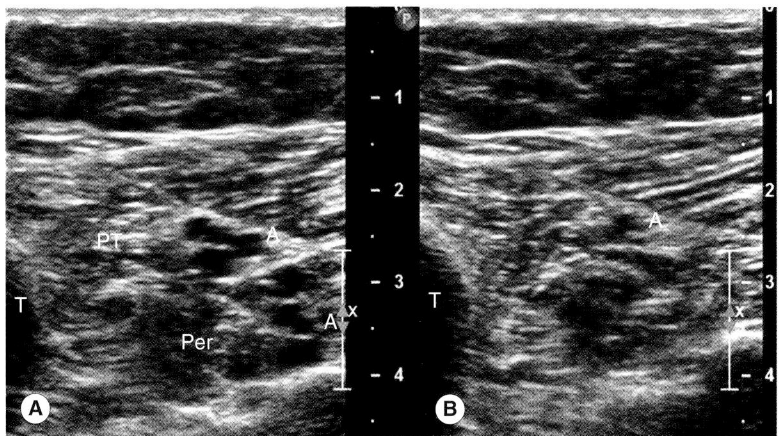

Figure 14.4 • (A) Transverse image of the calf demonstrating the posterior tibial (PT) veins and arteries and peroneal (Per) veins and arteries. The respective arteries (A) are shown between the paired veins. The border of the tibia is visible (T). (B) There is complete collapse of the veins with transducer compression but, in this image, the PT artery (A) is still visible. Note that it can sometimes be very difficult to differentiate the image of the veins from the surrounding tissue.

assessing. It is sometimes easier to locate a specific vein by looking for the adjacent artery, especially in the calf. The reader should also refer to Chapter 9 for more details on the probe positions for imaging the calf vessels and the main vessels in the thigh and pelvis.

1. Starting at the level of the groin, the common femoral vein is imaged in transverse section and will be seen to lie medial to the common femoral artery (Fig. 14.3A; see Fig. 9.8). The common femoral vein should be compressed to demonstrate patency and is followed distally beyond the saphenofemoral junction, to the junction of the femoral vein and deep femoral vein. The proximal segment of the deep femoral vein should also be assessed for patency if possible. With the transducer turned into the longitudinal plane, the flow pattern in the common femoral vein should be assessed with color flow imaging and spectral Doppler. Flow should appear spontaneous and phasic at this level if there is no outflow obstruction. A calf squeeze can provide evidence of good flow augmentation in the proximal femoral vein, which is a useful indirect indicator of probable femoral and popliteal vein patency. Alternatively, strong foot flexion will also normally augment flow.
2. The femoral vein is then followed in transverse section along the medial aspect of the thigh to the knee, using compression to confirm patency. The vein normally lies deep to the superficial femoral artery. In the adductor canal the vein may be difficult to compress. It is sometimes helpful to place a hand behind the back of the lower thigh and push the flesh toward the transducer, which will bring the vein and artery more superficial to the transducer. Color flow imaging can also be used to confirm patency in this segment, but areas of non-occluding thrombus could be missed. Remember that duplication of the femoral vein is relatively common, and both trunks should be examined.
3. The popliteal vein is examined by scanning the popliteal fossa in a transverse plane. Starting in the middle of the popliteal fossa, the vein is followed proximally as far as possible to overlap the area scanned from the medial lower thigh. The popliteal vein will be seen lying above the popliteal

artery when imaged from the popliteal fossa. The below-knee popliteal vein and gastrocnemius branches are then examined in the transverse plane. The popliteal vein can also be duplicated.

4 The calf veins are often easier to identify distally. They are then followed proximally to the top of the calf. The posterior tibial and peroneal veins can be imaged in a transverse plane from the medial aspect of the calf (Fig. 14.4A). From this imaging plane the peroneal veins will lie deep to the posterior tibial veins. It can sometimes be difficult to compress the peroneal veins from this position. Color flow imaging in the longitudinal plane may be useful for demonstrating patency (Fig. 14.5). The peroneal veins can frequently be examined from the posterolateral aspect of the calf (see Fig. 9.13). The common trunks of the posterior tibial and peroneal veins can also be very difficult to image, and medial and posterolateral transducer positions may be needed to examine this region at the top of the calf.

5 Examination of the anterior tibial veins is often not performed, as isolated thrombosis of these veins is rare (Mattos et al. 1996). However, assessment of the anterior tibial veins is usually easier with color flow imaging, in the longitudinal plane, as the veins are small and frequently difficult to identify with B-mode imaging.

6 The examination of the calf is completed with an assessment of the soleal veins and sinuses located in the soleus muscle, which lies deep to gastrocnemius. These veins are imaged from the posterior calf (Fig. 14.6). In practice, they can be very difficult to identify unless dilated with thrombus.

7 If there is a clinical indication, such as in pregnancy or abdominal carcinoma, then the iliac veins are examined. The patient

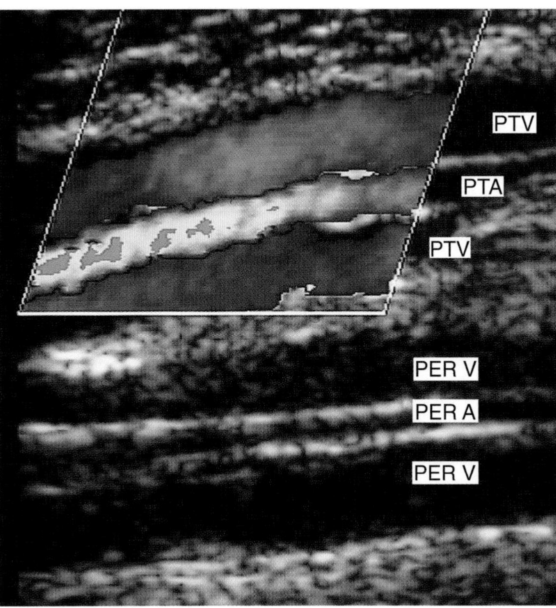

Figure 14.5 • A longitudinal color flow image from the medial calf demonstrates patency of the posterior tibial veins (PTV), which are seen lying on either side of the posterior tibial artery (PTA). Color filling is seen to the vein walls. The peroneal veins (PER V) and artery (PER A) are seen lying deep to the posterior tibial vessels. The peroneal vessels may not always be seen in the same scan plane.

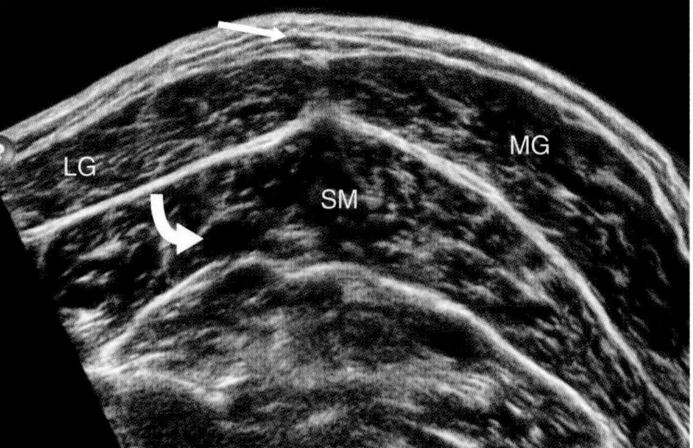

Figure 14.6 • A transverse B-mode panoramic image of the posterior aspect of the right mid-upper calf to demonstrate the position of the soleus muscle (SM). A soleal vein (curved arrow) is seen within the muscle. The lateral and medial gastrocnemius muscles (LG and MG respectively) lie above the soleus muscle, separated by a band of echogenic muscular fascia. The small saphenous vein is also visible in the saphenous compartment lying above the muscular fascia (arrow).

should be examined supine but as the iliac veins lie behind the bowel an oblique to lateral approach with the patient in the lateral decubitus position can prove advantageous. The iliac veins lie slightly deeper and medial to the iliac arteries. Compression of these veins is not possible, and patency should be confirmed using color flow imaging. In addition, spectral Doppler can be used to examine flow patterns with flow augmentation maneuvers. The main limitation of examining this area is incomplete visualization due to overlying bowel gas and the potential to miss partially occluding thrombus.

8 In some cases the vena cava may need to be examined. This vessel lies to the right of the aorta when imaged in transverse section. Color flow imaging can be used in the transverse plane to look for filling defects, but some transverse tilt may have to be applied to the transducer to produce a reasonable Doppler angle. Flow should also be assessed in longitudinal section with color flow and spectral Doppler ultrasound. Examination of this area should be undertaken by a sonographer with considerable experience. Other imaging modalities are generally preferable.

SCAN APPEARANCES FOR THE ASSESSMENT OF DVT

B-mode images

Normal appearance

The vein should appear clear, contain no echoes, and be easily compressible with transducer pressure. In practice, there are often speckle and reverberation artifacts in the image, but the experienced sonographer should have little difficulty in identifying these. Smaller veins can be difficult to distinguish from tissue planes. It is sometimes possible to image static or slowly moving blood as a speckle pattern within the lumen, owing to aggregation of blood cells, but the vein should collapse under transducer pressure (Figs 14.3 and 14.4). The deep calf veins can sometimes be difficult to identify without the help of color flow imaging. The common femoral vein should normally distend with a Valsalva maneuver if the venous outflow through the iliac veins is patent.

Abnormal appearance

> **Caution**
>
> Prudence should be exercised with transducer compression if free-floating thrombus is present, to avoid dislodging the thrombus.

In the presence of thrombus the vein will not compress (Figs 14.7 and 14.8). The varying ultrasonic appearances of acute and chronic thrombus are illustrated schematically in Figure 14.9. In the very early stages of thrombosis, the clot often has a degree of echogenicity due to the aggregation of red blood cells in the thrombus. Within 1–2 days, the clot becomes more anechoic, owing to changes occurring in the thrombus, and it can be difficult to define on the B-mode image. However, in practice, with advanced transducer technology, it is often possible to see subtle echoes. If the vein is totally occluded in the acute phase, it may appear distended. The thrombus can be free-floating, with large areas being nonadherent to the vein wall. It is usually possible to identify the upper limit of the thrombosis, and the thrombus tip often demonstrates slightly increased echogenicity (Fig. 14.10). The tip is much easier to identify if it extends to the popliteal or femoral veins. Smaller areas of nonocclusive thrombus may not cause the vein to distend, but they can be demonstrated by incomplete collapse of the vein during compression. Older thrombus, beyond 2 weeks in age, becomes more echogenic.

Color flow images

Normal appearance

Spontaneous phasic flow is usually seen in the larger proximal veins. There should be complete color filling of the lumen in both longitudinal and transverse planes during a calf squeeze. Color aliasing is sometimes observed if the distal

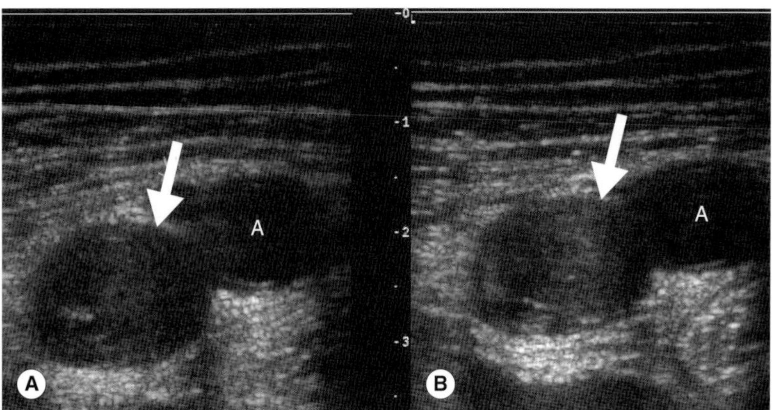

Figure 14.7 • (A) A transverse image of the left femoral vein (arrow) and superficial femoral artery (A). The femoral vein appears distended and contains some low-level echoes. (B) The femoral vein does not collapse during firm transducer pressure, confirming deep venous thrombosis.

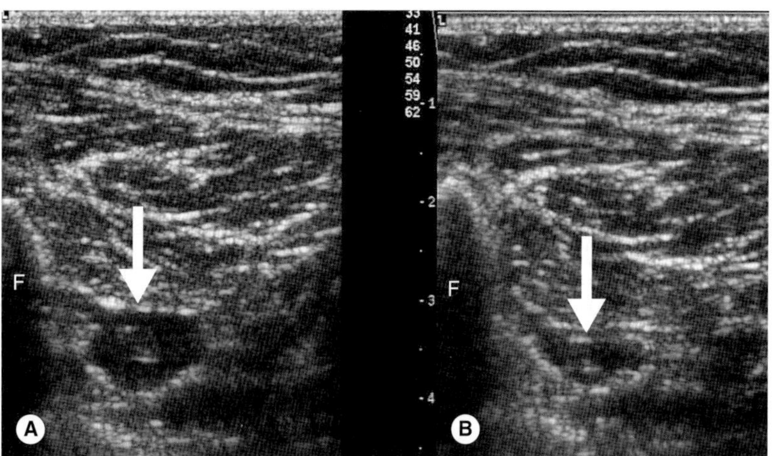

Figure 14.8 • (A) A transverse B-mode image of a peroneal vein thrombosis (arrow). The image is taken from the posterolateral aspect of the calf and the veins are lying adjacent to the fibula (F). (B) There is only partial collapse of the vein with transducer pressure (arrow) indicating a DVT.

augmentation causes a significant transient increase in venous flow. If it is difficult to squeeze the calf, owing to size or tenderness, it can be possible to augment flow by asking the patient to flex the ankle backward and forward, activating the calf muscle pump. The posterior tibial veins and peroneal veins are usually paired, which should be clearly demonstrated on the color flow image (Fig. 14.5). However, anatomical variations can occur. Color flow imaging of the gastrocnemius and soleal veins can be difficult, as blood flow velocities following augmentation can be low, especially if a degree of venous stasis is present.

Abnormal appearance

There is an absence of color filling in occluded veins, even with distal augmentation. Collateral veins may also be seen in the region of the occluded vein. The color flow pattern around free-floating thrombus is very characteristic, with flow seen

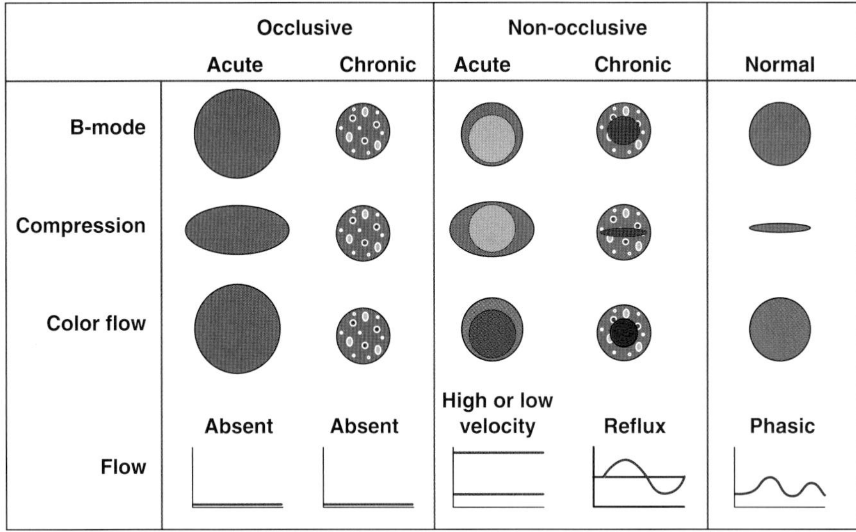

Figure 14.9 • A diagram showing transverse B-mode views of veins, their response to compression, and appearance on color flow imaging in the absence or presence of occlusive and nonocclusive DVT. The respective Doppler flow patterns are demonstrated at the bottom of the diagram.

between the thrombus and vein wall. This can be demonstrated in both longitudinal and transverse sections. Color flow imaging can be useful for demonstrating the position of the proximal thrombus tip as full color filling of the lumen will be seen just proximal to the tip (Fig. 14.11). Smaller areas of nonoccluding thrombus will be demonstrated as flow voids within the lumen. However, some care should be used in interpreting partially occluding thrombosis on the basis of color flow imaging alone, and probe compression should be used for confirmation if possible.

Spectral Doppler

Normal appearance

Spectral Doppler is the least-used modality in the assessment of venous thrombosis and should not be used as the only method of investigation. However, patent veins should demonstrate normal venous flow patterns. In our experience, it should be possible to augment flow velocity in the main trunks by at least 100% with a squeeze distal to the point of measurement. For example, there should be augmentation of flow in the femoral vein with a distal calf squeeze (see Ch. 13); however, this will not exclude small areas of nonoccluding thrombus. The Doppler signal at the level of the common femoral vein should exhibit a spontaneous phasic flow pattern, which temporarily ceases when the patient takes a deep inspiration or performs a Valsalva maneuver. This would suggest that there is no outflow obstruction through the iliac veins to the vena cava. However, the presence of small amounts of nonoccluding thrombus cannot be excluded on the basis of spectral Doppler alone.

Abnormal appearance

There is an absence of a spectral Doppler signal when the vein is completely occluded. When the vein contains a significant amount of partially occluding or free-floating thrombus, there is normally a reduced flow pattern that demonstrates little or no augmentation following distal compression. However, there are potential pitfalls when using this criterion, as there may be good collateral circulation between the point of distal calf compression and the position of the probe. An occlusive thrombosis in the iliac vein system usually results in a low-volume continuous flow pattern in the common femoral vein, with little or no response to a Valsalva maneuver (Fig. 14.12).

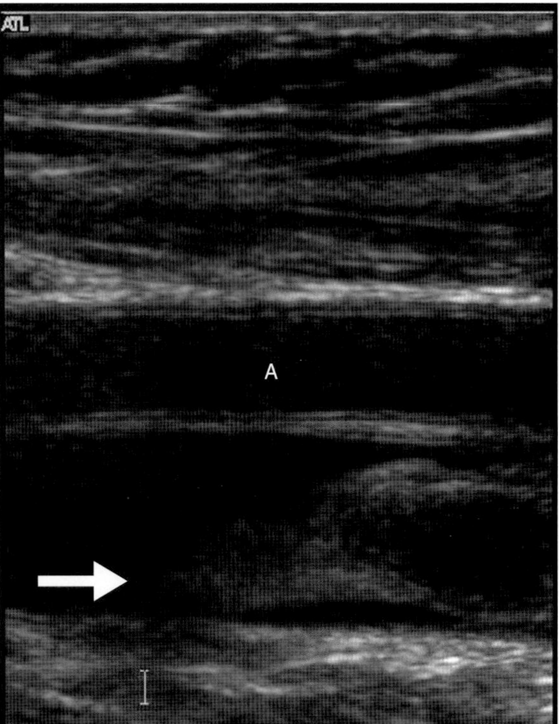

Figure 14.10 • The tip of a free-floating thrombus (arrow) is seen in the femoral vein. The thrombus is relatively anechoic. This appearance suggests an acute deep venous thrombosis. The superficial femoral artery (A) is seen in the image.

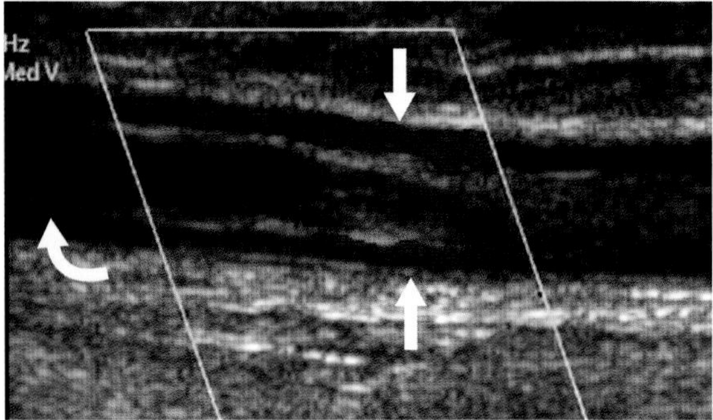

Figure 14.11 • A color flow image of free-floating thrombus. Flow is seen between the thrombus and vein wall (arrows). The proximal end of the thrombus towards the tip (curved arrow) is anechoic, which would indicate an acute thrombus. Note that the distal part of the thrombus in the image has a mild degree of echogenicity.

Diagnostic problems

Observation

It is possible to misidentify veins in the deep venous system and even confuse them with superficial veins. This occurs most commonly in the popliteal fossa and upper calf. The gastrocnemius vein can be mistaken for the popliteal vein or for the small saphenous vein. It is important to be able to identify the fascial layer that separates the superficial and deep venous systems to avoid this type of error (see Fig. 13.1).

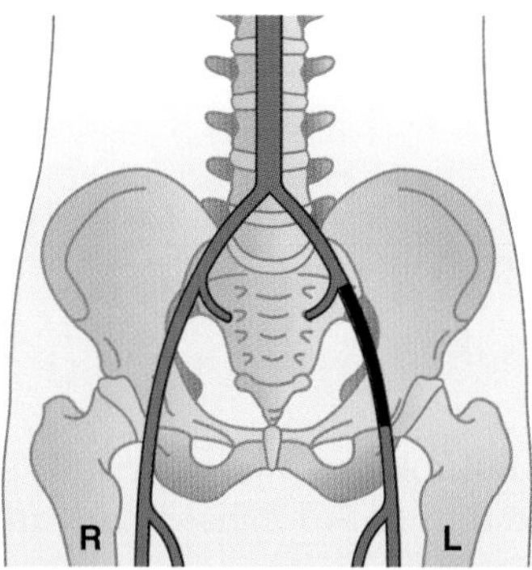

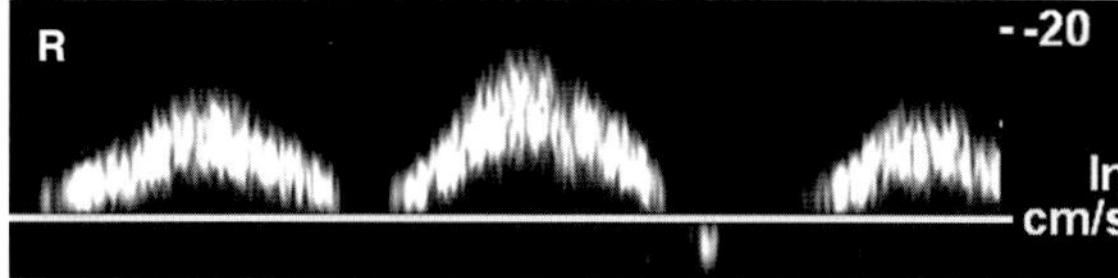

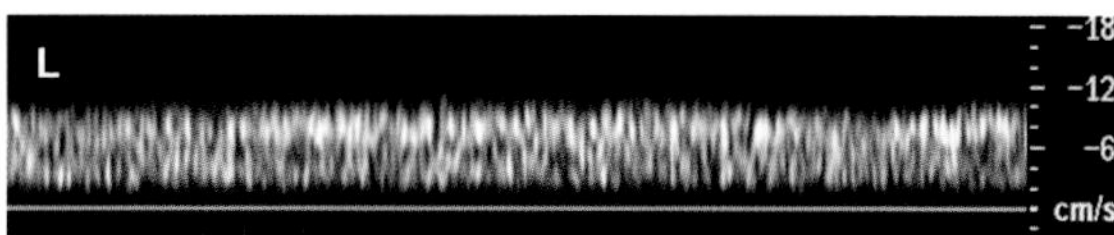

Figure 14.12 • The diagram demonstrates an occlusion of the left external iliac vein. The common femoral vein waveform distal to the obstruction demonstrates continuous low-velocity flow with a loss of phasicity, in contrast to the normal waveform shown on the right side.

The investigation of DVT can be very difficult, and it is important to use a logical protocol when performing the examination. There can be considerable variation in the anatomy of the venous system, as outlined in Chapter 13. Duplication of the femoral vein and popliteal vein is not uncommon. A study by Gordon et al. (1996) reported duplication of the femoral vein in 25% of healthy volunteers. This could lead to potential diagnostic errors if one-half of the system is occluded and the other is patent, as it is possible to miss the occluded system during the examination. Careful scrutiny of the transverse sectional image should demonstrate any bifid vein systems. The sonographer should also be highly suspicious of veins that appear small in calibre or that are located in abnormal positions with respect to their corresponding arteries, as this might indicate anatomical variation or evidence of post-thrombotic changes. Another potentially difficult situation occurs when there is a large deep-lying thigh vein running between the popliteal vein and the deep femoral vein, as the femoral vein may be unusually small. Both the femoral vein and the deeper vein should be carefully examined for defects.

Investigation of the iliac veins can be extremely difficult, especially in situations in which the vein may be under compression by structures in the pelvis, or by tumors, as this can be misinterpreted as a partially occluding thrombus. Compression of the iliac vein can also occur during pregnancy and is observed more frequently on the left side. This may lead to unilateral limb swelling and a reduction in the normal venous flow pattern in the femoral vein.

ACCURACY OF DUPLEX SCANNING FOR THE DETECTION OF DVT

Many studies have been performed to compare the accuracy of duplex scanning with venography. Miller et al. (1996) achieved sensitivities and specificities of 98.7% and 100%, respectively, at above-knee level, and corresponding values of 85.2% and 99.2% at below-knee level. A systematic review and meta-analysis by Goodacre et al. (2005) looked at various ultrasound methods and found duplex to have a sensitivity of 96% proximally and 75% distally. The authors noted that the current use of ultrasound is not solely based on diagnostic studies but also upon management studies in which cohorts of patients with negative ultrasound studies are not treated, but followed up to identify evidence of missed VTE; the moderate sensitivity in the calf does not appear to result in high rates of adverse outcome (Goodacre et al. 2005).

The variable results of different studies may reflect factors such as patient population, operator experience, or equipment quality. To implement a high-quality service, it is essential that staff are properly trained and a patient management protocol defined.

NATURAL HISTORY OF DVT

The natural history of a DVT is variable and is dependent on the position and extent of the thrombi (O'Shaughnessy & Fitzgerald 2001; Kearon 2003). In addition, the patient's age and physical condition will have a significant bearing on the final outcome. The thrombus can:

- Spontaneously lyse
- Propagate or embolize
- Recanalize over time
- Permanently occlude the vein.

Complete lysis of smaller thrombi can occur over a relatively short period of time due to fibrinolytic activity. Full recanalization of the vein will be seen, and the lumen will appear normal on the ultrasound image. Valve function can be preserved in these circumstances. If there is a large thrombus load, the process of recanalization can take several weeks (Fig. 14.13). The thrombus becomes more echogenic over time as it becomes organized. The vein frequently diminishes in size due to retraction of the thrombus. As the process of recanalization begins, the developing venous flow channel within the vein lumen may be tortuous due to irregularity of lysis in the thrombus. It is even possible to see multiple flow channels within the vessel. In cases of partial recanalization, old residual thrombus can be seen along the vein wall, producing a scarred appearance. It is sometimes possible to see fibrosed valve cusps, which appear immobile and echogenic on the B-mode image. Deep venous insufficiency is frequently the long-term outcome of slow or partial recanalization.

If the vein remains permanently occluded, the thrombus becomes echogenic due to fibrosis. The thrombus retracts over time, leading to shrinkage of the vein. It may even appear as a small cord adjacent to its corresponding artery, and in some cases the vein is difficult to differentiate from surrounding tissue. Color flow imaging frequently demonstrates the development of collateral veins in the region of the occlusion. In the case of chronic common femoral and iliac vein occlusion, visible distended superficial veins, which act as collateral pathways, are often seen across the pelvis and lower abdominal wall. The great saphenous vein can act as a collateral pathway in the presence of a femoral or popliteal vein occlusion. High-volume continuous flow recorded in the great saphenous vein should always be treated with suspicion.

There is considerable debate about the accuracy of duplex scanning for determining the age of thrombus, but it is generally accepted that it is possible to differentiate the acute phase, within the first week or two, from the post-acute and chronic phases of venous thrombosis. However, there is much less certainty about differentiating post-acute and chronic thrombus. This is due to the fact that the process of formation may not have been synchronous, and there are also irregularities in the process of lysis and fibrosis within the thrombus, producing a heterogeneous appearance.

Recurrent thrombosis

Recurrent thrombotic events are common after acute DVT (Meissner et al. 1995; Orbell et al. 2008). There are considerable diagnostic problems in attempting to detect fresh thrombus in a vein that has been damaged by a prior DVT. If the patient has had a previous scan or venogram, it is possible to check the extent of the thrombosis on the last report and compare it with the current scan. However, old reports may not be available, or the patient may not have had any previous investigations. In these situations, the vein should be examined carefully with B-mode and color flow imaging to look for areas of fresh thrombus. These will appear as anechoic areas on the B-mode image, and color flow imaging will demonstrate filling defects. In practice, this can be an extremely difficult examination to undertake. If there is a high degree of suspicion, a repeat scan can be performed a couple of days later to look for changes in the appearance of the vein or possible extension of thrombus.

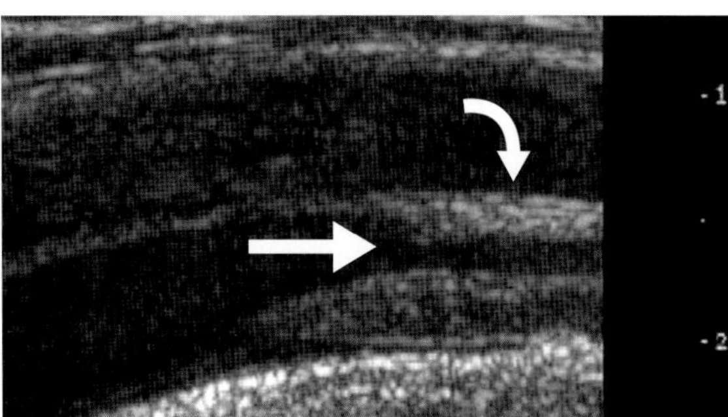

Figure 14.13 • A longitudinal B-mode image of a gastrocnemius vein showing a thrombus that has become adherent to the posterior vein wall. Some thrombus is also seen on the anterior wall (curved arrow). The flow lumen is in between the thrombus (straight arrow). The thrombus has a degree of echogenicity, suggesting that it is more than a week or two old.

OTHER PATHOLOGIC CONDITIONS THAT CAN MIMIC DVT

Other pathologic conditions that can clinically mimic deep venous thrombosis

- Abscesses
- Muscle tears
- Hyperperfusion syndrome following arterial bypass surgery or angioplasty for lower-limb ischemia
- Prolonged leg dependency resulting in edema
- Arteriovenous fistulas

A number of pathologic conditions produce symptoms similar to DVT, and the sonographer should be able to identify these disorders.

Thrombophlebitis

Thrombophlebitis occurs due to inflammation of the superficial veins, with thrombus forming in the great saphenous vein or small saphenous vein system (Fig. 14.14). It can be felt as a hard cord in the superficial tissues, often associated with erythema, localized heat, pain, and tenderness. Superficial thrombosis is generally not a serious condition compared with DVT. However, there are

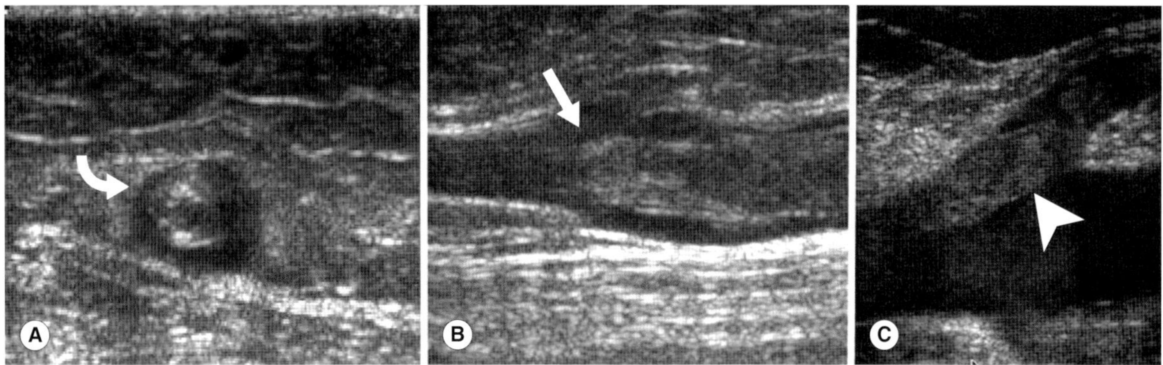

Figure 14.14 • Images of thrombophlebitis in the great saphenous vein. (A) A transverse image of the great saphenous vein (curved arrow). (B) A longitudinal image showing the proximal extent of the phlebitis (arrow) causing distension of the vein. The diameter of the vein is normal proximally. (C) There is extension of the phlebitis across the saphenofemoral junction (arrow head).

occasions when the thrombus tip extends along the proximal great saphenous vein and protrudes through the saphenofemoral junction into the common femoral vein. This situation can also occur in the small saphenous vein, with propagation across the saphenopopliteal junction. There is a reported risk of proximal embolization from the thrombus tip, and care should be used when examining any thrombus in this position (Blumenberg et al. 1998). It is essential to report this type of presentation as soon as possible, as this may require treatment.

Hematoma

Hematomas are accumulations of blood within the tissues that can clot to form a solid swelling. They can be caused by external trauma, or other mechanisms such as muscle tears, can be extremely painful, and can lead to limb swelling, especially in the calf. Blood in the hematoma may also track extensively along the fascial planes. The sonographic appearance of a hematoma is of a reasonably well-defined hypo echoic area in the soft tissues or muscles (Fig. 14.15). Hematomas can be very variable in size and shape. It is sometimes impossible to image the veins in the immediate vicinity, owing to the size of the hematoma or the pain the patient experiences. The hematoma may also partially or completely compress the deep veins in the local vicinity.

Lymphedema

Lymphedema is observed as chronic limb swelling due to reduced efficiency or failure of the lymphatic drainage system. This may be due to a primary abnormality of the lymphatic system or to secondary causes that lead to damage of the lymph nodes and drainage system in the groin and pelvis. These include damage following surgery, trauma, malignancy, and radiotherapy in the groin region. Lymphedema is usually most prominent in the calf but can extend throughout the leg, and two-thirds of cases are unilateral. Other sites can be affected by lymphedema, including the arms. The B-mode appearance of lymphedema demonstrates the subcutaneous layer to be thickened, and a fine B-mode speckle is observed in this region, making the image appear grainy (Fig. 14.16). The ultrasound image of lymphedema is usually different from that caused by simple fluid edema. Ultrasound can be used to confirm the patency of the deep veins, but unfortunately the presence of lymphedema degrades the ultrasound image, making many deep vein scans technically challenging.

Cellulitis

Cellulitis is caused by infection of the subcutaneous tissues and skin; it produces diffuse swelling in the lower limb, often associated with pain, tenderness, and redness. There is usually evidence of edema in the region of swelling. A duplex examina-

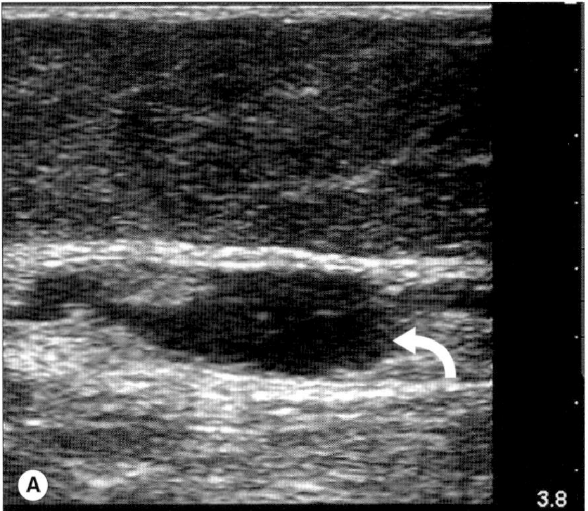

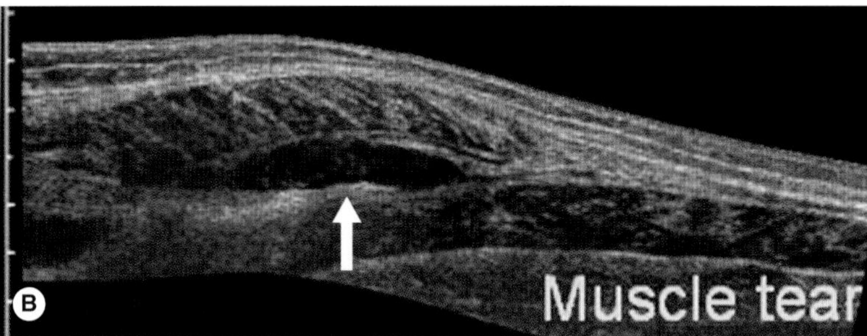

Figure 14.15 • Two images of hematomas. (A) An area of hematoma (arrow) is seen in a thigh muscle following a fall. (B) A large hematoma (arrow) has occurred due to a muscle tear.

tion can confirm patency of the deep veins. In addition, there may be hyperemic flow in the veins and arteries of the limb due to the infection (Fig. 13.36).

Edema

Patients can develop edema in the calf due to infection, leg ulceration, local trauma, or as a result of significant venous insufficiency. This is characterized as fluid or edema in the superficial tissues. The ultrasound appearance of edema demonstrates tissue splaying by numerous interstitial channels (Fig. 14.17). Patients with congestive heart failure often develop edema in the legs due to the increased pressure in the venous system and the right side of the heart. Another characteristic of congestive heart failure is the pulsatile flow pattern that is often observed in the proximal deep veins, which can be mistaken for arterial flow (Fig. 14.18). Careful attention to the color display will confirm the direction of flow.

Baker's cysts

A Baker's cyst is a distension of the semimembranosus-gastrocnemius bursa and normally originates on the medial side of the knee. This bursa usually communicates with the knee joint. Bursae are pouches containing synovial fluid that prevents friction between a bone joint or tendon. Baker's cysts occur due to a number of knee disorders, such as arthritis and repetitive trauma due to exercise. Baker's cysts can rupture, causing severe pain and symptoms similar to those of acute vein thrombosis. Large Baker's cysts can compress the popliteal vein or deep veins of the popliteal fossa, causing a DVT. It is always necessary to identify and confirm the patency of the deep veins in the popliteal fossa, even when a Baker's cyst has been diagnosed, as the Baker's cyst may be an incidental finding. Baker's cysts can also be clinically misdiagnosed as popliteal aneurysms.

Baker's cysts are easiest to define in a transverse scan plane from the popliteal fossa. They are normally anechoic due to the fluid in the cyst, but some may contain debris and osteocartilaginous fragments, which are echogenic. Many Baker's cysts have a typical oval or crescent shape, with a characteristic neck (Fig. 14.19). If the cyst is excessively large, it may distort the anatomy in the popliteal fossa. It is difficult to define a ruptured Baker's cyst with ultrasound.

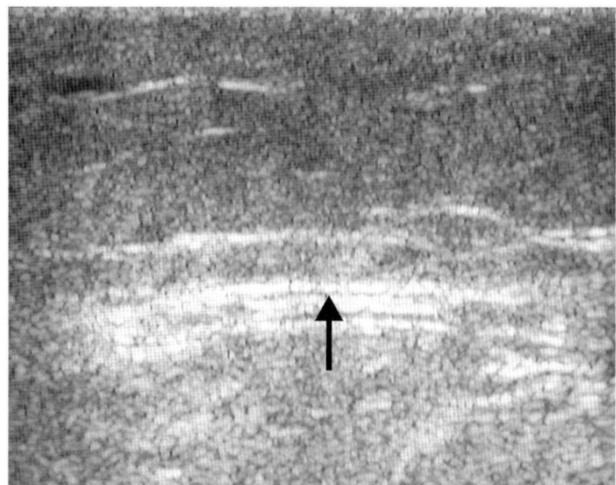

Figure 14.16 • Lymphedema produces a grainy appearance in the subcutaneous tissues, as demonstrated on this transverse B-mode image. The superficial tissue is relatively thick. The muscular fascia is demonstrated by the arrow. Note the degraded image quality, typical of this disorder.

Enlarged lymph nodes

Enlargement of lymph nodes can occur due to pathologic conditions such as infection and malignancy. The inflow of lymphocytes and other substances into the node exceeds the outflow leading to enlargement of the node. The main sites for enlargement visualized during venous duplex exams are the groin and axilla, and the nodes can become so large that they compress the adjacent vein. Enlarged nodes may be tender, and localized redness and heat (erythema) may be present. They can also be clinically misdiagnosed as femoral artery aneurysms if the pulsation of the artery is amplified to the skin surface by the enlarged node.

Enlarged lymph nodes are imaged as oval or spherical masses that are found in groups (Fig. 14.20). They are mainly hypoechoic in appearance but may contain stronger echoes within the center of the node and can be mistaken for a thrombosed vein. Color flow Doppler usually demonstrates blood flow in larger nodes, especially if infection is present.

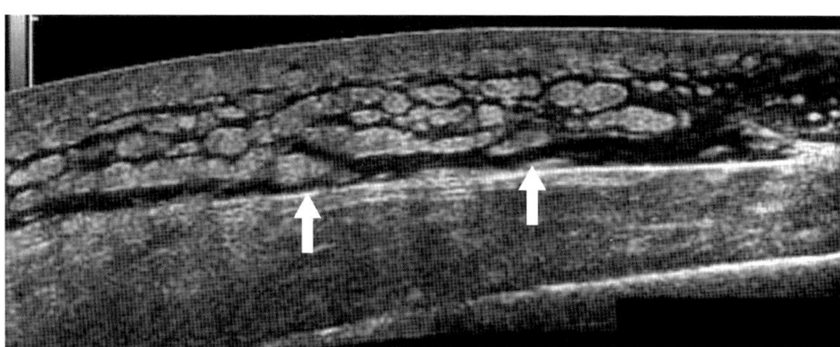

Figure 14.17 • In this panoramic image of the calf, fluid edema is demonstrated in the subcutaneous tissues as numerous anechoic channels (arrows) splaying the tissue.

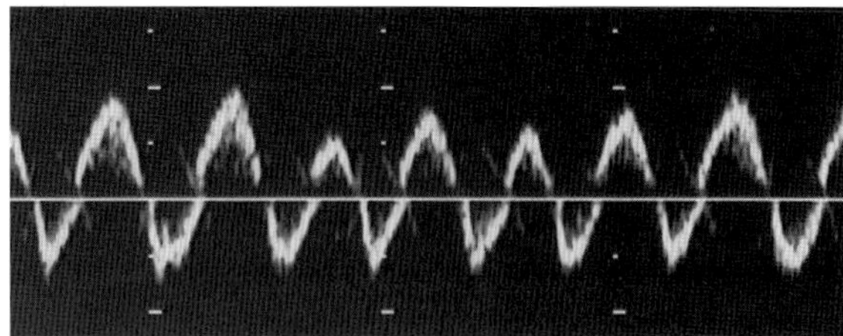

Figure 14.18 • The venous flow signals recorded from the common femoral vein of a patient with congestive cardiac failure demonstrate a pulsatile flow pattern.

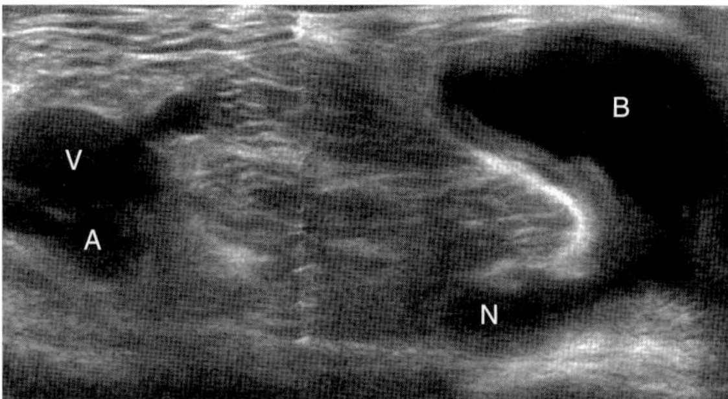

Figure 14.19 • A Baker's cyst (B) is demonstrated in this transverse image of the popliteal fossa. The popliteal artery (A) and vein (V) are also seen. The neck of the cyst (N) is clearly seen.

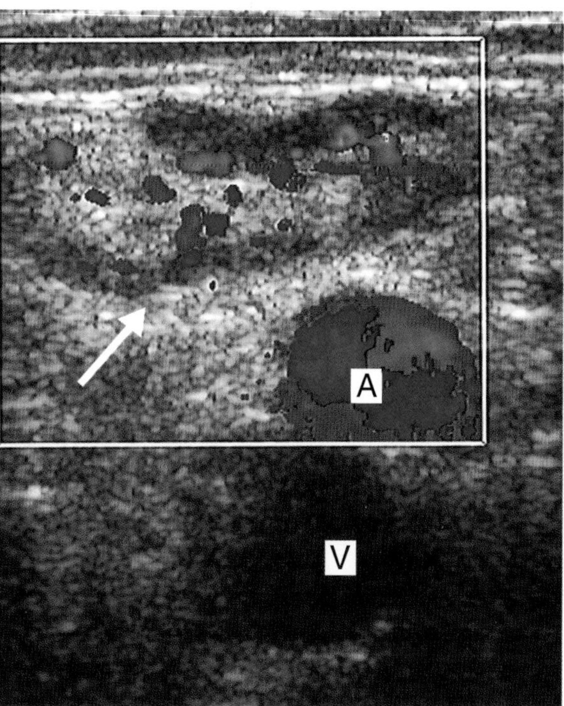

Figure 14.20 • An enlarged lymph node (arrow) is demonstrated in this transverse image at the top of the groin. Flow is demonstrated in the lymph node. The common femoral artery (A) and vein (V) are seen below the node.

UPPER-LIMB VEINS

Anatomy of the deep upper-limb veins

The upper-limb veins can also be divided into the deep and superficial veins (Fig. 14.21), and there are a number of anatomical variations. Usually, paired veins are associated with the radial and ulnar arteries. They normally join at the elbow to form the brachial vein but can run separately to form the brachial vein higher in the upper arm. The brachial vein is usually paired and associated with the brachial artery. At the top of the arm, the brachial vein becomes the axillary vein, which is usually a single trunk. The axillary vein becomes the subclavian vein as it crosses the border of the first rib. The subclavian vein enters the thoracic outlet but runs separately from the artery in front of the anterior scalene muscle. The internal jugular vein, from the neck, joins the proximal subclavian vein, which then drains via the brachiocephalic vein to the superior vena cava. The left brachiocephalic vein is longer than the right brachiocephalic vein. It is very difficult to image the brachiocephalic veins clearly with ultrasound.

Anatomy of the superficial upper-limb veins

The cephalic vein and the basilic vein are the two major superficial veins in the arms (Fig. 14.21). The cephalic vein drains the dorsal surface of the hand and runs up the lateral (radial) aspect of the forearm to the antecubital fossa at the elbow and then continues in a subcutaneous path along the lateral aspect of the biceps muscle. Toward the shoulder, it runs in the deltopectoral groove between the deltoid and pectoralis muscles and

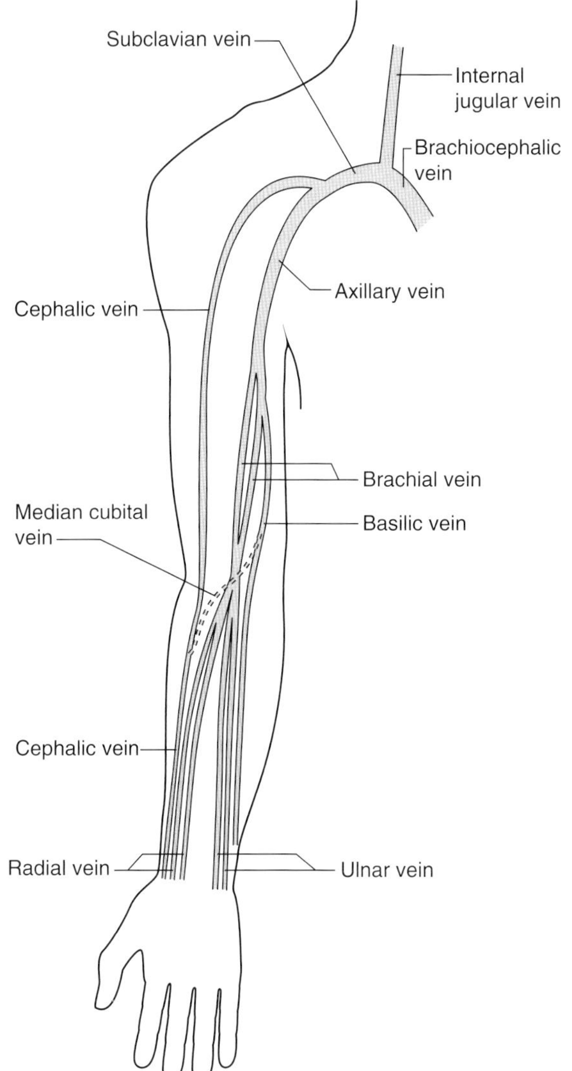

Figure 14.21 • The venous anatomy of the arm.

then pierces the clavipectoral fascia to join the axillary vein in the infraclavicular region. The basilic vein drains blood from the palm and ventral aspects of the hand and runs along the medial (ulnar) side of the forearm to the medial aspect of the antecubital fossa. The basilic vein then penetrates the fascia in the lower aspect of the upper arm to join the brachial vein. However, its insertion can be variable, and sometimes the basilic vein may run directly into the distal axillary vein.

Thrombosis of the upper limbs

DVT is the main pathology that affects the upper-limb venous system. The subclavian and axillary veins are the commonest sites for thrombosis. This can lead to upper-limb swelling with distension of the superficial veins. The causes of upper-limb thrombosis are similar to many of those that lead to lower-limb DVT. In addition, long-term catheter access for feeding and drug administration can damage the axillary and subclavian veins. Venous thoracic outlet syndrome can also cause thrombosis of the subclavian vein. Effort-induced thrombosis of the subclavian vein, referred to as Paget–Schroetter syndrome, is associated with strenuous upper-body exercise or repetitive movements and is mainly seen in younger patients.

The appearance of thrombosis in the upper extremities is similar to that seen in the lower extremities. A combination of compression, color flow imaging, and spectral Doppler is required to confirm patency, as it is sometimes difficult to apply satisfactory probe compression, particularly in the supraclavicular fossa. However, duplex scanning provides good results when compared to contrast venography in areas where compression can be applied, but caution should be used when attempting to diagnose DVT on the basis of Doppler flow patterns (Baarslag et al. 2002). Upper-limb swelling can also be caused by lymphedema, following mastectomy with removal of lymph nodes in the axilla and the effects of radiotherapy.

TECHNIQUE FOR ASSESSING THE BRACHIAL, AXILLARY, AND SUBCLAVIAN VEINS

The patient should lie supine so that the subclavian and axillary veins are distended. The scan normally takes 10–15 min for each arm. Remember, it can be useful to compare the scan appearance from both sides in cases of suspected unilateral thrombosis. It should also be noted that the color flow image of the proximal subclavian vein can look rather confusing and cluttered because of the proximity of other vessels and the often pulsatile appearance superimposed on the venous flow pattern, due to atrial contractions (Fig. 16.8). Imaging of the subclavian vein is also discussed in Chapter 16.

1 The arm should be abducted and placed on a comfortable support. It is easier to start the examination distally in the brachial vein, which will be seen lying adjacent to the brachial artery in the upper arm.
2 The brachial vein is imaged in transverse section and should be compressible with relatively light transducer pressure. Color and spectral Doppler recordings should demonstrate flow augmentation with manual compression of the forearm.
3 The axillary vein can be imaged using a combination of transaxillary and infraclavicular transducer positions (see Fig. 16.3 and Ch. 10) (see Ch. 10 and Ch. 16). The vein will be seen lying adjacent to the artery, but color flow imaging can aid identification, particularly if B-mode imaging is poor. A combination of compression and color flow imaging may be needed to confirm patency in this region. The cephalic vein may act as a collateral pathway to the subclavian vein in the presence of a distal axillary vein thrombosis.
4 The distal end of the subclavian vein is initially imaged from the infraclavicular fossa in transverse section, where it will be seen lying inferior to the subclavian artery. The mid subclavian vein is imaged from the supraclavicular fossa. A large acoustic shadow will be seen as the subclavian vein runs under the clavicle. Compression of the subclavian vein is extremely difficult, owing to the contour of the neck and the presence of the clavicle, and color flow imaging in transverse and longitudinal planes is used to confirm patency. In addition, spectral Doppler should demonstrate spontaneous phasic flow with respiration if there is no outflow obstruction. It is also usual to observe a pulsatile flow pattern superimposed on the phasic flow pattern due to atrial contractions of the heart (see Ch. 5). It should be noted that it is extremely easy to miss a proximal thrombosis in the subclavian vein, owing to poor visualization of this area, especially if it is a partially occluding thrombus. It is possible to image indwelling catheters, such as Hickman lines, in the subclavian vein. Always state any limitations or doubts about the scan in this region, as other imaging tests, may be required.
5 Two breathing maneuvers can be used for assessing flow in the subclavian vein. The first is a Valsalva maneuver, in which there should be cessation of flow or flow reversal during Valsalva. This is followed by an enhancement in flow toward the heart during expiration. The second involves multiple sniffing through the nose. During continued sniffing the subclavian vein will be seen to contract. Neither of these maneuvers can exclude DVT, as there may be nonoccluding thrombus present. However, if an abnormal flow pattern or response is recorded, it may indicate a potential abnormality.
6 Occasionally, a thrombosis may involve the internal jugular vein in the neck. This can be imaged in cross-section.
7 It is usually diffcult to image the brachiocephalic veins (see Fig. 16.4), but a thrombosis may be indirectly suggested if there is an abnormality in the subclavian and axillary vein flow patterns.

Other upper-limb venous disorders

Phlebitis of the superficial veins can occur due to repeated catheter access or intravenous drug abuse. Arteriovenous malformations are sometimes found in the arms and hands, and in some cases can be very extensive, leading to upper-limb swelling.

REPORTING

The report should indicate the scan to be normal or abnormal, and, if it is abnormal, the level and extent of the thrombosis should be stated. The report should also clearly specify which veins were examined and which were omitted due to technical limitations. This avoids any confusion or assumption that veins not mentioned on the report are normal. Other pathologic conditions that may mimic the symptoms of DVT should also be reported. The report of a positive DVT should be brought to the attention of the appropriate medical staff as soon as possible, in order that the appropriate management can be implemented.

References

Anderson F A, Spencer F A 2003 Risk factors for venous thromboembolism. Circulation 107: I-9–I-16

Aschwanden M, Labs K H, Jeanneret C et al. 1999 The value of rapid D-dimer testing combined with structured clinical evaluation for the diagnosis of deep vein thrombosis. Journal of Vascular Surgery 30: 929–935

Baarslag H J, Van Beek E J, Koopman M M et al. 2002 Prospective study of color duplex ultrasonography compared with contrast venography in patients suspected of having deep venous thrombosis of the upper extremities. Annals of Internal Medicine 136: 865–872

Beyer J, Schellong S 2005 Deep vein thrombosis: current diagnostic strategy. European Journal of Internal Medicine 16: 238–246

Bjorgell O, Nilsson P E, Jarenros H 2000 Isolated nonfilling of contrast in deep leg vein segments seen on phlebography, and a comparison with color Doppler ultrasound, to assess the incidence of deep leg vein thrombosis. Angiology 51: 451–461

Blumenberg R M, Barton E, Gelfand M L et al. 1998 Occult deep venous thrombosis complicating superficial thrombophlebitis. Journal of Vascular Surgery 27: 338–343

Bradley M, Bladon J, Barker H 2000 D-dimer assay for deep vein thrombosis: its role with color Doppler sonography. Clinical Radiology 55: 525–527

Cayley W E 2007 Preventing deep vein thrombosis in hospital inpatients. British Medical Journal 335: 147–151

Cogo A, Lensing A W, Koopman M M et al. 1998 Compression ultrasonography for diagnostic management of patients with clinically suspected deep vein thrombosis: prospective cohort study. British Medical Journal 316: 17–20

Cranley J J, Canos A J, Sull W J 1976 The diagnosis of deep vein thrombosis: fallibility of clinical symptoms and signs. Archives of Surgery 111: 34–36

Fowkes F G, Evans C J, Lee A J 2001 Prevalence and risk factors of chronic venous insufficiency. Angiology (Suppl. 1):S5–S15

Fowkes F J, Price J F, Fowkes F G 2003 Incidence of diagnosed deep vein thrombosis in the general population: systematic review. European Journal of Vascular and Endovascular Surgery 25: 1–5

Goodacre S, Sampson F, Thomas S et al. 2005 Systematic review and meta analysis of the diagnostic accuracy of ultrasonography for deep vein thrombosis. BMC Medical Imaging 5:6. Available online at: www.biomedcentral.com/1471-2342/5/6

Gordon A C, Wright I, Pugh N D 1996 Duplication of the superficial femoral vein: recognition with duplex ultrasonography. Clinical Radiology 51: 622–624

Haenen J H, Janssen M C, Wollersheim H et al. 2002 The development of postthrombotic syndrome in relationship to venous reflux and calf muscle pump dysfunction at 2 years after the onset of deep venous thrombosis. Journal of Vascular Surgery 35: 1184–1189

Jongbloets L M, Lensing A W, Koopman M M et al. 1994 Limitations of compression ultrasound for the detection of symptomless postoperative deep vein thrombosis. Lancet 343: 1142–1144

Kearon C 2003 Natural history of venous thromboembolism. Circulation 107: I22–I30.

Khaw K 2002 The diagnosis of deep vein thrombosis. In: Beard J D, Murray S (eds) Pathways of care in vascular surgery. TFM Publishing, Shrewsbury, pp 161–169

Labropoulos N, Kang S S, Mansour M A et al. 2002 Early thrombus remodelling of isolated calf deep vein thrombosis. European Journal of Vascular and Endovascular Surgery 23: 344–348

Lohr J M, Kerr T M, Lutter K S et al. 1991 Lower extremity calf thrombosis: to treat or not to treat? Journal of Vascular Surgery 14: 618–623

Mattos M A, Melendres G, Sumner D S et al. 1996 Prevalence and distribution of calf vein thrombosis in patients with symptomatic deep venous thrombosis: a color-flow duplex study. Journal of Vascular Surgery 24: 738–744

Meissner M H, Caps M T, Bergelin R O et al. 1995 Propagation, rethrombosis and new thrombus formation after acute deep vein thrombosis. Journal of Vascular Surgery 22: 558–567

Meissner M H, Caps M T, Bergelin R O et al. 1997 Early outcome after isolated deep vein thrombosis. Journal of Vascular Surgery 26: 749–756

Miller N, Satin R, Tousignant L et al. 1996 A prospective study comparing duplex scan and venography for the diagnosis of lower-extremity deep vein thrombosis. Cardiovascular Surgery 4: 505–508

National Institute for Clinical Excellence 2007 Venous thromboembolism: reducing the risk of venous thromboembolism (deep vein thrombosis and pulmonary embolism) in inpatients undergoing surgery. Available online at: www.nice.uk/CG046

Nicolaides A N, Belcaro G, Bergqvist D et al. 1994 Prevention of thromboembolism: European consensus statement. In: Bergvist D, Comerota A J, Nicolaides A N et al. (eds) Prevention of venous thromboembolism. Med-orion, London, pp 445–446

Orbell J H, Smith A, Burnand K G et al. 2008 Imaging of deep vein thrombosis British Journal of Surgery 95: 137–146

O'Shaughnessy A M, Fitzgerald D E 2001 The patterns and distribution of residual abnormalities between the individual proximal venous segments after an acute deep vein thrombosis. Journal of Vascular Surgery 33: 379–384

Sampson FC, Goodacre S, Kelly A-M et al. 2005 How is deep vein thrombosis diagnosed and managed in UK and Australian emergency departments? Emergency Medicine Journal 22: 780–782

Virchow R. Die Verstopfung den Lungenarteries und ihre Folgen. Beitr Exp pathol physiol 1846; 21

Wells P S 2007 Integrated strategies for the diagnosis of venous thromboembolism. Journal of Thrombosis and Haemostasis 5: 41–50

White R H 2003 The epidemiology of venous thromboembolism. Circulation 107 (Suppl. 1): I4–I8

Further reading

Zwiebel W J, Pellerito J S 2005 Introduction to vascular ultrasonography. 5th edn. Elsevier Saunders, Philadelphia

Graft surveillance and preoperative vein mapping for bypass surgery

CONTENTS

INTRODUCTION

Patients with significant lower-limb ischemia or threatened limb loss usually require arterial bypass surgery if no other option is available to improve blood flow in the leg. Vascular surgeons are able to perform an extensive range of arterial bypass procedures to restore circulation to the extremities. Bypass grafts can be made of synthetic materials, such as polytetrafluoroethylene (PTFE), or constructed from native vein, which can be assessed and marked preoperatively as described at the end of this chapter. Failure of a bypass graft due to the development of a graft stenosis is a serious complication that can result in amputation if it is not possible to unblock the graft. It is therefore common practice for vascular laboratories to perform regular graft surveillance scans to detect the development of graft defects. The majority of surveillance scans are performed for native vein bypass grafts below the groin (infrainguinal grafts). The surveillance of synthetic grafts is equivocal and benefits are less clear-cut (Lundell et al. 1995). Ultrasound can also be used to image areas of potential infection following graft surgery, to see if the region of infection is in contact with the graft. The emphasis of this chapter will be on infrainguinal vein graft surveillance.

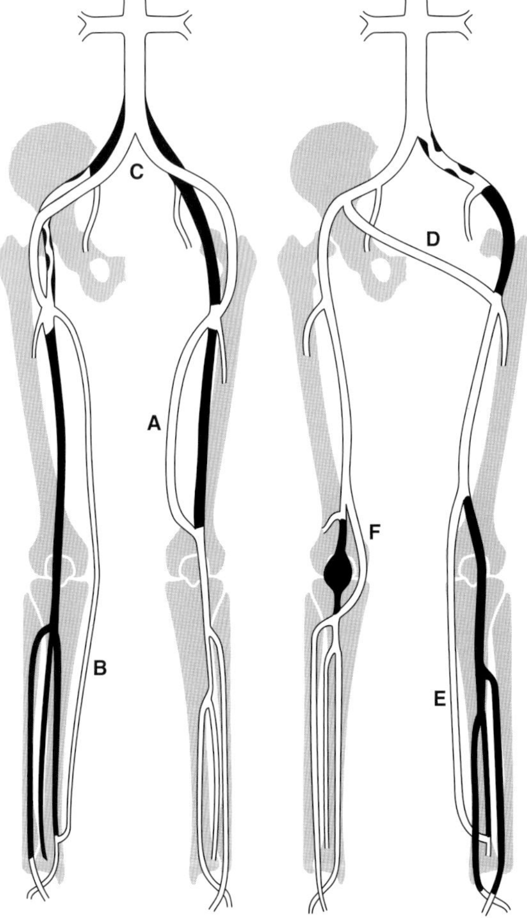

Figure 15.1 • Examples of bypass grafts. (A) Above-knee femoropopliteal graft. (B) Femoroposterior tibial artery graft. (C) Aortobifemoral graft. (D) Iliofemoral cross-over graft. (E) Superficial femoral artery to peroneal artery graft. (F) Popliteal artery bypass graft for a thrombosed popliteal aneurysm.

ANATOMY

The routes of grafts vary considerably and depend on the level and extent of the native arterial disease that has been bypassed. Synthetic grafts are mainly used to bypass inflow disease (aortoiliac segment), whereas vein grafts are frequently used for distal procedures below the inguinal ligament. The different types of graft frequently encountered in the graft surveillance clinic are shown in Figure 15.1.

Vein grafts

Whenever possible, native vein is used for femoral distal bypass surgery, as it offers good long-term patency rates and there is less risk associated with infection compared to synthetic grafts. The great saphenous vein is the vein of choice for infrainguinal bypass surgery, although an arm vein or the small saphenous vein can also be used if the great saphenous vein is unsuitable in part or all of its length. Vein grafts composed of more than one segment of vein are known as composite vein grafts. Femoral distal bypass surgery is performed using three common types of surgical procedure (Fig. 15.2).

The first is the in situ technique, in which the great saphenous vein is exposed but left in its native position and side branches are ligated to prevent blood shunting from the graft to the venous system. As the vein contains valves which would prevent blood flow toward the foot, they have to be removed or disrupted using a device called a valvulotome. The main body of an in situ vein graft lies superficially along the medial aspect of the thigh. In the second technique, called a non-reversed vein graft, the vein is removed from its bed and can be tunnelled or positioned elsewhere in the leg. The proximal anastomosis of a vein graft is usually located at the common femoral artery, although the position can vary and it may be sited at the superficial femoral artery or, less commonly, at the popliteal artery. The position of the distal anastomosis is variable and depends on the distal extent of the native arterial disease. The distal anastomosis may lie very deep in the leg, particularly if the graft is anastomosed to the tibioperoneal trunk or peroneal artery. The natural taper of the vein along the leg matches the naturally decreasing diameter of the arteries as they run to the periphery.

In the third type of procedure, the great saphenous vein is completely removed and turned through 180° so that the distal end of the vein will form the proximal anastomosis. This is called a reversed vein graft. One particular advantage of this technique is that, in this orientation, the valves will not prevent blood flow toward the foot and do not need to be removed (Fig. 15.2B). Reversed vein grafts are often tunneled deep in the thigh beneath the sartorius muscle, which can make imaging difficult. As the vein is reversed, the diameter of the proximal segment of the graft is usually smaller than the distal segment. This can result in a size mismatch between the proximal inflow artery and proximal graft that is evident on the scan. When there is insufficient length of native vein available,

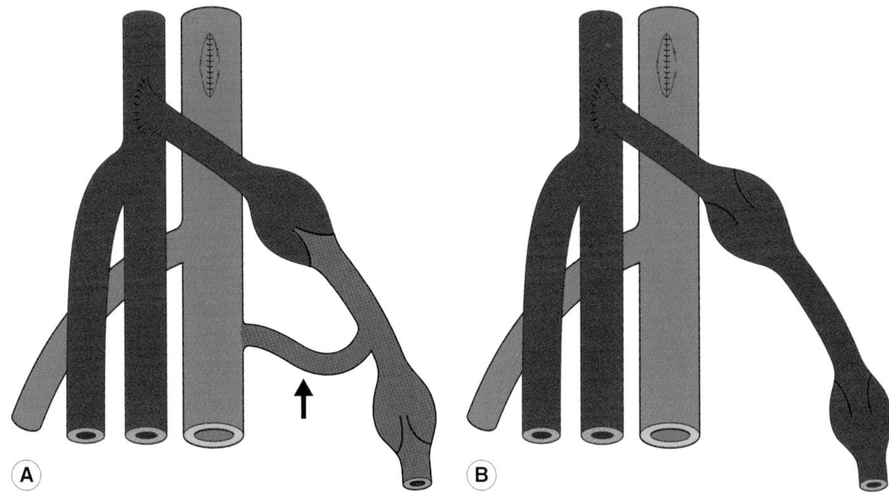

Figure 15.2 • Diagrams of two different types of vein graft at the proximal anastomosis to the common femoral artery. (A) An in situ vein graft. Blood will not flow beyond the first valve and therefore the valves in the great saphenous vein have to be removed (see text). The tributaries must be ligated to prevent blood flowing directly back into the femoral vein (arrow). (B) A reversed vein graft. The valves will open in the direction of flow.

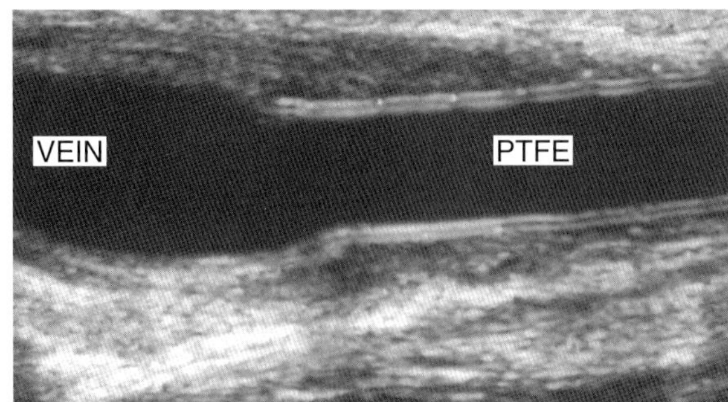

Figure 15.3 • An example of a composite polytetrafluoroethylene (PTFE) and vein graft.

a combination of synthetic material and vein may be used to form a composite graft (Fig. 15.3).

Synthetic grafts

Synthetic grafts are used for aortobifemoral, iliofemoral, axillofemoral, and femorofemoral crossover grafts. Synthetic PTFE grafts are also used for femoropopliteal bypass, but the long-term patency rates are not as good as grafts constructed from native vein (Klinkert et al. 2003). Vein cuffs or collars are sometimes used to join the distal end of a synthetic femoral distal graft to the native artery. They produce a localized dilation at the anastomosis, which is thought to reduce the risk that a stenosis will occur.

PURPOSE OF GRAFT SURVEILLANCE

Vein grafts

The development of an intrinsic vein graft stenosis is a major source of vein graft failure (Grigg et al. 1988; Caps et al. 1995). An angiogram demonstrating a graft stenosis is shown in Figure 15.4. Early graft failure, within the first month, is attributed to technical defects or poor patient selection. Such an example would be a patient with very poor run-off below the graft, resulting in increased resistance to flow and eventual graft thrombosis. Graft failure beyond 1 month is attributed to the development of intimal hyperplasia that can occur when there is damage to the endothelium of the vessel wall. This causes smooth-muscle proliferation into the vessel lumen and subsequent narrowing. Stenoses can occur at any point along the graft and can sometimes be extremely short, web-like lesions. Incomplete removal of valve cusps during in situ bypass surgery can also cause localized flow disturbance and narrowing. Late graft failure, beyond 12 months, can also be due to progression of atherosclerotic disease in the native inflow or outflow arteries, above and below the graft.

Patients are normally scanned at regular intervals in the first 12 months following bypass surgery. The program used by our unit is shown in Box 15.1.

Some vascular units also continue to scan patients indefinitely beyond the first year at 6-month intervals to detect late graft problems. The time interval between scans is shortened to 1–2 months if a patient shows signs of developing a moderate stenosis. Patients requiring angioplasty or surgical revision of a significant graft defect recommence the surveillance program from the beginning. It can be seen that graft surveillance programs require considerable commitment from the vascular laboratory. There therefore remains considerable debate about the usefulness of such programs. The principal results of the Vein Graft Surveillance Randomised Trial (Davies et al. 2005) indicated that intensive surveillance with duplex scanning did not show any additional benefit in terms of limb salvage rates for patients undergoing bypass surgery, but it does incur extra costs. Other studies suggest that they are effective in maintaining patency rates and are less costly than surgical revision after a graft thrombosis, or rehabilitation following amputation (Lundell et al. 1995; Wixon et al. 2000). There is also evidence that an early postoperative scan, 6 weeks after surgery, can predict which lesions will require continuing duplex surveillance (Mofidi et al. 2007), enabling the effective targeting of resources to selected patients. In practice, many departments have developed local protocols that are a hybrid of published studies.

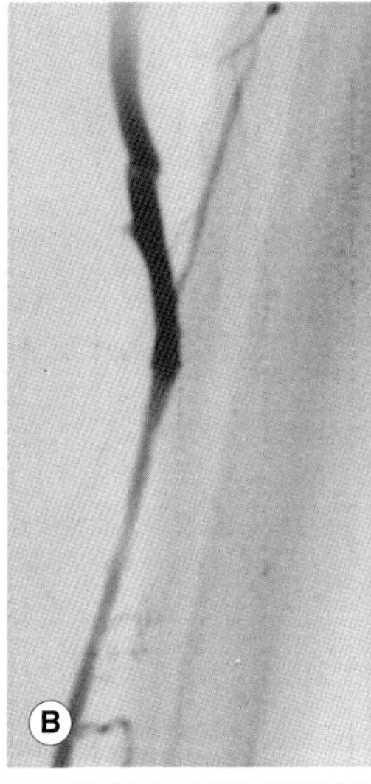

Figure 15.4 • (A) An angiogram demonstrating a significant graft stenosis (arrow) at the distal anastomosis of a vein graft. (B) The stenosis has been successfully dilated by balloon angioplasty.

BOX 15.1 Suggested program for graft surveillance following discharge from hospital; time intervals are shown in months (M)

PROGRAM IF NO SIGNIFICANT ABNORMALITY IS DETECTED, PEAK SYSTOLIC VELOCITY (PSV) RATIO <2

1 M, 3 M, 6 M, 9 M, 12 M, 18 M and 24 M when patient is discharged

PROGRAM IF STENOSIS IS DETECTED

PSV ratio 2–2.5: reduce follow-up to 2 months

PSV ratio 2.6–2.9: reduce follow-up to 4–6 weeks

PSV ratio ≥3: angioplasty or graft revision

If the scan has remained normal for 24 M following angioplasty the patient is discharged.

Synthetic grafts

The surveillance of synthetic grafts remains debatable, as many synthetic graft occlusions occur due to spontaneous graft thrombosis. Some vascular centers perform surveillance of iliofemoral crossover grafts and aortobifemoral grafts, particularly if there have been problems with disease in the inflow or outflow arteries. Synthetic grafts are more likely to become infected, and fluid collections or pus are sometimes found surrounding the graft at the site of infection, which frequently occurs at the groin. Graft infection is a serious complication and can cause the breakdown of the graft anastomosis, leading to uncontrollable hemorrhage. Duplex scanning has proved a useful technique for detecting and monitoring potential graft infections.

SYMPTOMS AND TREATMENT OF GRAFT STENOSIS OR FAILURE

Advice

Issue the patient with an information card giving the details of the type of graft and useful phone numbers to contact if problems or symptoms are encountered. These can include the vascular laboratory and vascular ward.

Most patients experience no symptoms in the presence of a developing graft stenosis, and grafts may fail without any prior warning. However, symptoms that can be attributable to imminent graft failure are the sudden onset of severe claudication or a sensation of coldness involving the foot. Urgent intervention is required in this situation to prevent graft occlusion. Most graft stenoses are treated successfully by balloon angioplasty. However, recurrent stenoses sometimes require surgical revision involving local patching of a defect or partial graft replacement using a new segment of vein. Early graft occlusion can be treated by thrombolysis or graft thrombectomy. There is often an underlying cause for the occlusion that requires correcting, such as a graft stenosis, inflow stenosis, or run-off occlusion. Conversely, some grafts develop a local aneurysm that may become so large that a segment of graft has to be replaced.

PRACTICAL CONSIDERATIONS FOR SCANNING BYPASS GRAFTS

What does the clinician want to know?

- Is the graft patent?
- Is there a graft stenosis and where is it located?
- What is the peak systolic velocity (PSV) across the stenosis?
- What is the PSV ratio across the stenosis?
- Estimate the degree of stenosis
- Does flow appear compromised in the graft (damped flow, low-velocity flow, or very high-resistant flow)?
- Is there evidence of inflow or outflow obstruction?
- Are there any graft aneurysms? Measure their size and position
- Is there evidence of graft entrapment? State the position
- Are there abnormal fluid collections associated with the graft? State the position
- Are there any significant changes since the previous scan? If so, what are they?

If a significant problem is suspected, it is advisable to seek senior medical advice before letting the patient go home as this can make arrangements for admission or treatment easier.

Problems finding the graft?

Beware: in some situations the great saphenous vein is removed and tunneled elsewhere in the leg and may follow an unusual route. Check the operation notes before starting the scan.

No special preparation is required for the examination, and the vast majority of graft scans can be completed within half an hour. The majority of bypass scans are performed with the patient lying supine or semisupine. When scanning vein grafts, the leg should be externally rotated and the knee gently flexed and supported. It is sometimes necessary to roll the patient over to one side in order to scan the posterior lower thigh, popliteal fossa, or upper posterior calf if the graft is anastomosed to the popliteal artery. Positions for scanning the tibial arteries are discussed in Chapter 9. The scanner should be configured for a graft scan, or in the absence of a specific preset, a lower-limb arterial investigation. Adjustment of the controls is frequently necessary, especially if there is low-volume flow in the graft (see Ch. 7).

Before beginning the scan, it is important to know the position and type of graft that is to be examined. The examination request card or operation notes should indicate this information. A potentially confusing situation can occur if a previous graft has been performed, and this has since occluded. An old thrombosed graft might be mistakenly identified as the new graft, which would then be reported as occluded. A combination of mid- and high-frequency, flat linear array transducers are most suited for graft surveillance in the thigh and calf. A low-frequency probe is required for imaging grafts above the inguinal ligament or for grafts that have been tunneled very deep in the thigh.

SCANNING TECHNIQUES

Advice

Don't apply excessive probe pressure when scanning superficial grafts as it is possible to compress the graft, especially if more pressure is applied to one end of the transducer, giving the false impression of a stenosis or narrowing. This is particularly important if the graft is close to or running over a bony surface.

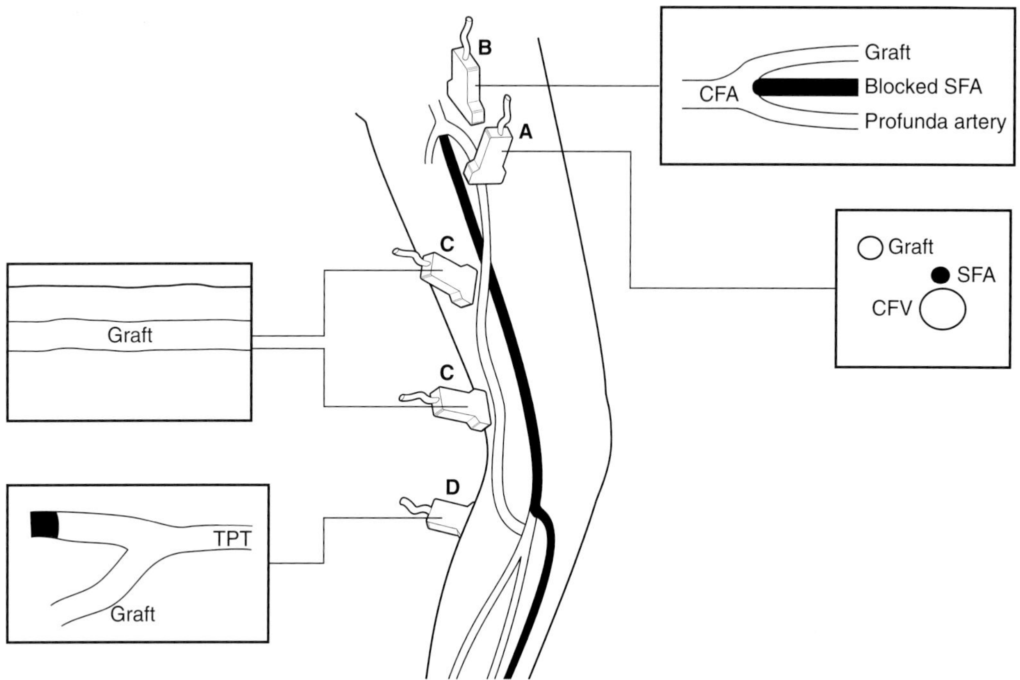

Figure 15.5 • Transducer positions for assessing a femoral to tibioperoneal trunk (TPT) in situ vein graft. (A) Proximal graft, transverse section. (B) Proximal anastomosis, longitudinal section. (C) Main body of the graft, longitudinal section. (D) Distal anastomosis below the popliteal fossa, longitudinal section. Scanning from a medial position below the knee may also provide a good image of the distal anastomosis. CFA, common femoral artery; SFA, superficial femoral artery.

In situ vein graft

The main body of an in situ vein graft remains superficial in the leg and runs along the medial aspect of the thigh (Fig. 15.5). It is often easier to locate the graft in the upper medial thigh using a transverse imaging plane and then to follow the graft up to the proximal anastomosis (Fig. 15.5A).

The transducer is rotated into a longitudinal scan plane at the proximal anastomosis (Fig. 15.5B). Ideally, a minimum 5 cm length of the inflow artery above the graft origin should be examined to exclude any disease. For instance, damped waveforms at this level are likely to indicate significant inflow disease. The proximal anastomosis should be carefully interrogated using color flow imaging and spectral Doppler for any signs of stenosis.

The graft is then carefully followed in longitudinal section along the thigh (Fig. 15.5C) with the color pulse repetition frequency (PRF) optimized to use the full color scale to demonstrate any flow disturbances. A high-frequency transducer provides the best image of the main body of an in situ graft. Spectral Doppler measurements should be made along the length of the graft, looking for waveform changes, especially in areas demonstrating color flow changes. It is often difficult to obtain good Doppler angles when scanning superficial vein grafts, and gentle 'heel-toeing' of the transducer may be required. A wedge of ultrasound gel can help if a specific region needs close examination.

The distal portion of many in situ vein grafts run deep to join a native artery at the distal anastomosis (Fig. 15.5D). This is especially true for grafts joined to the popliteal or peroneal arteries. It is often necessary to use a mid-frequency transducer in this region. The distal anastomosis should be scrutinized very closely with color flow imaging and spectral Doppler. Grafts that are anastomosed to the anterior tibial artery are commonly tunneled through the interosseous membrane (Fig. 15.6). The graft is imaged on the medial or posteromedial aspect of the calf, where it is seen to drop away very sharply and disappear through the membrane. The

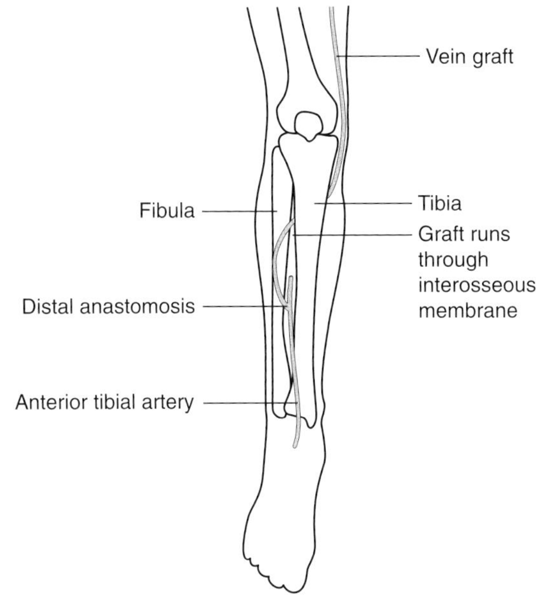

Figure 15.6 • Grafts to the anterior tibial artery are usually tunneled through the interosseous membrane between the tibia and fibula.

graft can then be relocated by scanning over the anterolateral aspect of the calf, where it will be seen to rise toward the transducer, and followed distally to locate the anastomosis. There should be a longitudinal scar on the anterior aspect of the calf in the region of the anastomosis. Transducer positions for locating the distal anastomosis are shown in Table 15.1.

Reversed and non-reversed vein grafts

The imaging techniques are similar to those for in situ grafts, but reversed and non-reversed vein grafts are frequently tunneled deep in the thigh and, consequently, are more difficult to image. A mid-range transducer is usually required for imaging such grafts. The graft is best located in transverse section as it divides from the native artery. The graft may drop away deeply from the proximal anastomosis. If the proximal anastomosis is located at the common femoral artery, the graft can be mistaken for the profunda femoris artery, or vice versa. If the graft lies deep, it may be very difficult to follow from the medial aspect of the thigh, and it can be easier to image from a posterior thigh position. If the graft is proving very

LEVEL OF ANASTOMOSIS	TRANSDUCER POSITION
Above-knee popliteal artery	Medial aspect of lower thigh or posterior lower thigh just above popliteal fossa
Below-knee popliteal artery and tibioperoneal trunk	Popliteal fossa or posterior, lateral and medial aspects of upper calf
Posterior tibial artery	Medial aspect of calf
Peroneal artery	Medial aspect of calf or from a lateral posterior position
Anterior tibial artery	Anterolateral aspect of calf

Table 15.1 Common transducer positions for imaging the distal anastomosis of an infrainguinal graft

difficult to locate in the thigh, attempt to find a more distal segment around the level of the knee in the popliteal fossa and work upward. In extreme cases, it may be necessary to use a low-frequency transducer to locate a deep segment of graft in the thigh or calf (Fig. 15.7).

Synthetic grafts

The majority of problems occurring in synthetic grafts are located at the proximal or distal anastomosis. It is rare for problems to develop in the main body of the graft, and a surveillance scan can often take the form of a spot check for patency combined with a more detailed assessment of the anastomosis. It is necessary to perform a detailed assessment of the inflow and outflow of the graft when abnormal graft flow is recorded in the absence of any obvious graft defect.

For inflow grafts anastomosed to the common femoral arteries, the proximal profunda artery and superficial femoral artery should be checked for any stenoses or occlusions that might compromise flow in the graft due to increased outflow resistance.

Femoropopliteal PTFE grafts

These are scanned in a similar fashion to vein grafts. The graft is often tunneled deep in the leg.

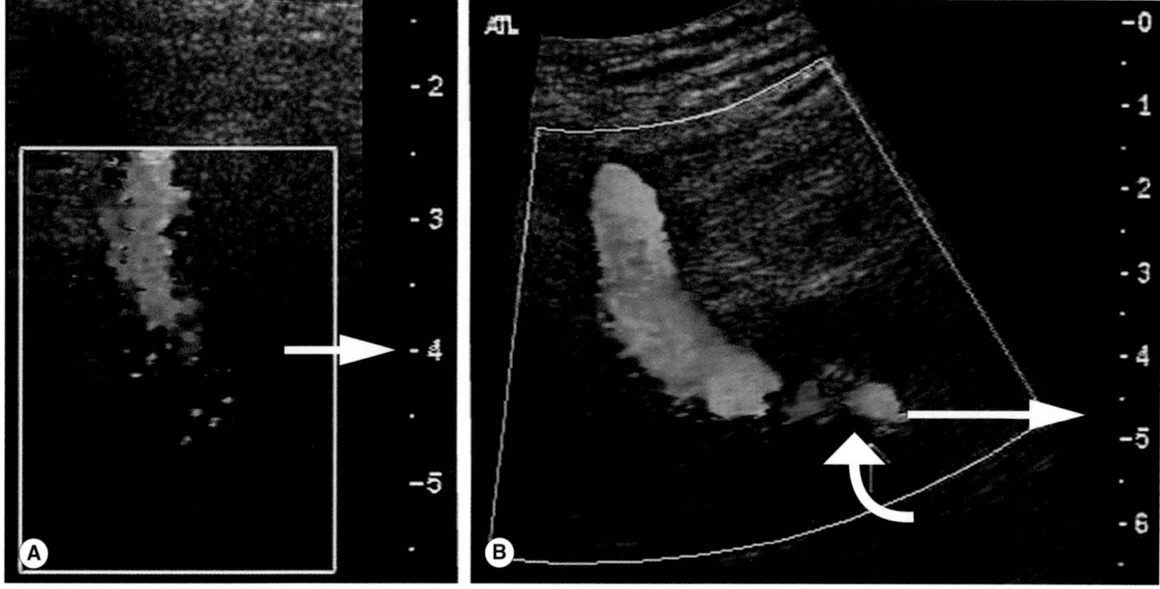

Figure 15.7 • Two images of the same graft towards the distal anastomosis, located in the lower thigh of a patient with healing wounds. (A) A mid-range transducer is unable to show flow in the distal section of the graft below 4 cm depth (arrow). (B) A low-frequency transducer demonstrates flow to the anastomosis (curved arrow) which is located at a depth of 4.5 cm.

Aortobifemoral grafts

These are imaged by locating the graft at the level of the groin and following it proximally to the aorta. A combination of low- and mid-frequency transducers is required for this examination.

Femorofemoral cross-over grafts

These can be imaged by starting at either groin and following the graft across the pubic region to the opposite side. This can normally be achieved with a mid-frequency transducer.

Iliofemoral cross-over grafts

These grafts are easier to scan by starting at the distal anastomosis at the level of the femoral artery and following the graft back to the proximal anastomosis in the contralateral iliac artery. A combination of mid-frequency linear and low-frequency curvilinear transducers is needed for this assessment. It is usually worth scanning the iliac artery above the proximal anastomosis to identify any inflow disease.

Axillobifemoral grafts

These usually remain relatively superficial along their length. The cross-over section of the graft can be scanned from the distal anastomosis at the femoral artery to its bifurcation from the main segment of the graft on the opposite side of the body. The remainder of the graft is then imaged from the ipsilateral groin, along the lateral wall of the abdomen and chest, to the infraclavicular fossa, where the anastomosis to the axillary artery can be imaged.

B-MODE IMAGES

Normal appearance

Vein grafts

The graft lumen should be clear and of a reasonably even caliber. Some gentle tapering is often seen in the lower portion of an in situ vein graft or non-reversed graft, as the native great saphenous vein is smaller in the lower leg. In contrast, the proximal lumen of a reversed vein graft may be smaller in caliber than the distal graft. It is common to see slight areas of dilation along a vein graft at points corresponding to valve sites. The proximal and distal anastomoses are sometimes difficult to image clearly, due to surrounding scar tissue or depth. It may be difficult to image a deep reversed vein graft without color flow imaging.

Synthetic grafts

Synthetic grafts made of PTFE produce a characteristic image, with the anterior and posterior walls displaying a 'double line' appearance due to the strong reflection of ultrasound (Fig. 15.3). Some PTFE grafts are externally supported by rings that can be seen on the image (see Fig. 7.3). The corrugated structure of Dacron grafts, used mainly for aortobifemoral bypass surgery, is usually easy to see (see Fig. 15.18). Vein cuffs or collars are sometimes used to join the graft to the distal native artery, and these are often seen as a short dilation at the anastomosis.

Abnormal appearance

Many vein graft stenoses are difficult to identify with B-mode imaging alone, as they can be short or web-like and poorly echogenic. Larger areas of hyperplasia can appear as moderately echogenic regions in the vessel lumen (Fig. 15.8). It is sometimes possible to see remnant valve cusps flapping in the lumen of in situ vein grafts due to inadequate stripping with the valvulotome. Areas of vein grafts may become tortuous and dilated over time, and changes in graft diameter should be recorded. In some cases large areas of thrombus or hyperplasia can be seen in aneurysmal segments, and the B-mode image may show partial stagnation or stasis of blood flow in these areas. This will be visualized as strong specular reflections in the dilated region, swirling in time with arterial pulsation. True and false aneurysms of vein or synthetic grafts can be easily seen and are discussed later in this chapter.

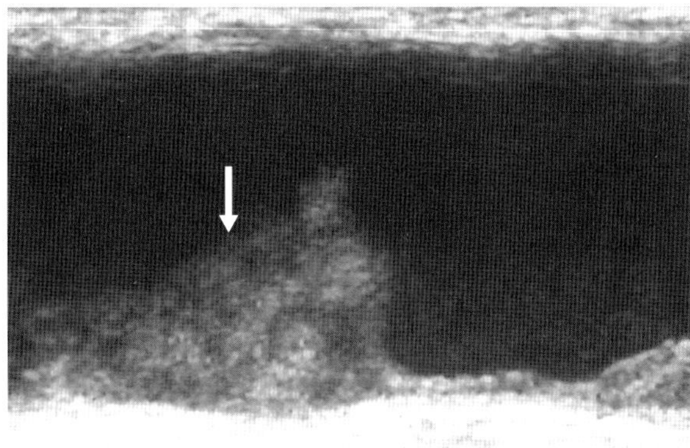

Figure 15.8 • In this magnified B-mode image, a large area of intimal hyperplasia (arrow) is seen in a vein graft.

COLOR DOPPLER IMAGES

Normal appearance of vein grafts

An ultrasound montage of an in situ vein graft is shown in Figure 15.9. The color flow image often demonstrates areas of marked flow disturbance and flow reversal at the proximal anastomosis due to the size, geometry, and orientation of the graft origin from the native artery. This may also be seen at the level of the distal anastomosis and should not be considered abnormal unless spectral Doppler recordings demonstrate significant velocity changes. Beyond the proximal anastomosis, the color flow image should demonstrate an undisturbed flow pattern. Grafts with well-established biphasic or triphasic flow will display normal reversal of flow (from red to blue or vice versa) during the diastolic phase. New grafts may demonstrate hyperemic flow due to peripheral dilation and the flow requirements of healing tissue, exhibited as constant forward flow throughout the cardiac cycle. If the graft has a large lumen, the flow velocity may be very low, and the PRF or color scale may have to be significantly lowered to demonstrate color filling. Some areas of flow reversal may be seen in areas of vein grafts corresponding to valve sites. In rare instances in which the vein is found to be bifid for a short segment, it is possible to see two flow lumens. The distal anastomosis of a femoral distal graft is usually easier to identify with color flow imaging than with B-mode imaging. It is common to see the graft supplying a patent segment of the native artery above the anastomosis as well as distally, and retrograde flow will be seen in the native vessel above the anastomosis, producing a Y-shaped junction (Fig. 15.9). There is often a considerable size discrepancy between the distal end of a vein graft, which can be quite large, and the outflow artery, which may be a smaller tibial vessel. This will cause a natural velocity increase due to the change in vessel diameter, possibly producing color aliasing at the position of the anastomosis and proximal run-off vessel, but this should not be assumed to indicate a significant stenosis without close interrogation with spectral Doppler.

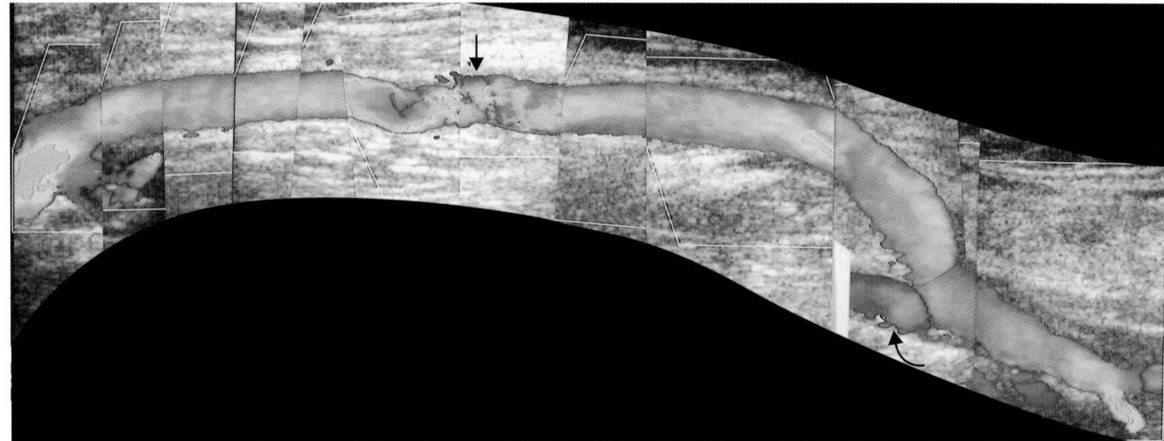

Figure 15.9 • A color montage of an in situ vein graft. Areas of color flow aliasing and flow disturbance within the body of the graft may indicate a graft stenosis (arrow). These areas should be closely checked with spectral Doppler. There is retrograde filling of a short segment of the popliteal artery (curved arrow) above the distal anastomosis.

Normal appearance of synthetic grafts

Flow in synthetic grafts can sometimes be difficult to demonstrate using color flow imaging, as the graft material attenuates the Doppler signal, requiring an increase in the color gain. Significant flow disturbance can be seen at the origins and ends of synthetic iliofemoral or femorofemoral cross-over grafts, as the graft is often joined at a 90° angle to the native artery.

Abnormal appearance of vein grafts

A significant graft stenosis will produce marked flow disturbance, which is usually associated with aliasing on the color flow image (Fig. 15.9; see Fig. 15.14), and there may be considerable flow disturbance beyond the stenosis. Failing grafts may demonstrate very low volume flow, which can sometimes be difficult to demonstrate with color flow imaging, and the graft may be mistakenly reported as occluded. If no flow is detected in the graft, the color PRF and high-pass filter setting should be reduced to confirm the occlusion, which should also be checked with spectral Doppler. Arteriovenous fistulas and aneurysms are other graft abnormalities that are visible with color flow imaging, as discussed below.

SPECTRAL DOPPLER WAVEFORMS

Normal appearance

Caution

Remember, when comparing peak systolic velocities in adjacent segments of a vessel with differing diameters, the respective velocities will be different even in the absence of a stenosis as flow velocity is inversely proportional to cross-sectional area (Figs 5.3. and 15.13)

The waveform shapes in normal vein grafts can vary considerably depending on the age of the graft. New grafts may demonstrate a hyperemic monophasic flow profile because of sustained peripheral vasodilation that can be due to a combination of the previous ischemia and healing tissue (Fig. 15.10A). Over time, the flow pattern should become pulsatile, and biphasic or triphasic waveforms are usually recorded (Fig. 15.10B). It is good practice to take spectral Doppler measurements at regular intervals along a graft, even in the presence of a normal color flow display, as changes in the waveform shape can indicate an approach-

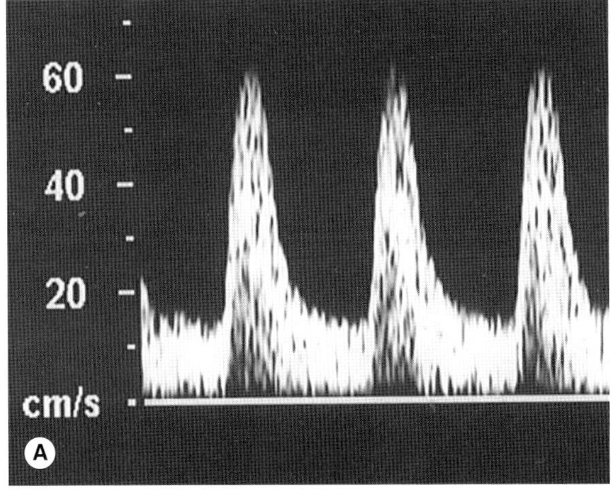

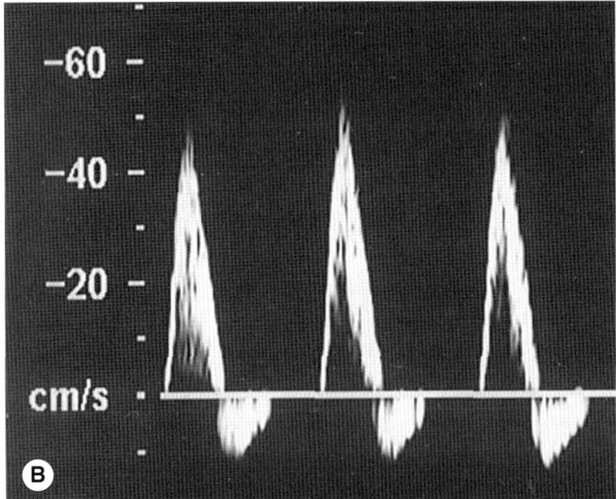

Figure 15.10 • (A) Hyperemic flow is often seen in the early postoperative period. (B) Over time, the flow normally assumes a pulsatile flow pattern.

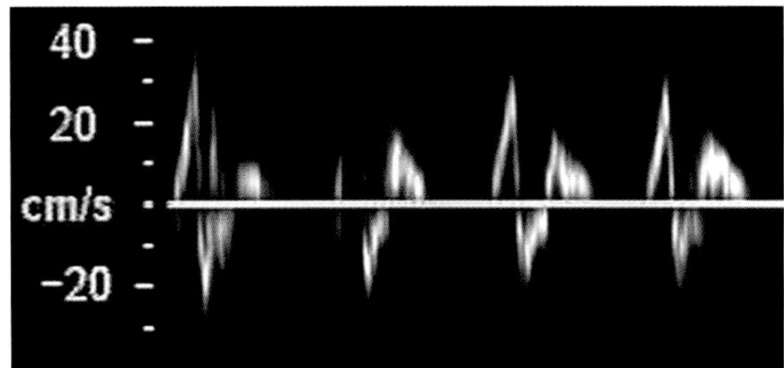

Figure 15.11 • A Doppler waveform taken from the origin of a vein graft indicates a slightly disturbed flow pattern due to the geometry of the anastomosis but there is no evidence of stenotic flow.

ing problem. Disturbed flow, including areas of flow reversal, is usually encountered around the proximal anastomosis, but there should be no significant increase in systolic velocity (Fig. 15.11). Natural changes in the diameter of the graft will produce changes in the peak systolic velocity (PSV), which should not automatically be assumed to represent a stenosis. In this situation, velocities should be compared in adjacent areas of similar vessel diameter. Perhaps the most difficult assessment to make during graft surveillance is the estimation of the degree of narrowing at the distal anastomosis, where there is often a large-diameter vein graft joined to a smaller outflow artery, producing a natural velocity increase. In this situation, it is possible to see a significant increase in the PSV in the absence of a stenosis. However, flow velocities just below the distal anastomosis should be similar to those several centimeters downstream, provided that the vessel diameter is the same. A significant stenosis would be indicated if the velocities at the anastomosis were found to be substantially higher (i.e., 3–4 times) than distal velocities. It is also important to ensure that the spectral Doppler angle is set correctly at the distal anastomosis, as flow is not always parallel to the vessel walls, and this can lead to errors in velocity measurements.

Abnormal appearance

Graft stenoses are categorized using a similar method to that for grading lower-limb arterial disease. The PSV across the stenosis is divided by the PSV in a normal segment of graft just proximal to the stenosis (Figs 15.12–15.14). The criteria for grading graft stenoses are shown in Table 15.2. Intervention by angioplasty or surgical revision is usually performed when the PSV ratio is equal to or greater than 3 (London et al. 1993; Olojugba et al. 1998; Landry et al. 2002). Stenoses producing a PSV ratio of 2–2.9 are kept under close surveillance. In addition, a PSV of less than 45 cm/s within the graft has been suggested to indicate a graft defect (Mills et al. 1990). Care must be exercised in the use of this criterion as patients with large-diameter grafts may have relatively low velocity flow within the graft, because velocity

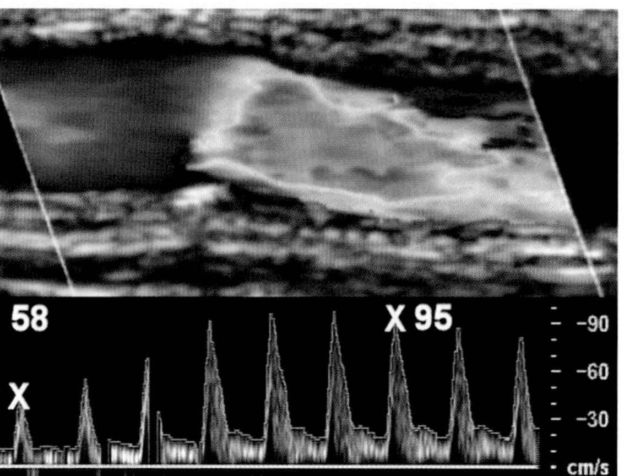

Figure 15.12 • A stenosis is indicated in the body of a vein graft by an area of color aliasing. Spectral Doppler measurements show a mild to moderate velocity increase across the stenosis from 58 to 95 cm/s, equivalent to 1.7 times velocity ratio. This is not considered significant.

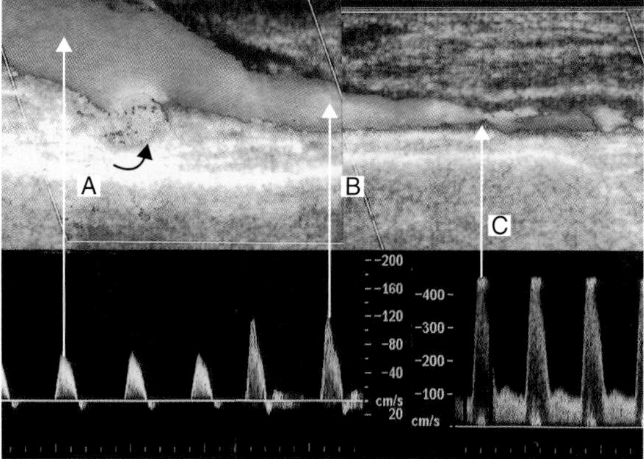

Figure 15.13 • Problems in interpreting flow velocities in a vein graft anastomosed to the posterior tibial artery. At point A, the peak systolic velocity (PSV) in the distal graft is 65 cm/s. At point B the PSV in the posterior tibial artery, just distal to the anastomosis, is 120 cm/s. This represents a near doubling in velocity, suggesting a stenosis. However, the diameter of the posterior tibial artery is significantly smaller than that of the distal graft, leading to a natural increase in systolic velocity, as flow velocity is inversely related to cross-sectional area, and in this example no narrowing is indicated. Unfortunately, at point C, a significant stenosis is demonstrated in the posterior tibial artery, 2 cm distal to the anastomosis, by color flow aliasing and there is a significant increase in the PSV, >400 cm/s. In this image there is some retrograde filling of the native vessel above the anastomosis (curved arrow).

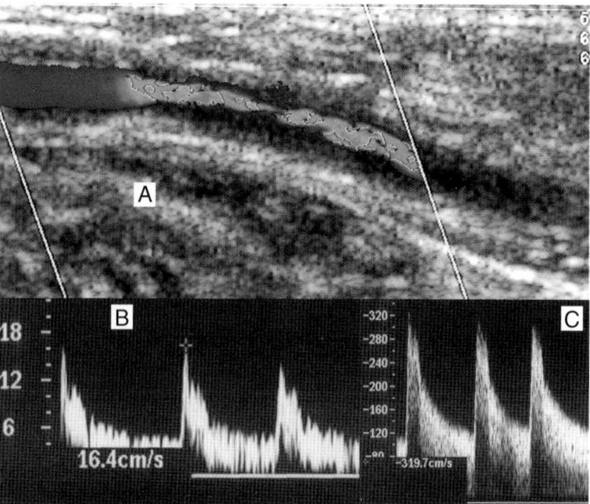

Figure 15.14 • The peak systolic velocity (PSV) ratio is used to estimate the degree of narrowing across a graft stenosis. (A) Color flow imaging demonstrates a severe graft stenosis. (B) The PSV just proximal to the stenosis is 16.4 cm/s. (C) The PSV across the stenosis is 319 cm/s, associated with marked spectral broadening. This represents a 19 times velocity ratio, indicating a critical stenosis.

DIAMETER REDUCTION	SPECTRAL DOPPLER CRITERIA
<50%	PSV ratio < 2
50–69%	PSV ratio 2–2.9; increased spectral broadening and turbulence just beyond the stenosis; waveform becomes more monophasic
70–99%	PSV ratio ≥3; marked turbulence distal to the stenosis; waveform may be monophasic
Occlusion	No flow signal present

A peak systolic velocity (PSV) > 300 cm/s across a stenosis is also considered significant (Bandyk 2007).

Table 15.2 Spectral Doppler criteria for grading a graft stenosis

is inversely related to cross-sectional area. In our experience, many normal grafts with velocities below this level do not occlude. Poor spectral Doppler angles may produce considerable errors in one-spot velocity measurements, and it is therefore important to select an area of the graft where a good Doppler angle can be obtained for accurate velocity measurement. Damped flow in the artery proximal to the proximal anastomosis often indicates an inflow stenosis, and this should be examined with duplex, as poor inflow can lead to graft occlusion. A stenosis of the outflow artery below the distal anastomosis can also dramatically reduce flow in the graft by increasing distal resistance. For this reason, it is important to scan the run-off artery below the graft. However, it is interesting to note that some grafts remain patent for years, despite occlusion of the run-off vessel. This is due to retrograde flow into a patent segment of artery above the anastomosis, filling collateral vessels (Fig. 15.15).

GRAFT FAILURE AND OCCLUSION

Despite the most aggressive surveillance programs, some grafts will occlude for a variety of reasons. Occluded vein grafts can be difficult to identify by B-mode imaging, especially if the graft lies deep, as it may merge into the tissue planes. When it is possible to identify the graft, there is usually thrombus seen within the lumen. An occluded graft is usually easiest to identify by scanning at the level of the proximal anastomosis. The most obvious signs of graft occlusion are an absence of color flow and spectral Doppler signals. Ankle–brachial pressures will also be reduced. A thrombosing graft may contain clot at the distal end, and spectral Doppler will demonstrate a characteristic low-volume, high-resistance flow pattern in the patent lumen above this area with no net forward flow (Fig. 15.16). In this situation the B-mode image may demonstrate slight backward and forward pulsation of the blood, exhibited as a speckle pattern. This indicates imminent graft occlusion and should be reported immediately. Conversely, a low-volume damped waveform in the proximal graft would indicate an inflow stenosis.

COMMONLY ENCOUNTERED PROBLEMS

Large and obese patients can be difficult to examine, and it may be necessary to use a lower-frequency transducer (Fig 15.7). Early postoperative scans can be difficult if the wounds are still healing, and scanning over a sterile transparent plastic dressing is useful in this situation. Having no prior knowledge of the type and position of graft can lead to considerable problems. For example, a popliteal to tibial vein bypass graft may require the great saphenous

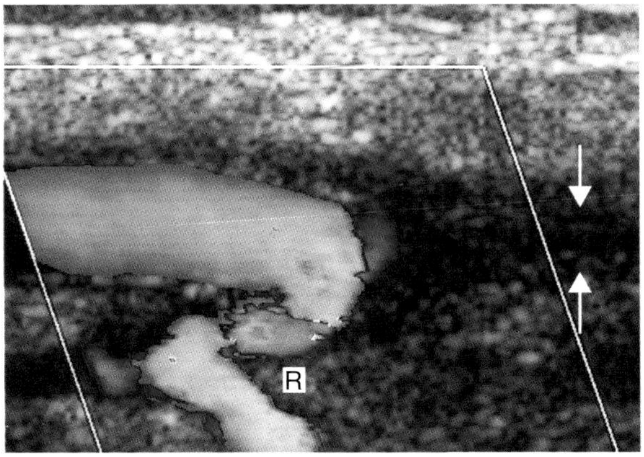

R

Figure 15.15 • A color flow image of the distal end of a vein graft demonstrates occlusion of the posterior tibial artery (arrows) at the distal anastomosis. However, the graft remains patent due to retrograde flow (R), filling a segment of native vessel above the anastomosis.

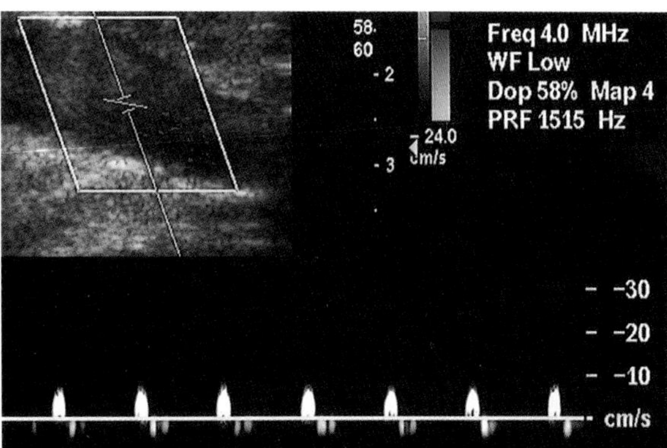

Figure 15.16 • Extremely low-volume flow recorded from an in situ vein graft indicates imminent graft occlusion. In this example the distal end of the graft had already thrombosed and the Doppler waveform demonstrates no net forward flow.

vein to be harvested from the thigh, as it is larger at this level. Therefore, a large scar will be seen in the thigh, but the graft will not be located at this level; however, the sonographer may automatically assume that this corresponds to the position of the proximal graft. A copy of the operation notes is a useful aid to locating the graft.

It is also possible for grafts to be routed in unusual directions, such as across the anterolateral thigh to join the anterior tibial artery in the calf. Some patients may have had a previous graft that has since occluded, and this could be mistaken for the new graft, which may still be patent. It is also possible for segments of native vessels to be patent, such as the superficial femoral artery, and this may cause some confusion or may even be mistaken for the graft.

TRUE AND FALSE ANEURYSMS

Vein grafts can develop true aneurysmal dilations over time, particularly at valve sites or at the anastomoses (Fig. 15.17). This can occur if the vein wall becomes structurally weak. A localized doubling in the graft diameter indicates the development of an aneurysm, and this should be reported and kept under regular surveillance to monitor progression. It is not uncommon to see thrombus in aneurysmal areas. Color flow imaging and spectral Doppler usually demonstrate areas of flow reversal in the aneurysmal regions. Large true aneurysms are repaired surgically by replacing the aneurysmal area with a new segment of vein.

False aneurysms are caused by blood flowing into and out of a defect in the vessel wall (see Ch. 11). They are typified as swirling areas of flow in a contained cavity outside the true flow lumen and may contain thrombus. They can occur if the suture line at the anastomosis fails or as a complication of balloon angioplasty, due to splitting of the graft wall following high-pressure balloon inflation (Fig. 15.18). False aneurysms also occur at catheter puncture sites (see Ch. 11).

ENTRAPMENT OF GRAFTS

Entrapment of grafts can occur around the knee level, especially where in situ vein grafts run from superficial to deep, through a tunnel in the muscles. In this situation, normal flow may be recorded with the leg extended, but mild to moderate flexion of the knee joint produces pinching of the graft between muscle groups, causing a temporary ste-

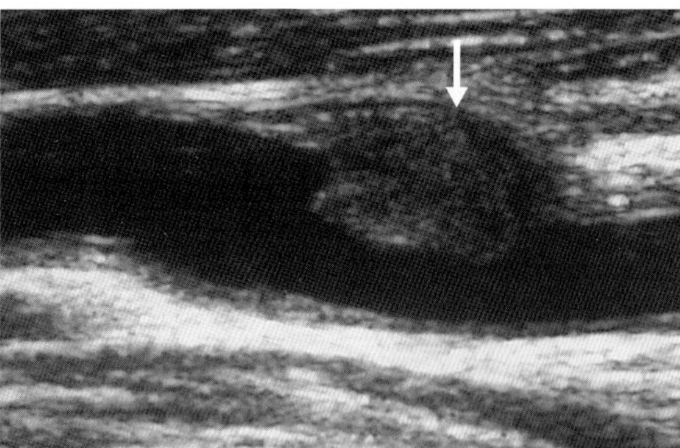

Figure 15.17 • An aneurysmal area in a vein graft corresponding to a valve site. Note the area of hyperplasia or thrombus (arrow) in the area of dilation.

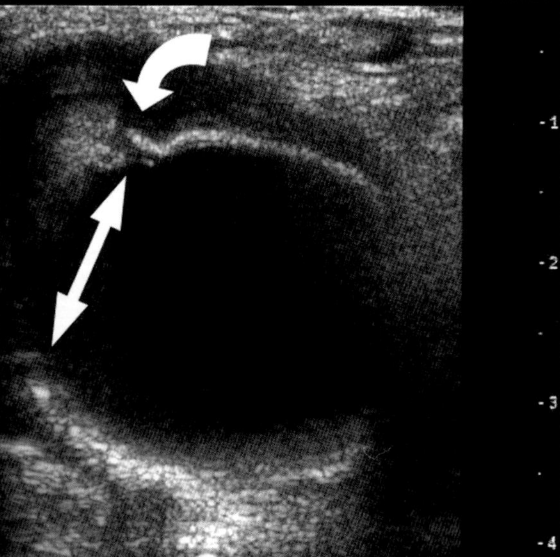

Figure 15.18 • The suture line at the distal anastomosis of an aortobifemoral graft has failed and a large gap is now visible between the graft material (double-headed arrow), creating a false aneurysm, which in this case mainly contains thrombus (curved arrow).

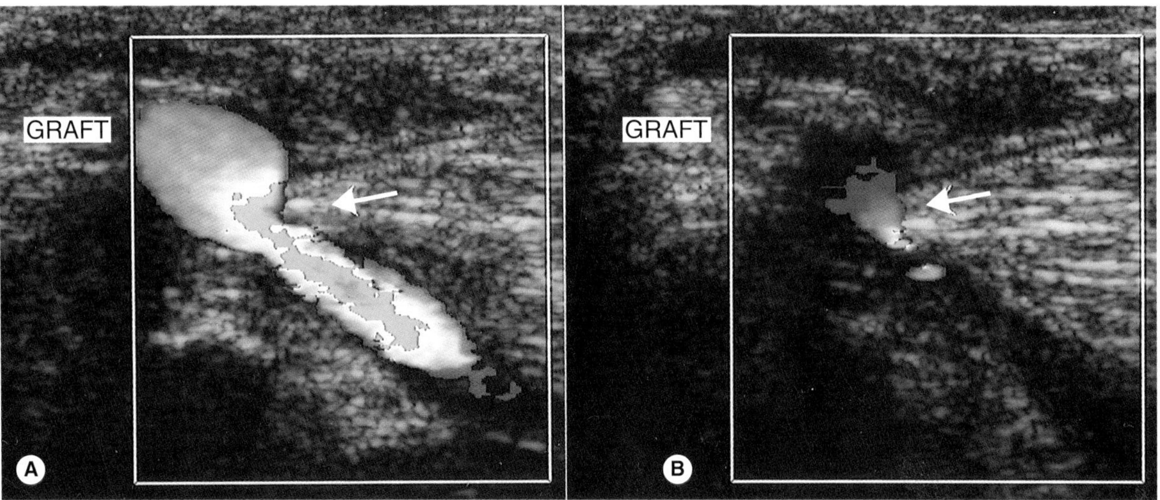

Figure 15.19 • An example of graft entrapment. (A) A vein graft is running between two muscles in the lower thigh, and a moderate stenosis is seen (arrow). (B) During leg flexion the graft is compressed between the muscles, causing a virtual occlusion (arrow).

nosis (Fig. 15.19). Conversely, some grafts become temporarily obstructed during full knee extension. This is a relatively rare problem, but it will be seen from time to time in a busy laboratory. If the problem is significant, the muscle can be divided or the graft re-routed.

ARTERIOVENOUS FISTULAS

Arteriovenous fistulas occur in in situ vein grafts where there has been incomplete ligation of a great saphenous vein side branch, allowing blood to short-circuit from the graft directly into the venous system (Fig. 15.20). Arteriovenous fistulas are characterized by hyperemic or high-volume flow in the graft proximal to the fistula, with an area of marked color flow disturbance at the site of the fistula (Fig. 15.21). Spectral Doppler also demonstrates turbulent high-volume flow with a low-resistance waveform at this site. The veins leading from the fistula also demonstrate a high-volume flow pattern. Flow in the graft distal to the fistula is usually lower in volume and more pulsatile. In some circumstances, the graft below the site of the fistula may be totally occluded. Arteriovenous fistulas can be ligated or embolized. It is useful to mark the level of the defect using duplex so that the surgeon can easily locate the fistula.

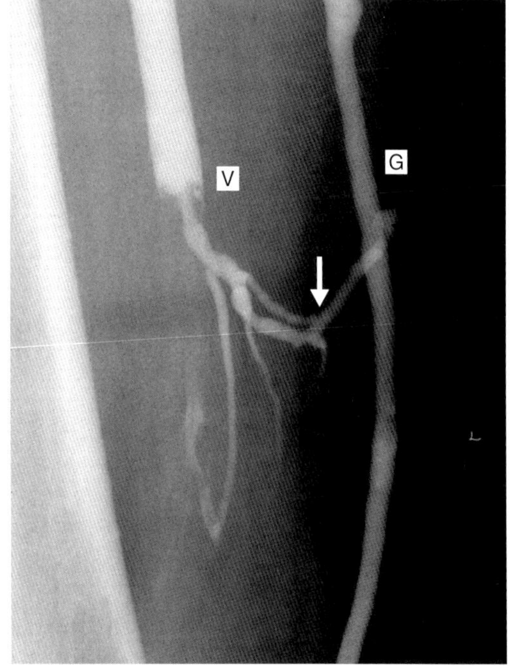

Figure 15.20 • An arteriogram demonstrates an arteriovenous fistula (arrow) between a vein graft (G) and the venous system (V).

SEROMAS, FLUID COLLECTIONS, AND GRAFT INFECTIONS

Seromas are fluid-filled collections that are occasionally seen adjacent to vein grafts, particularly at the level of the groin. They can be mistaken for false aneurysms on B-mode imaging, but color flow imaging will demonstrate an absence of flow (Fig. 15.22A). Fluid collections around synthetic grafts can be due to local reaction of the surrounding tissues, but they can also be due to graft infection (Fig 15.22B). Graft infections are a serious complication and are more frequently associated with synthetic grafts. The outcome for patients with synthetic graft infections is often poor (Mertens et al. 1995). Infections at the level of the groin are common due to the rich source of bacteria in this region, and aortobifemoral, iliofemoral, and axillobifemoral grafts are especially at risk. Complications of infection can lead to the disintegration of a graft anastomosis, resulting in severe hemorrhage. Failure of wound healing is also a frequent complication. Ultrasound imaging can be useful for investigating wound infections, as the B-mode image can show whether the graft is in direct contact with suspected areas of infection, especially if the suspected region tracks to discharging wounds or openings on the skin surface (Fig. 15.23). It is essential to image any suspected area of graft infection in cross-section to see how it relates to the graft and surrounding structures. It can be difficult to differentiate areas of infection from simple hematomas, and bacterial cultures are often required to isolate infective organisms. Ultrasound can be used to guide the needle puncture during the sampling of fluid collections to avoid accidentally puncturing the graft. Computed tomography and magnetic resonance imaging are also commonly used for investigating graft infections, especially in the abdomen. Methicillin-resistant *Staphylococcus aureus* (MRSA) is now endemic in most hospitals. Graft infections caused by MRSA are difficult to treat, requiring prolonged use of powerful antibiotics. In some cases, graft removal is necessary to remove the focus of infection, but this may lead to inevitable amputation of the limb, due to poor blood flow. In extreme situations, the patient may be overwhelmed by the infection and die.

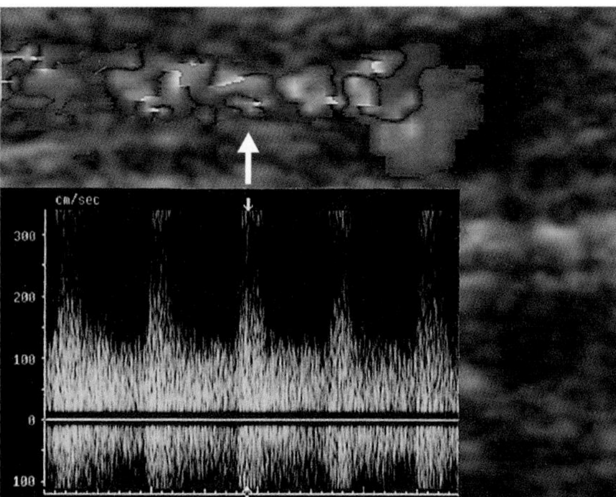

Figure 15.21 • A transverse color flow image of a vein graft demonstrating an arteriovenous fistula (arrow). The Doppler waveform displays low-resistance, high-volume flow across the fistula.

REPORTING

The easiest method of reporting the scan results is by the use of diagrams. The graft position can be drawn on to the diagram with velocity measurements and other relevant information recorded (Fig. 15.24). It is also useful to keep a file for each patient in the graft surveillance program in the vascular laboratory, as this makes comparison of serial follow-up scans easier. Any significant graft problems must be reported to the appropriate medical staff immediately. In addition, many vascular units combine the duplex assessment with a measurement of the ankle–brachial pressure index (ABPI). An ABPI <1 can indicate a problem. A serial reduction <0.1 in ABPI readings is indicative of a significant problem (Brennan et al. 1991).

SUPERFICIAL VEIN MAPPING FOR ARTERIAL BYPASS SURGERY

A preoperative duplex scan can determine the suitability of a superficial vein for use as a bypass graft (Bagi et al. 1989). Careful marking of its path avoids undermining of skin flaps during surgery and possible wound necrosis. The great saphenous vein is the most commonly used vein for arterial bypass surgery, due to its length. Arm veins and the small saphenous vein can also be used for bypass

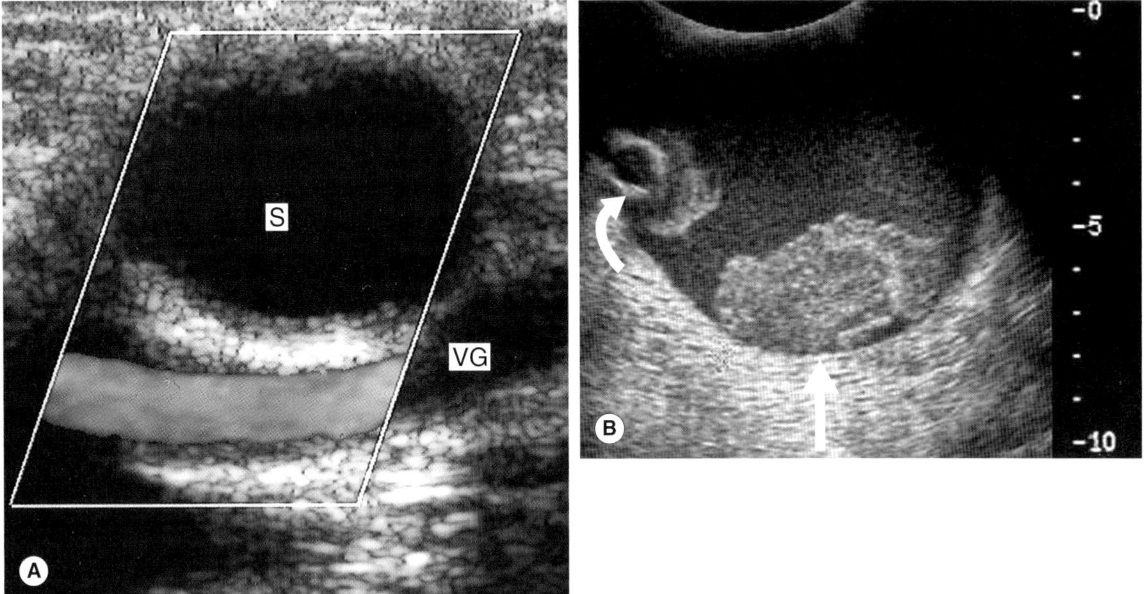

Figure 15.22 • (A) A fluid-filled seroma (S) adjacent to a vein graft (VG). (B) A femorofemoral cross-over graft (curved arrow) is running through a large region of fluid, with echogenic debris shown by the straight arrow. This appearance does not necessarily represent an infection but can be due to tissue reaction to the graft.

grafts, provided that their lumens are of sufficient diameter.

Technique for assessing the great saphenous vein

> **OBSERVATION**
>
> Normal non-varicose great saphenous veins having a borderline diameter (2.5–3 mm) in younger patients can be relatively compliant and will dilate to a larger diameter when exposed to arterial pressure. Try examining the leg in a dependent position. Any doubts about vein suitability should be discussed with the surgeon.

The patient should be positioned with the feet tilted down to distend the veins. A high-frequency, flat linear array transducer should be used to image the veins. Starting at the top of the leg, the great saphenous vein should be identified in transverse section at the level of the saphenofemoral junction and followed distally down the thigh and into the calf. Scanning the vein in transverse section is important, because it is easier to assess its diameter and to identify any large tributaries dividing from the vein, or duplicated or bifid systems. The diameter of the vein should be recorded at frequent intervals throughout its length. Ideally, the diameter should be greater than 3 mm to be suitable as a graft. Veins of less than 2 mm in diameter are regarded as too small to be used for femoral distal bypass grafting. Veins that become excessively large (0.8 cm diameter) or grossly varicose may also be unsuitable, and this should be drawn to the attention of the surgeon. The common femoral vein, femoral vein, and popliteal vein should be examined when vein mapping to ensure deep venous patency, as the great saphenous vein can act as an important collateral pathway if the deep veins have been obstructed and, in such circumstances, should not be harvested for a graft. In this situation, other sources of vein can be assessed.

Arm vein mapping

It is not uncommon to find that part or all of the great saphenous vein is unsuitable for use as a graft

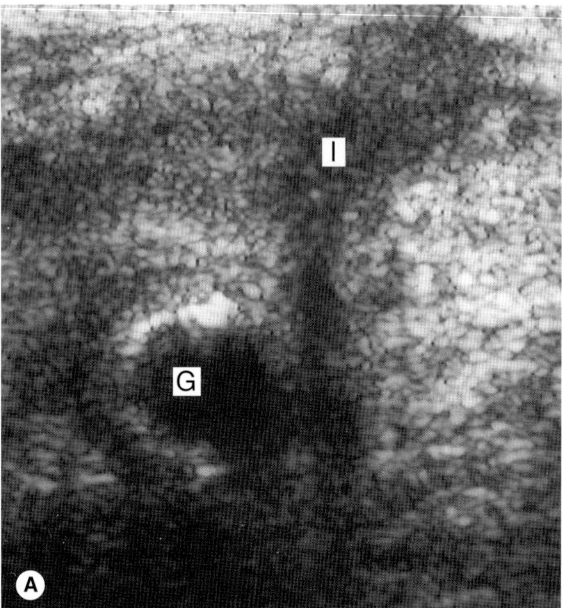

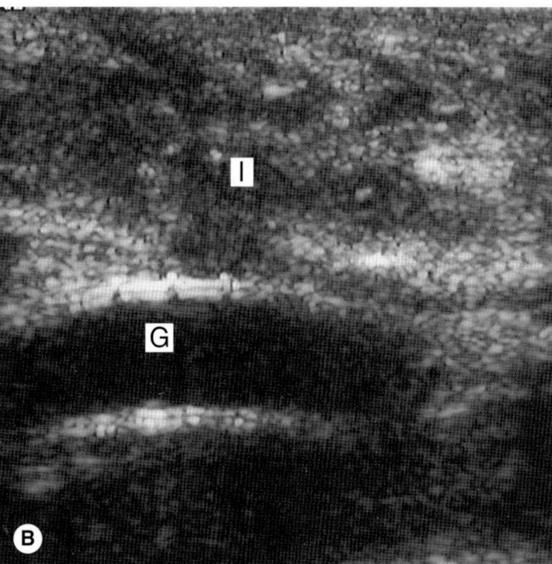

Figure 15.23 • (A) A transverse image of a polytetrafluoroethylene (PTFE) graft (G) demonstrating an echo region (I) tracking to the skin surface that is in contact with the graft, indicating a potential graft infection. (B) A longitudinal image of a graft, indicating a suspicious area (I) lying over the graft (G). Note that the ring supports of the graft can be seen in this image.

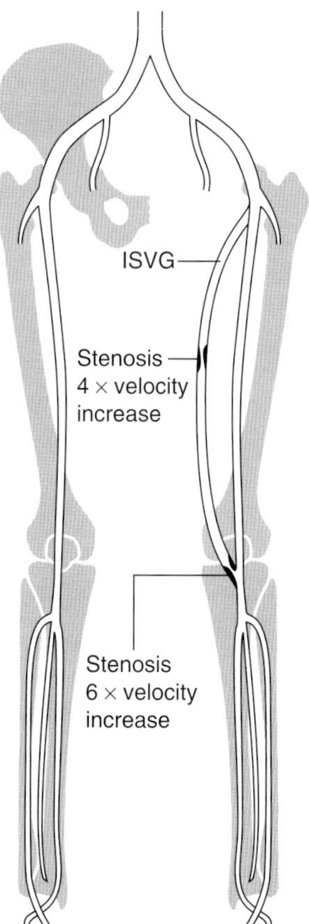

Figure 15.24 • Diagrams are the simplest method of reporting the results of graft surveillance scans. ISVG, in situ vein graft.

because it is too small, because it is varicose, or because the deep veins are obstructed. In addition, the great saphenous vein may have already been removed for coronary artery bypass surgery. The cephalic or basilic veins of the arm can be harvested for bypass grafts provided they are of adequate diameter. The cephalic vein is the vein of choice, as it is longer than the basilic vein, and the anatomy of the basilic vein is more variable in its proximal segment. To image the veins, the arm should be in a comfortable dependent position with the palm facing upward. The cephalic vein can be located in transverse section along the outer aspect of the forearm 2–3 cm above the wrist, lateral to the radial artery and followed proximally. Alternatively, it can be located in the anterior aspect of the upper arm, lying superficial to the biceps muscle and then followed proximally toward the shoulder and then distally into the forearm (see Figures 16.6 and 16.7). The vein can be difficult to follow as it crosses the antecubital fossa, as there are a number of superficial veins crossing this area.

The basilic vein is easiest to locate with the arm extended outward (abducted) and the palm facing upward. The probe is placed on the medial aspect of the arm 2–3 cm above the elbow joint. Imaging in cross-section, the basilic vein should be seen as separate from the brachial vein and artery (Fig. 15.25). The vein can then be followed proximally, where it is usually seen to course toward the proximal brachial vein or the axillary vein, although there can be anatomical variation of the veins in this region. Following the basilic vein distally into the forearm can be confusing, as it sometimes joins the cephalic vein in the forearm via the median cubital vein, but it usually runs toward the medial (ulnar) aspect of the wrist. One potential pitfall of mapping the basilic vein is accidentally confusing it with the brachial artery, but use of probe compression to collapse the vein and color flow imaging should avoid this error.

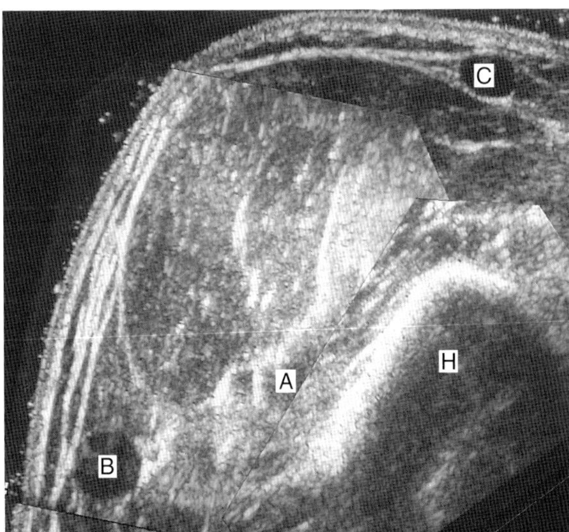

Figure 15.25 • A transverse B-mode montage of the left upper arm demonstrating the position of the basilic vein (B), cephalic vein (C), and brachial artery and veins (A). The arm was positioned with the palm up so that the cephalic vein lies on the anterior aspect of the arm and the basilic vein and brachial vessels on the medial aspect. The humerus is also seen (H).

Technique of marking the vein

There are two techniques for marking leg or arm veins (Fig. 15.26). Using the first method, the vein is imaged in transverse section with the vein appearing in the center of the image. Using a marker pen, a dot is then placed on the skin surface against the middle of the probe. It is easier to start by marking the vein in the upper thigh, rather than at the level of the saphenofemoral junction, and then to work toward the saphenofemoral junction. The vein should be marked with a dot at frequent intervals along the thigh and calf. Finally the gel is completely removed and the dots joined up with

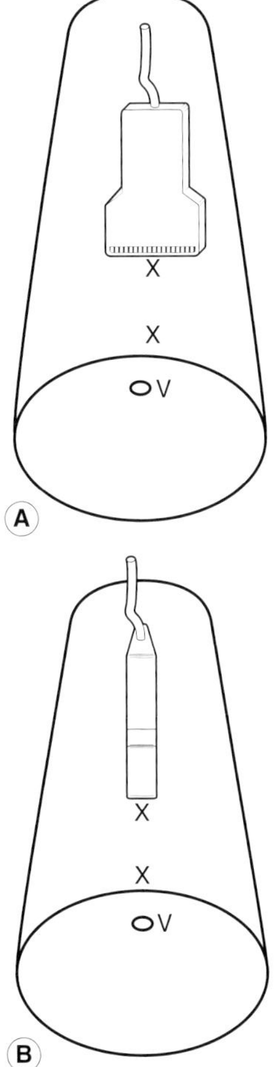

Figure 15.26 • Two methods can be used for vein mapping. (A) The vein (V) can be marked (X) in the transverse plane. (B) The vein can also be marked in a longitudinal plane.

a continuous line using a permanent felt-tipped marker pen.

The second technique involves assessing the vein in transverse section for its size and position, and then marking the vein with the transducer turned into a longitudinal plane and the vein imaged in this direction. A dot is placed against the end of the transducer to correspond to the position and direction of the vein. This technique is more difficult in terms of imaging, as it is easy to 'slip off' the image of the vein and follow a tissue plane, but it does seem to produce a more accurate map of the vein. When the position of the vein has been marked using this technique, it is wise to run down the length of marking with the transducer in transverse section to ensure that the dots follow the main trunk, in case a smaller side branch in the lower leg may have accidentally been followed using this method.

Problems encountered during vein mapping

One major practical problem of vein mapping is trying to mark the position of the vein with a felt-tipped pen through the ultrasound gel, as the pen quickly becomes clogged with gel and no longer works. Many vascular units have their own personal preferences for overcoming this problem. A charcoal pencil can be useful for dotting in the position of the vein and the dots joined up later with a felt-tipped pen once the gel has been removed. Alternatively, using small amounts of gel and frequently wiping the gel away from the probe edge before marking prevents the pen tip from becoming saturated in ultrasound gel. It is also useful to place a non-sterile probe cover over the transducer when vein mapping, as this prevents the probe from becoming covered in ink from the marker pen.

If the patient has very poor muscle volume and the superficial tissues are baggy, it can be very difficult to ensure that the marking is accurate. If in any doubt, tell the surgeon. In obese patients, the vein may be very deep, and it can be difficult to mark it in the correct incision plane.

References

Bagi P, Schroeder T, Sillesen H et al. 1989 Real time B-mode mapping of the greater saphenous vein. European Journal of Vascular Surgery 3: 103–105

Bandyk D F 2007 Surveillance after lower extremity arterial bypass. Perspectives in Vascular Surgery and Endovascular Therapy 19: 376–383

Brennan J A, Walsh A K, Beard J D et al. 1991 The role of simple non-invasive testing in infrainguinal graft surveillance. European Journal of Vascular Surgery 51: 13–17

Caps M T, Cantwell-Gab K, Bergelin R O et al. 1995 Vein graft lesions: time of onset and rate of progression. Journal of Vascular Surgery 22: 466–475

Davies AH, Hawdon AJ, Sydes MR et al. 2005 Is duplex surveillance of value after leg vein bypass grafting? Principal results of the Vein Graft Surveillance Randomised Trial (VGST). Circulation 112: 1985–1991

Grigg M J, Nicolaides A N, Wolfe J H 1988 Femorodistal vein bypass graft stenoses. British Journal of Surgery 75: 737–740

Klinkert P, Schepers A, Burger D H C et al. 2003 Vein versus polytetrafluoroethylene in above-knee femoropopliteal bypass grafting: five-year results of a randomized controlled trial. Journal of Vascular Surgery 37: 149–155

Landry G J, Moneta G L, Taylor L M et al. 2002 Long-term outcome of revised lower-extremity bypass grafts. Journal of Vascular Surgery 35: 56–63

London N J M, Sayers R D, Thompson M M et al. 1993 Interventional radiology in the maintenance of infrainguinal vein graft patency. British Journal of Surgery 80: 187–193

Lundell A, Lindblad B, Bergqvist D et al. 1995 Femoropopliteal-crural graft patency is improved by an intensive surveillance program: a prospective randomized study. Journal of Vascular Surgery 21: 26–34

Mertens R A, O'Hara P J, Hertzer N R et al. 1995 Surgical management of infrainguinal arterial prosthetic graft infections: review of a thirty-five-year experience. Journal of Vascular Surgery 21: 782–791

Mills J L, Harris E J, Taylor L M Jr et al. 1990 The importance of routine surveillance of distal bypass grafts with duplex scanning: a study of 379 reversed vein grafts. Journal of Vascular Surgery 12: 379–389

Mofidi R, Kelman J, Berry O et al. 2007 Significance of the early postoperative duplex result in infrainguinal vein bypass surveillance. European Journal of Vascular and Endovascular Surgery 34: 327–332

Olojugba D H, McCarthy M J, Naylor A R et al. 1998 At what peak velocity ratio should duplex-detected infrainguinal vein graft stenoses be revised? European Journal of Vascular and Endovascular Surgery 15: 258–260

Wixon C L, Mills J L, Westerband A et al. 2000 An economic appraisal of lower extremity bypass graft maintenance. Journal of Vascular Surgery 32: 1–12

Ultrasound of hemodialysis access

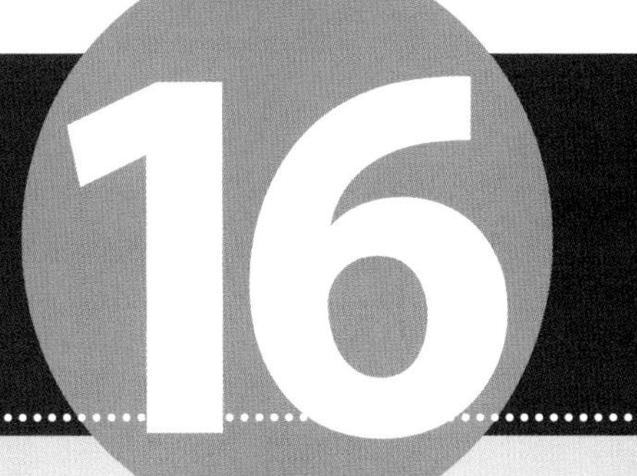

Colin Deane

CONTENTS

INTRODUCTION

Ultrasound has an important role in planning temporary and permanent hemodialysis access, for examining permanent access fistulas and grafts prior to first use, and in the investigation of complications in these fistulas and grafts. Ultrasound may be used for routine monitoring of access flow, although other methods are also available.

Portable ultrasound scanners may be used in dialysis units to aid needling where access is difficult. For a more detailed examination of the access, radiology departments and vascular laboratories are equipped to undertake ultrasound investigation of the whole access circuit. The high flows, unusual hemodynamics, and anatomy of fistulas and grafts can make this a challenging investigation but it is potentially a rewarding one. Ultrasound is a quick, safe, and effective means to identify existing and impending problems, enabling early radiological or surgical intervention to prolong the use of the existing access and to plan effective alternatives.

HEMODIALYSIS ACCESS

Hemodialysis requires high blood flow, from 250 to 400 ml/min, to the extracorporeal dialyzer. Hemodialysis is used in both acute and chronic renal failure.

Acute renal failure

Following a sudden loss of renal function, dialysis is usually via a central venous catheter. Ultrasound is used to examine central, neck, and arm veins and to guide catheter placement. In patients with reversible failure, dialysis is discontinued as the kidneys recover. In kidneys with irreversible failure, permanent access is planned, since central venous catheters have a limited life.

Chronic renal failure

Once chronic end-stage renal failure is identified, measurement of the patient's creatinine levels and estimated glomerular filtration rate (eGFR) are used to determine the impending need for dialysis. Ideally, as the prospect of dialysis approaches, permanent access is planned and surgery undertaken so that the access is ready in time for first use.

Permanent access, through a fistula or graft, requires high flows through a superficial vein or graft that can be repeatedly needled (Fig. 16.1), is easy to keep clean, and is comfortable for the patient during periods of dialysis – typically 4 hours three times a week. American and European reviews and guidelines have been produced and are regularly updated to foster good hemodialysis practice (National Kidney Foundation 2006; Tordoir et al. 2007). Both contain comprehensive bibliographies. Amongst challenges for the clinical teams that may involve ultrasound investigation are the need to increase the number of patients with a permanent access in place when they first present for dialysis, identifying the most appropriate access site for patients, and maintaining effective surveillance to reduce the incidence of complications and access failure.

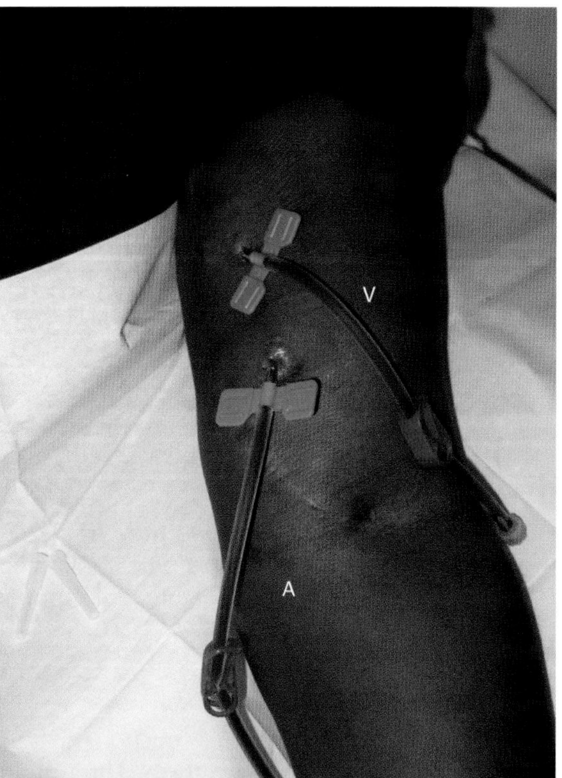

Figure 16.1 • Needles inserted into the basilic vein of a brachial artery/transposed basilic vein fistula prior to dialysis. The distal, upstream, needle is referred to as the arterial needle (A) from which blood is drawn for dialysis. Blood is returned through the venous needle (V).

Access sites

Permanent hemodialysis accesses can be either an arteriovenous fistula where the vein is used for needle access or a prosthetic graft between an artery and vein. Fistulas generally have a lower incidence of complications than grafts (0.2 events/patient per year versus 0.8–1.0 events/patient per year for European Best Practice Guidelines) and superior long-term patency. Grafts can be used earlier following surgery whereas fistulas need more time for the vein to develop and diameter to increase, typically 6 weeks postoperatively. Recommendations are to use fistulas where possible initially.

There are several possible sites for fistulas and grafts in the arms. Once arm accesses are exhausted, femoral artery to femoral vein grafts may be used. Several unusual variations of grafts and veins are possible where access is difficult, depending on the preference of the surgeon and the availability and access of suitable arteries and veins.

The main sites for fistulas and grafts are listed in Box 16.1 and shown diagrammatically in Figure

BOX 16.1 Main sites for arteriovenous fistulas and grafts in approximate order of preference

- Radial–cephalic fistula (ulnar basilic is possible in some patients)
- Brachial–cubital or brachial–cephalic fistula
- Brachial artery–transposed basilic vein fistula
- Forearm graft from radial artery–cubital fossa vein or looped graft from brachial artery–cubital fossa vein
- Upper-arm graft brachial artery–axillary vein
- Femoral–femoral loop graft
- Axillary artery–contralateral axillary vein graft

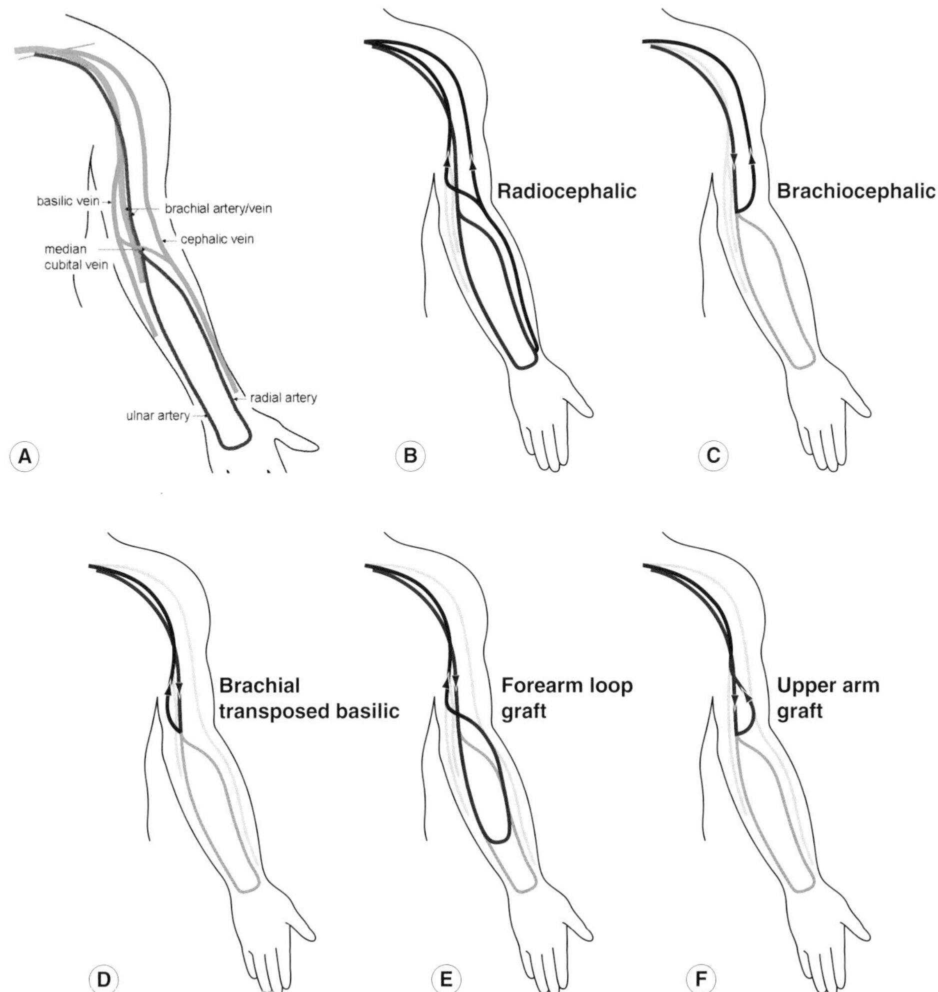

Figure 16.2 • Diagram of common arm fistula and graft sites. (A) Main arm vessels. In the other images, the arterial supply and venous drainage for the high-flow dialysis access circulation are shown in bold. (B) Radiocephalic. (C) Brachiocephalic. (D) Brachial transposed basilic. (E) Forearm loop graft. (F) Upper-arm graft.

16.2. The nondominant arm is generally used initially. Box 16.1 shows an approximate order of preference; the choice for an individual patient depends on many factors. For example, a young patient with good peripheral arm vessels may be a better candidate for a radiocephalic fistula whereas an elderly patient with diabetes and known peripheral vascular disease might start dialysis with a more proximal access. A major advantage of a peripheral fistula is that it may leave more proximal vessels available for future access.

Temporary access – role of ultrasound

Ultrasound is useful to assess central veins to ensure patency for emergency central dialysis catheter placement in patients with acute renal failure or failed permanent access. The patient should be lying flat so that the central veins are not collapsed. The internal and external jugular veins are examined using a low-frequency (4–8 MHz) linear array in B-mode and with color and pulsed Doppler to ensure patency and normal venous flow patterns. The subclavian veins may be imaged in long section either supraclavicularly or infraclavicularly (Fig. 16.3). The subclavian vein often collapses during the cardiac cycle or in response to breathing. The right and left proximal internal jugular vein and subclavian veins may be difficult to image with a linear array due to clavicle, sternum, and ribs which restrict ultrasound access. A small footprint phased or tightly curved array (Fig. 16.4) aids in color flow imaging of these veins (Fig. 16.5) and the brachiocephalic veins, although B-mode images are poor and compression of all these veins, to rule out deep-vein thrombosis, is impossible.

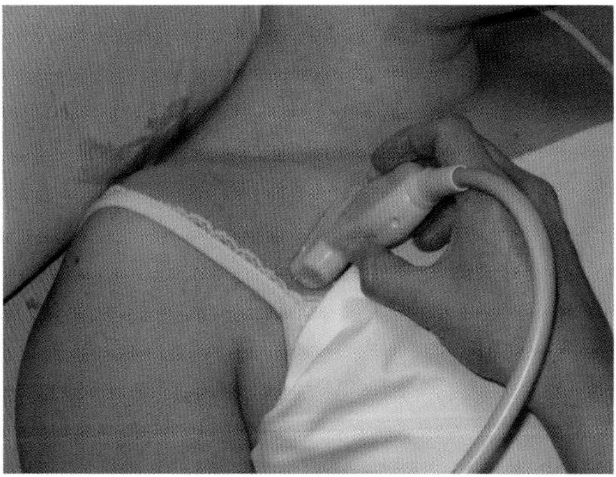

Figure 16.3 • Infraclavicular approach for imaging the subclavian vein with a linear array.

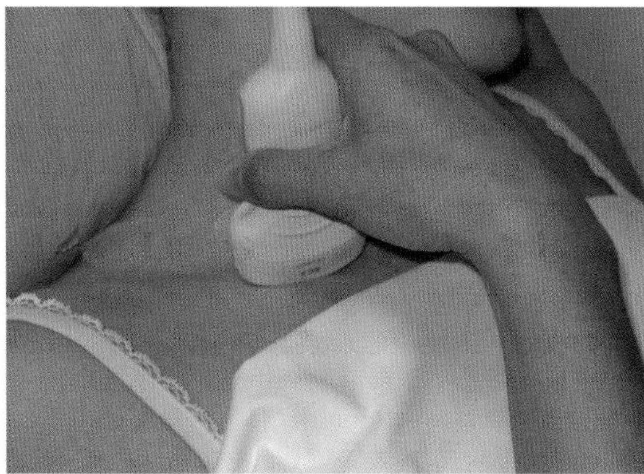

Figure 16.4 • High-frequency curvilinear array used to image the brachiocephalic vein.

PERMANENT ACCESS

Preassessment

A successful dialysis access requires good inflow and outflow. Poor selection of vessels for permanent access is associated with high failure rates. As dialysis is increasingly offered to older patients and those with diabetes and arterial disease, ultrasound has an important role to complement physical examination in identifying the most suitable site for access surgery. Trials have shown that ultrasound measurement of arterial and venous diameters can be predictive of likely success of a radiocephalic fistula. In reviewing the results of published investigations, European recommendations are that the minimum diameter of radial artery and cephalic vein at the wrist level should be 2 mm.

Technique for assessing arm veins and arteries

The arm to be imaged is supported comfortably with the palm of the hand uppermost (Fig. 16.6). For the superficial veins, a high-frequency (for example, 8–14 MHz) linear array is used. A tourniquet is applied proximal to the measurement sites to occlude venous return and the veins are allowed to expand (Fig. 16.7).

It is important to use very light pressure; even with a tourniquet, veins are readily compressed

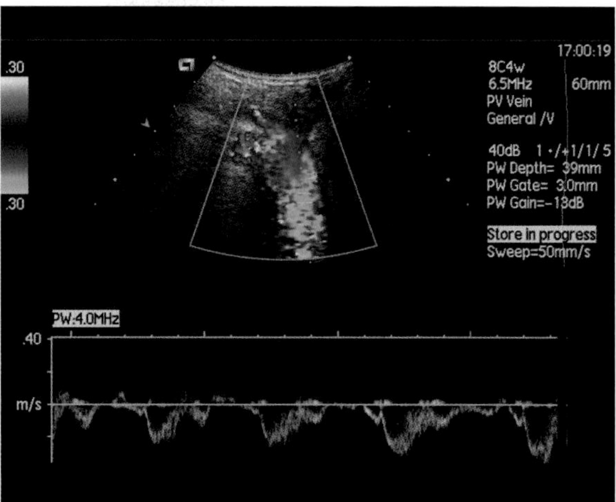

Figure 16.5 • Color flow and spectral Doppler image of the right brachiocephalic vein. The B-mode image is poor but contiguous color flow and venous waveform fluctuations indicate normal venous return.

and the diameter may be underestimated. The veins are measured in transverse section and are scanned through their length to check for patency, narrowing, particularly near confluences/bifurcations, anatomical variations (for example, large veins communicating with the deep veins), and continuity of flow. The proximal cephalic vein may be compressed extrinsically by surrounding tissue just before its insertion to the subclavian vein. This is sometimes relieved by relaxation of the arm.

The deep veins are imaged to ensure patency for the outflow of the fistula. For the proximal arm veins, axillary and subclavian veins, a lower-frequency transducer may be required. Color filling of the deep veins is helpful where compression is impossible (Fig. 16.5). Flow waveforms in the proximal veins should show phasicity with respiration (Fig. 16.8). Lack of or reduced phasicity is an indication of possible proximal occlusion or stenosis; compare the waveforms with those on the contralateral side. A phased or curvilinear array may be helpful to determine central vein patency.

Figure 16.6 • Imaging the cephalic vein. A proximal tourniquet causes the vein to enlarge.

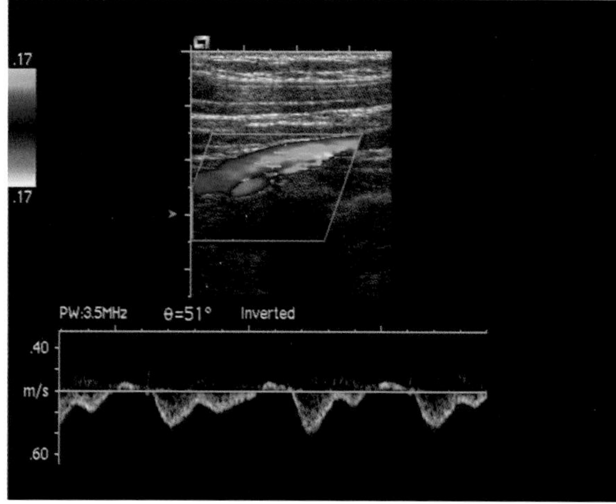

Figure 16.8 • Subclavian vein imaged from an infraclavicular approach. The flow waveform is phasic with changes in right atrial pressure, indicative of unimpeded venous return.

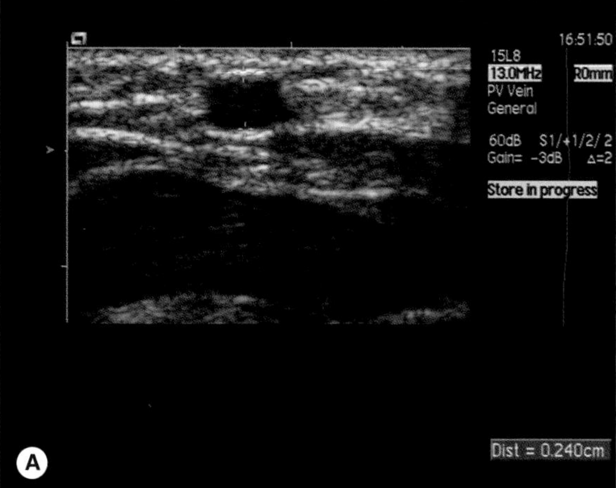

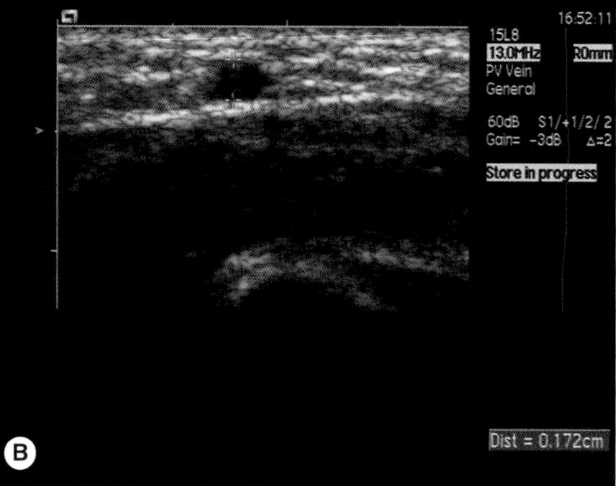

Figure 16.7 • Transverse image of cephalic vein with (A) and without (B) a proximal tourniquet.

The arteries should be examined for normal pulsatile flow to wrist level. Radial artery internal diameter should be measured and note is taken of arterial disease, including general calcification in the arm arteries. Even moderate stenoses should be noted as they can become more hemodynamically significant with the larger flow volumes after fistula creation. It is important to identify the brachial bifurcation level if surgery in the cubital fossa is contemplated. For patients with evidence of arterial disease, measurement of right and left brachial artery blood pressure may reveal proximal disease.

For radiocephalic fistulas, it has been suggested that measurement of flow waveform changes in an induced hyperemic response in the radial artery prior to surgery is a good measure of the likelihood of success of the fistula. A low resistance index (< 0.7) in the initial period of hyperemia was associated with a markedly improved outcome when compared with fistulas formed from arteries with an index ≥ 0.7 (Malovrh 2002) (Fig. 16.9), although others have been unable to show the same discrimination between fistula success and failure (Lockhart et al. 2004).

A checklist of observations and measurements made is given in Box 16.2.

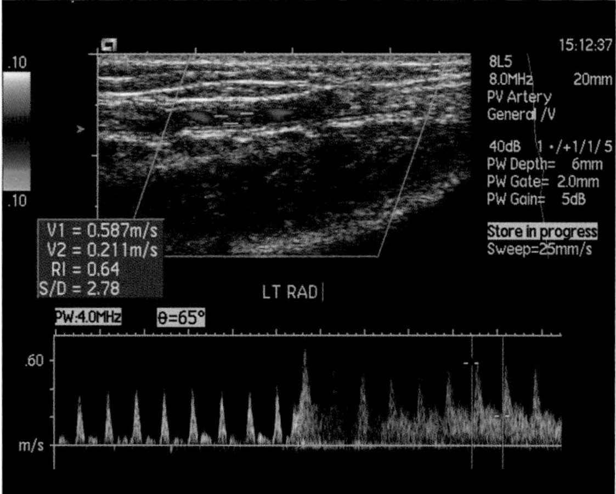

Figure 16.9 • Radial artery flow waveform changes following a 2-minute hand clench. The hyperemic response is evidence of higher velocities throughout the cardiac cycle, with a marked change in diastolic flow which can be measured by a resistance index of 0.64.

BOX 16.2 Measurements and checklist for arm preassessment scan for hemodialysis access

- Cephalic vein diameter upper arm/lower arm*
- Basilic vein diameter upper arm/lower arm*
- Anomalies (thrombus/stenosis/unusual anatomy) of superficial veins
- Patency of deep veins, including brachial, axillary, subclavian, and brachiocephalic veins
- Radial artery internal diameter at wrist
- Normal flow waveforms in major arm arteries (including radial/ulnar/brachial)
- Normal flow augmentation in radial artery in response to hyperemia
- Level of brachial artery bifurcation
- Anomalies (calcification/occlusion/unusual anatomy) of arm arteries

Note: It should be stated whether the measurements (indicated with an asterisk) of superficial vein diameters are made with or without a proximal tourniquet.

Postoperative assessment of dialysis access

Postoperatively, flow through the fistulas causes the vein to enlarge. There is an initial large increase of flow into the vein followed by a gradual further increase for several weeks. The fistula is examined clinically to determine its readiness for dialysis, which occurs typically from about 6 weeks postoperatively onwards. Grafts have a higher initial flow and can be used earlier. It is our practice to measure flow by duplex ultrasound at 2 weeks postoperatively and to record the size and depth of the fistula vein as a baseline record. This early scan also shows potential difficulties, including multiple venous returns, venous occlusions, and abnormal flows, particularly low flows. In radiocephalic fistulas, early postoperative flows < 400 ml/min have a high incidence of nonmaturation and failure (Tordoir et al. 2003).

If the fistula fails to mature at this stage or the dialysis staff have concerns then a full ultrasound investigation is completed. Complications can include use of inappropriate vessels, stenosis at the anastomosis, supplying arteries or draining veins (possibly due to undiagnosed pre-existing stenosis or perioperative clamp injuries), thrombosis, or venous return through communicating veins to deep veins.

Once in use, later complications of fistulas and grafts include:

- Stenosis: in fistulas this occurs most commonly in the vein or more central veins but may also occur in the artery or anastomosis. In grafts the most common site is the venous anastomosis
- Thrombosis
- Aneurysms/pseudoaneurysms
- Infection, which may lead to poor dialysis access function,
- Steal
- Venous hypertension
- Congestive heart failure, which may require revision of the fistula or graft.

In grafts the most common complication is thrombosis; in fistulas the most common is reduced flow from stenosis. Stenosis in the access circuit is commonplace, even in fistulas and grafts with good function. The presence of a stenosis without other clinical or hemodynamic anomalies is not sufficient to classify the access as a dysfunctional access. These stenoses can usually be left untreated but can be monitored by ultrasound.

Ultrasound investigation of dialysis access

It is important to record complete details for the patient's referral; good communication with the dialysis nursing staff is essential. For example, the cause of steal in the hand distal to fistula is more likely to be from arterial insufficiency, possibly due to proximal stenosis. The reason for high venous pressures is more likely to be a venous complication. Nurses' experience of the most recent dialysis sessions may be helpful and, for scans booked several days in advance, discussion with the patient can sometimes reveal that a problem has now resolved.

Volume flow

Volume flow is an important indication of the health of the access. The ultrasound examination should always include a measurement of flow through the fistula or graft. Flows may range from 300–400 to 3000 ml/min in fistulas and grafts, although most fall in the range 600–1500 ml/min. Fistulas tolerate lower flows than do grafts.

Other techniques are available to measure flow at the time of dialysis and there is a close correlation of these methods with duplex ultrasound. Volume flow is affected by severe stenoses anywhere in the access circuit. There is a high risk of thrombosis if flow falls below 300 ml/min in a fistula or 600 ml/min in a graft. Low flows lead to recirculation where blood leaving the dialyzer is drawn back into it leading to inefficient dialysis (Fig. 16.10). Recommendations are that investigations for the cause of low or reduced flow should be made if flows fall below a certain level or show a reduction in consecutive scans. Recommended criteria are given in Box 16.3.

Ultrasound measurement of volume flow is fraught with possible errors but the high flows in dialysis accesses and large changes in a failing access make this a practical and useful measurement in clinical practice. The volume flow is calculated by:

$$\text{Volume flow (ml/min)} = \text{cross-sectional area } (\text{cm}^2) \times \text{mean velocity (cm/s)} \times 60$$

The cross-sectional area is obtained from the diameter (area = diameter$^2 \times \pi/4$) and mean velocity by obtaining the weighted time-averaged velocity over several cardiac cycles (Fig. 16.11). Many scanners offer volume flow calculations from individual measurements made.

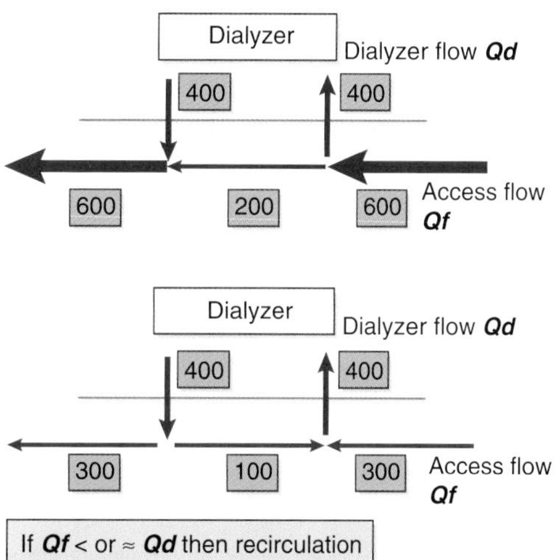

Figure 16.10 • Diagram of (A) adequate and (B) inadequate access flow. If access flow falls to less or close to dialyzer flow, recirculation of blood from the venous needle back into the arterial needle leads to inefficient dialysis.

Flow should be measured in the supplying subclavian or brachial artery even for wrist fistulas for the following reasons:

- The subclavian and brachial arteries have a circular cross-section, enabling measurement of area to be obtained from diameter. Flow velocities are predominantly axial in the direction of the vessel, allowing good approximation of mean velocity to be measured. The arteries are relatively straight, permitting accurate Doppler angle correction. Turbulent and nonaxial flows in the access vein or graft preclude accurate flow measurement at these sites.
- Most of the flow through the brachial artery is to the fistula/graft with only a small proportion supplying the forearm and hand.
- In radiocephalic fistulas, flow to the fistula is usually from both the radial artery and ulnar artery via the arch (see Fig. 16.2). Measuring flow in the subclavian or brachial artery accounts for all of the flow to the fistula/graft.
- Measurements in the vein are prone to error from turbulent nonaxial flow velocities and noncircular cross-sectional area (Fig. 16.12).

When making measurements of diameter and mean velocity, ensure the following:

- Obtain a longitudinal image of the artery, scanning through the plane of maximum diameter, and measure the diameter in B-mode from inner edge to inner edge. Some users recommend a transverse scan where area can be measured

BOX 16.3 Criteria for further investigation/intervention of access

EUROPEAN BEST PRACTICE GUIDELINES RECOMMENDATIONS	
Grafts	<600 ml/min >20% reduction in flow/month
Forearm fistulas	<300 ml/min
NATIONAL KIDNEY FOUNDATION/KIDNEY DISEASE OUTCOMES QUALITY INITIATIVE GUIDELINES	
Grafts	<600 ml/min Flow 1000 ml/min with decrease >25% over 4 months
Fistulas	No absolute measure recommended. Flows should be considered for individuals. It is noted that levels of <400 ml/min and <650 ml/min have been proposed

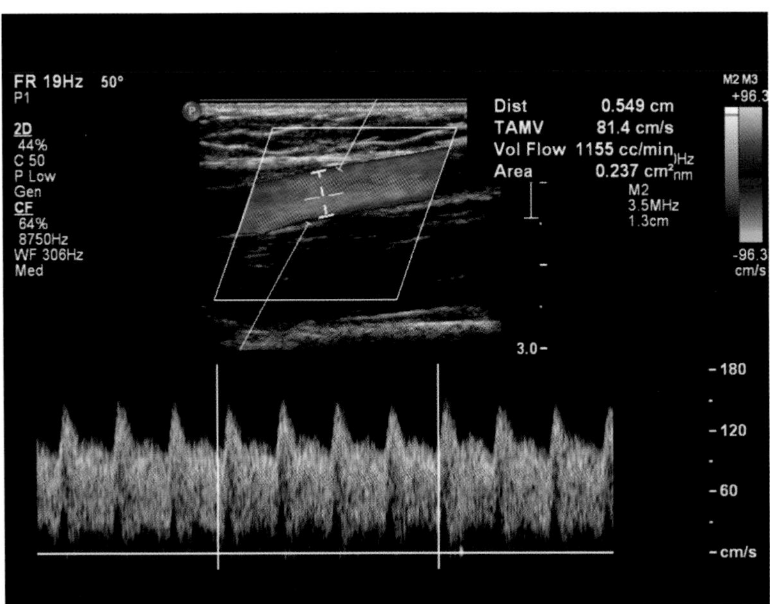

Figure 16.11 • Measurement of volume flow. The flow waveform is regular; the sample volume spans the artery. The scanner uses the measured diameter and mean velocity to calculate flow as 1155 ml/min.

directly but the site may not be identical to the Doppler measurement of velocity.

- When measuring mean velocity, scan longitudinally where there is a straight portion of artery. Ensure that the sample volume covers the entire width of the artery and that the beam/vessel angle is 60° or less (Fig. 16.13). If the sample volume only insonates the center of the vessel, mean velocity is overestimated with consequent errors in volume flow (see Ch. 6).
- Ensure that the flow waveform is regular and that it does not contain evidence of flow disturbances or low-frequency bruits. Ensure that the spectrum only displays signal from the artery; venous velocities below the baseline may subtract from the arterial signals and reduce the calculated mean velocity in the spectrum. Measure the time-averaged velocity over several cardiac cycles.
- Ensure that the patient is resting. Experience has shown us that flow is stable within 3 min of a change of posture.

It is worth repeating flow measurements to determine/ascertain the reproducibility of your technique. We routinely take three separate measurements to ensure consistency.

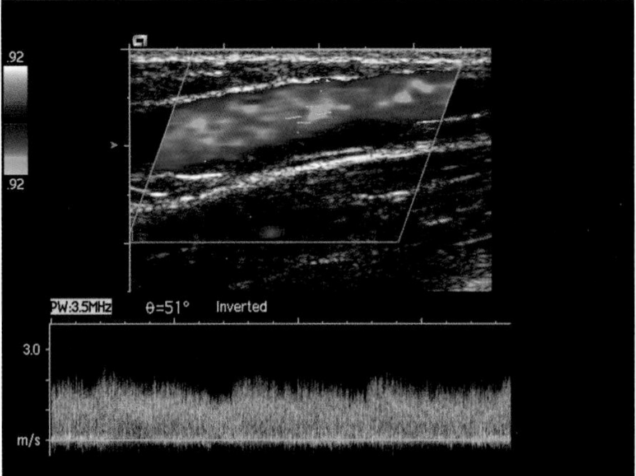

Figure 16.12 • Flow in the cephalic vein in a fistula. The irregular 'feathered' peaks are indicative of velocity fluctuations in the center of the vessel. Flow is unlikely to be completely axial along the vessel direction and mean velocity measurements will be inaccurate.

Scanning the access

Ensure that the patient is comfortable with the arm supported to allow ultrasound access to the major arteries and veins from neck to wrist level. Use an appropriate linear array. For access work there is a compromise to be made between the need for

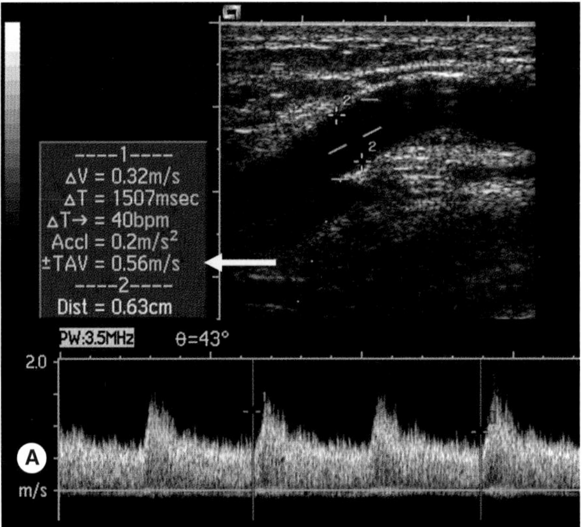

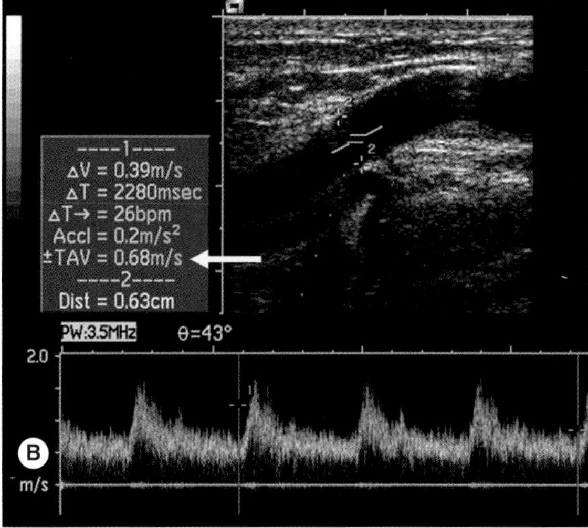

Figure 16.13 • Mean velocity measured with a sample volume in the center of the vessel 68 cm/s (right) and across the vessel 52 cm/s (left). By omitting lower velocities near the vessel wall the mean velocity value is artificially raised when the sample volume only insonates the center of the artery.

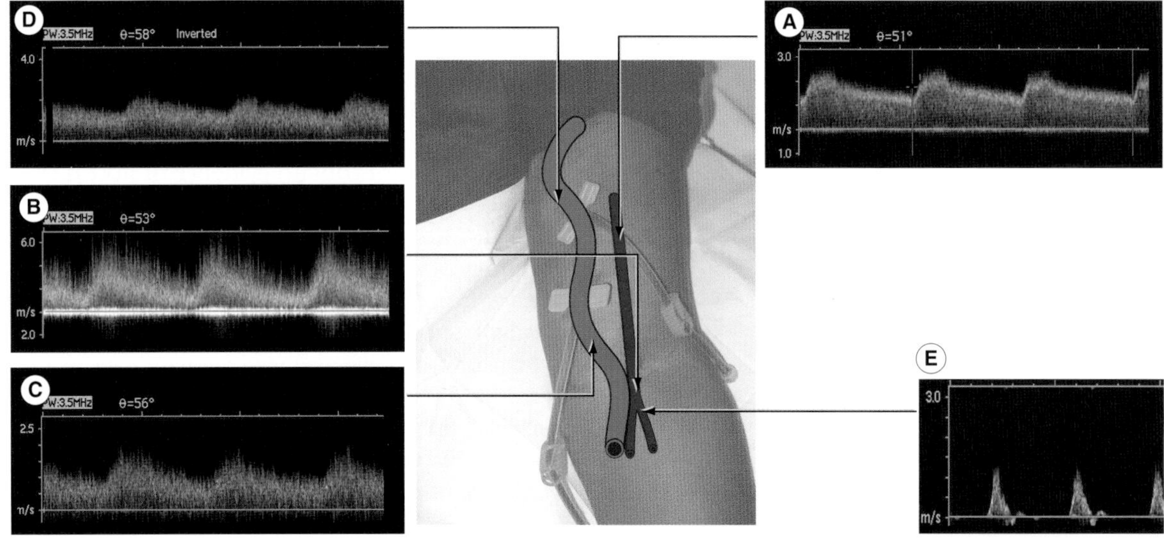

Figure 16.14 • Typical flow waveforms in arterial fistula. (A) Arterial supply, high velocities, low resistance. (B) Fistula site: high flows with turbulence and changes in flow direction. (C) Fistula vein close to the fistula; flow disturbances from the fistula site are evident. (D) Fistula vein. The flow becomes more ordered downstream. Damped arterial-like waveforms are evident. (E) Distal arteries exhibit normal triphasic flow waveforms.

good B-mode imaging in the near field, for which a high-frequency linear array (7–15 MHz) is best, and the need to image very high velocities, for which lower Doppler frequencies, found in lower-frequency transducers (3–8 MHz), are less prone to aliasing.

Measure volume flow as described above. If flow has decreased significantly since the last scan then it is imperative to identify possible causes.

The entire circuit is scanned for evidence of abnormality. An initial rapid transverse scan of the vessels with color flow can identify major anomalies, including aneurysms, partial thrombus, and collections, and can ascertain the presence of multiple unsuspected venous returns or venous occlusions.

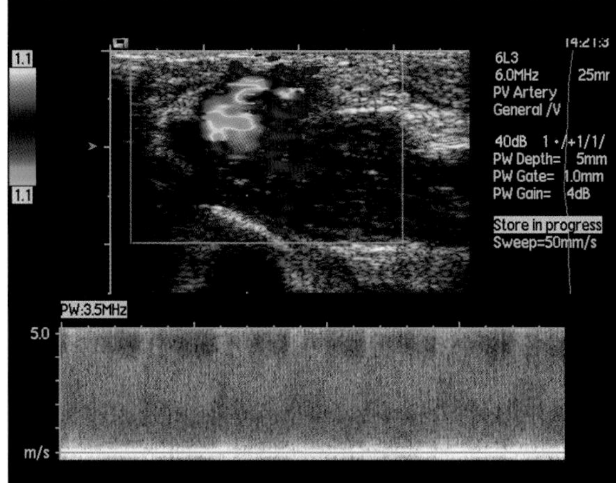

Figure 16.15 • At the fistula site, flow velocities are very high and change direction over a short distance. Accurate measurement of velocity is difficult. Here there is no angle correction made and measured velocities are at least 5 m/s. Aliasing and noise in the color flow image and spectral trace are evident.

Normal characteristics

Typical flow waveforms in the circuit are illustrated in Figure 16.14. Flow in the supplying artery is characterized by high-velocity, low-pulsatility flow. At the site of a fistula, velocities are usually very high with sudden changes in direction; velocities may be difficult to measure accurately (Fig. 16.15). Close to the anastomosis venous flows may be turbulent and exhibit nonaxial flow (Fig. 16.14C) which reorganizes more proximally downstream. The vein normally exhibits arterial-like pulsations up to axillary/subclavian vein level. More proximally, venous pulsations become more evident. Pressure in the vein at the needling site is high (typically) and light pressure from the transducer should not cause visible compression. The vein diameter should be adequate for repeated needling; diameters of at least 5 mm are recommended.

In radiocephalic fistulas, flow to the vein is commonly from antegrade flow in the radial artery and retrograde flow from the radial artery distal to the anastomosis from the ulnar artery via the palmar arches (Fig. 16.16).

Abnormalities and complications

Thrombosis. Occlusive thrombosis most commonly occurs in the vein or graft, initially at the site of needling. In grafts, thrombosis rapidly extends along the entire length of the graft. In veins the length of thrombosis depends on collateral flow which may keep sections of the vein patent. In cases of vein and graft thrombosis, flow in the supplying artery shows a high distal resistance, usually triphasic, flow waveform (Fig. 16.17A). Thrombus is evident in the vein; there may be a small channel of flow around it (Fig. 16.17B). Thrombosis may occur in the artery leading to the fistula; this is common in the radial artery in radiocephalic fistulas. It is important to determine the site and length of thrombus so that the clinical team can plan for surgical or radiological intervention. Venous diameter must be reported as aneurysms can affect management strategy for the thrombosed native fistula. It is also helpful to establish the age of the thrombus if possible; for example, if the thrombus is still 'fresh' such that it is still partially compressible. The patient may be able to give a useful guide as to when the access stopped 'buzzing' – a vibration at the site of the fistula caused by the high-velocity hemodynamics.

Stenoses, aneurysms, pseudoaneurysms. Accesses frequently contain stenoses, aneurysms, and pseudoaneurysms or hybrid aneurysms/ pseudoaneurysms. By themselves they do not necessarily preclude successful dialysis. Older fistulas can develop multiple aneurysms at the needling sites yet may still be viable for dialysis (Fig. 16.18). These pose challenges for imaging and Doppler measurement, not least from maintaining good transducer contact (Fig. 16.19). Other anomalies can include partial thrombus which may be evident particularly at the needling site. Aneurysms, stenoses, and the presence of partial thrombus give rise to complex flows with turbulence and areas of recirculation which may promote thrombus formation around the dialysis needle. Aneurysms and pseudoaneurysms are visible on B-mode and color flow imaging. The lumen, size of the aneurysm/pseudoaneurysm, and the presence of thrombus can be imaged and measured (Figs 16.20 and 16.21).

Stenoses may be evident on B-mode but are determined by their peak systolic velocity (PSV) and the PSV ratio of prestenotic or poststenotic flow to in-stenosis flow. High PSVs are indicative of pressure loss at the stenosis. Typical criteria used are PSVs > 400 cm/s and/or PSV ratios of > 3:1 (Older et al. 1998). The following points are useful when considering stenoses:

- When reporting stenoses we combine measurement of PSV ratios with absolute measure of PSV to give an assessment of the anatomy and severity and functional importance of the stenosis (Figs 16.22 and 16.23).
- It is essential to view the stenosis in the context of the flow measurement or changes in flow from a previous scan and from the clinical indications for the scan. Moderate stenoses (for example twice PSV increase, maximum velocity 200 cm/s, may be incidental findings) and even more severe stenoses may be found in fistulas with good function.
- The cephalic vein is often narrowed close to its insertion to the subclavian vein and may be compressed by pressure from the transducer. True stenoses have high velocities with little extrinsic pressure, in a range of arm positions.
- The presence of bruits can obscure the color flow image of a stenosis. Severe bruits and very elevated velocities are indicative of pressure-reducing and flow-limiting stenoses (Fig. 16.24).
- Flow waveform changes are useful in identifying severe stenosis with more pulsatile flow upstream of a narrowing and damped flow downstream and turbulent flow in the poststenotic region.

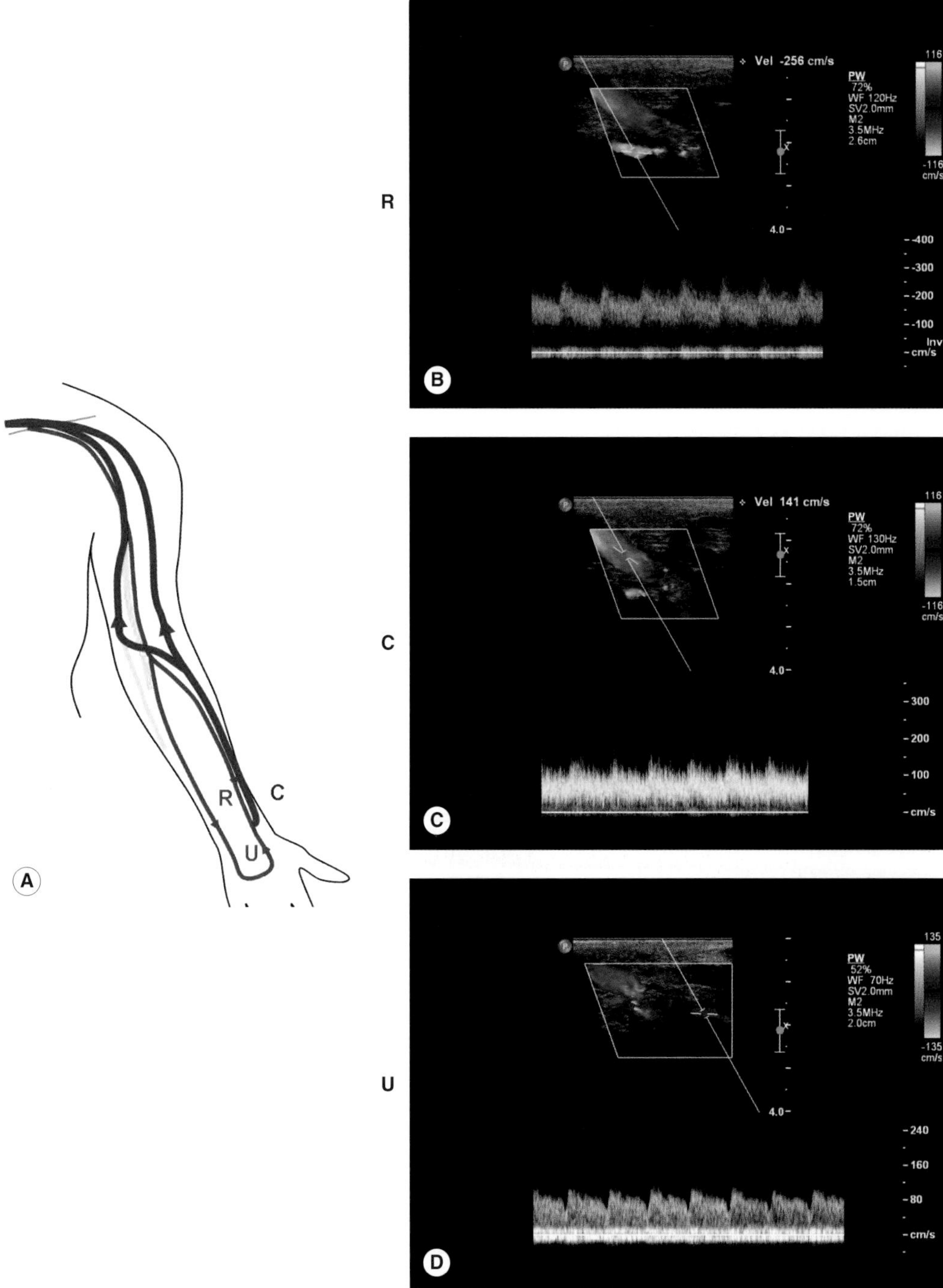

Figure 16.16 • Flow waveforms in a radiocephalic fistula. Flow in the radial artery distal to the fistula shows flow back towards the fistula from the ulnar artery and palmar arch. R, radial artery; U, flow from ulnar artery; C, cephalic vein.

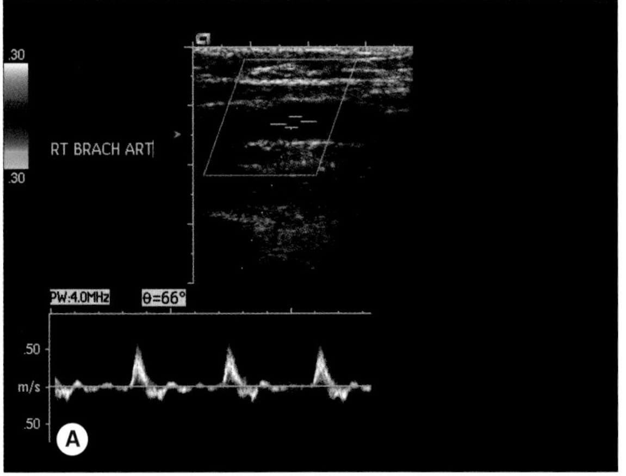

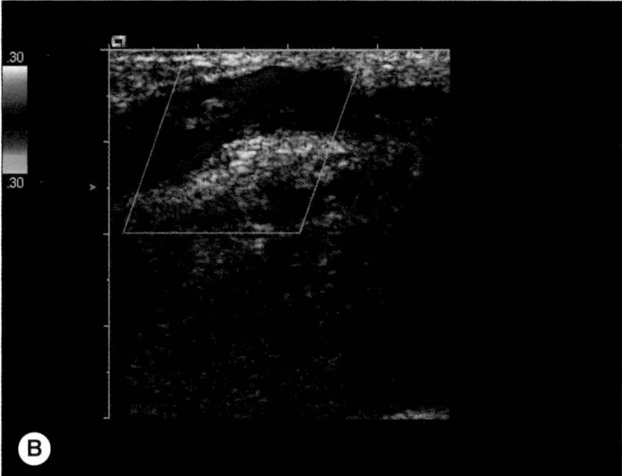

Figure 16.17 • (A) Flow waveform in the brachial artery leading to an occluded fistula showing high distal resistance. (B) Color flow imaging shows a vein with thrombus almost completely occluding the lumen.

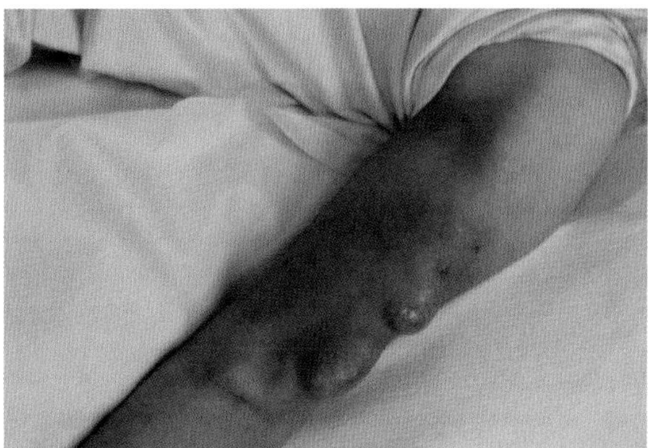

Figure 16.18 • Aneurysms visible in a brachiocephalic fistula.

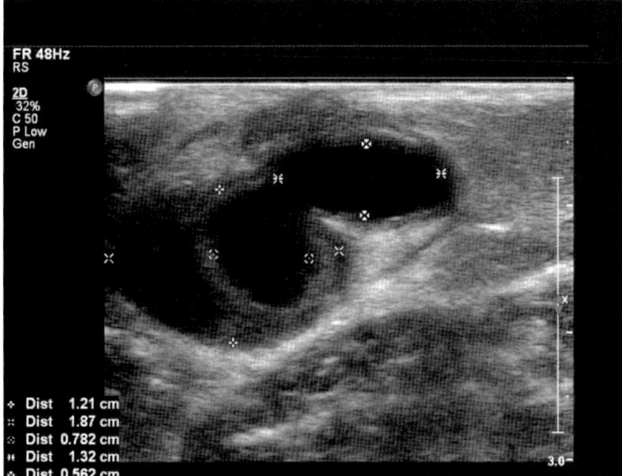

Figure 16.20 • Transverse image of a fistula vein with pseudoaneurysm partially filled with thrombus.

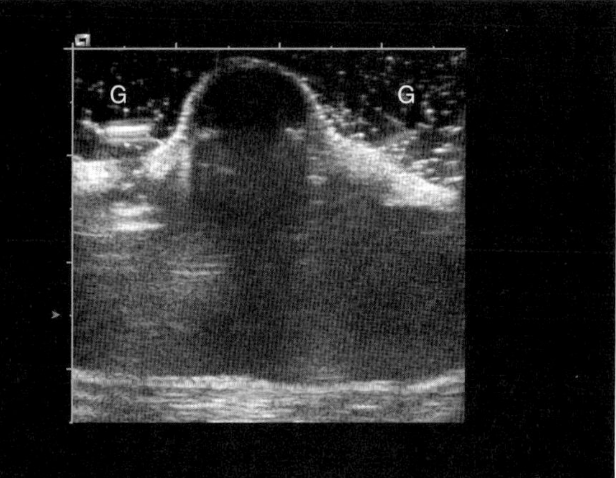

Figure 16.19 • Superficial aneurysm in a cephalic vein. Large quantities of ultrasound gel (G) are needed to maintain ultrasound contact with the skin.

- A qualitative measure of venous pressure can be gained by observing the ease of vein compression with pressure from the transducer. Low-pressure veins are indicative of upstream stenosis. High-pressure veins with low flow are indicative of downstream stenosis. Pressure loss across the stenosis in a fistula vein may be evident as a marked difference in compressibility of the vein pre- and poststenosis.

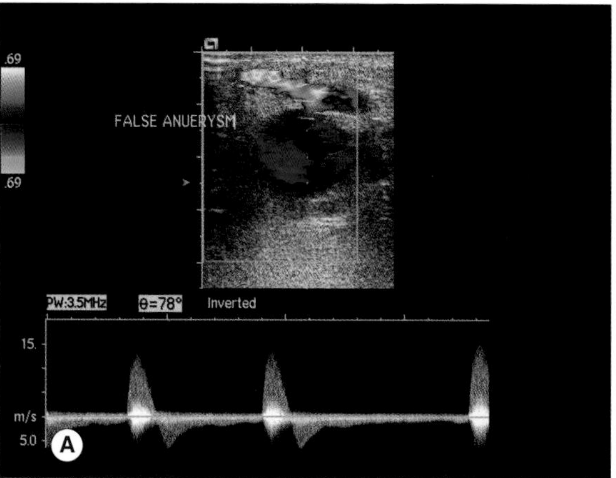

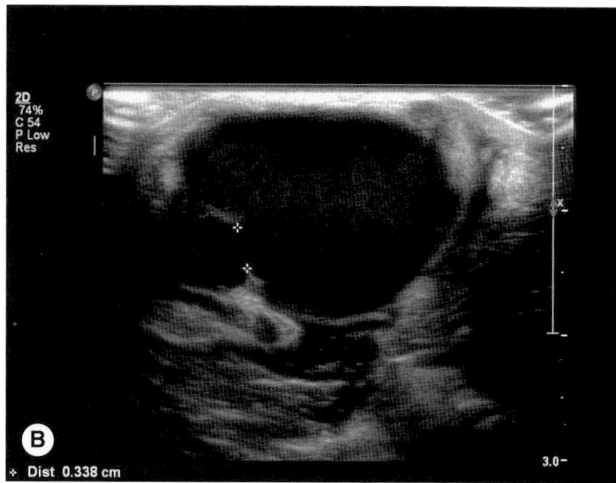

Figure 16.21 • Ultrasound in pseudoaneurysms. (A) Doppler spectrum of flow through a tract into a pseudoaneurysm, caused by needling through the deep wall of the vessel. (B) Ultrasound measurement of the size of the breach in the vein wall can help in planning intervention.

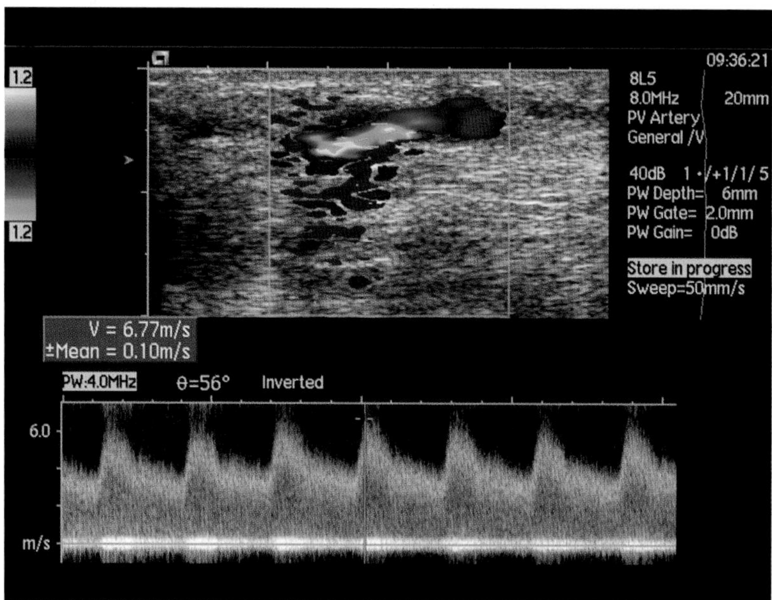

Figure 16.22 • Severe stenosis in a cephalic vein. Color flow and spectral Doppler show severe narrowing. Peak velocities exceed 6 m/s, at the upper limit of velocities possible in the circulation and indicative of low pressures at this point.

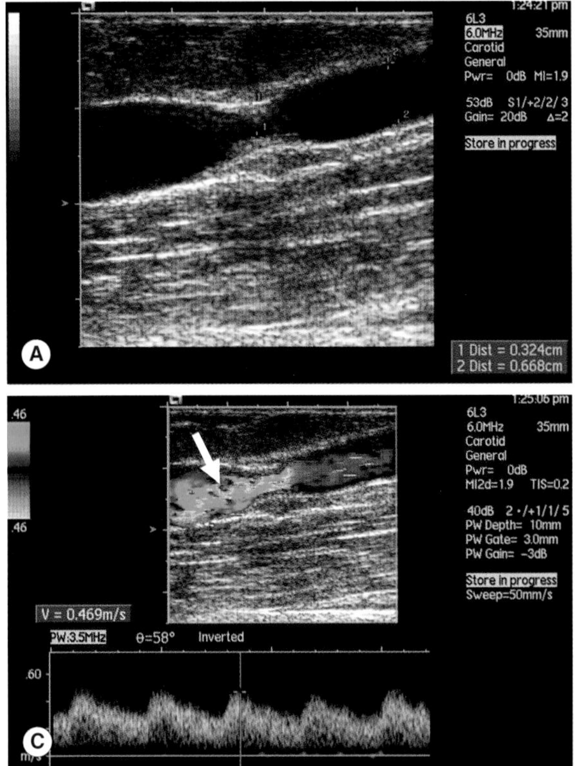

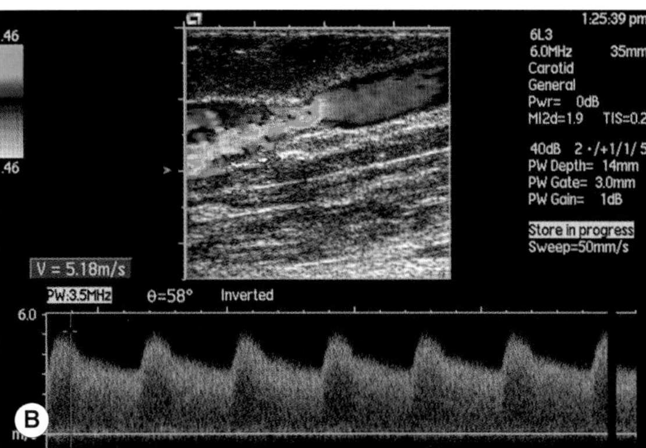

Figure 16.23 • Stenosis in a fistula vein. (A) The B-mode image shows the site of a stenosis. (B, C): The color flow image shows velocity changes through the stenosis with disordered turbulent flow downstream (arrow). Peak systolic velocity changes through the stenosis exceed 10 times, indicating severe narrowing.

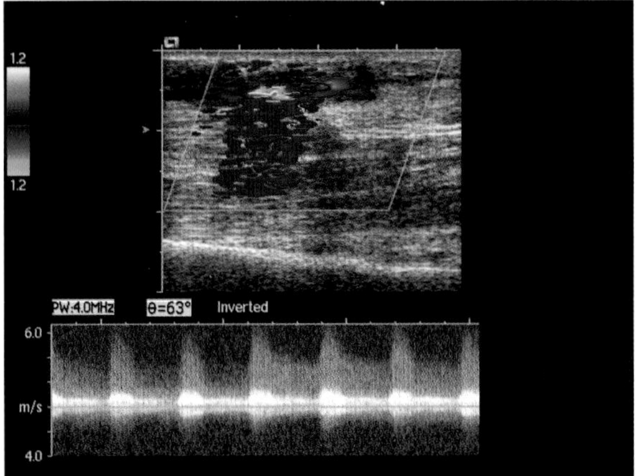

Figure 16.24 • High velocities through a stenosis lead to a bruit, vibration of the tissue which is evident as color flow noise, and high-intensity, low-velocity spectral traces.

A protocol for postoperative imaging of permanent access is given in Box 16.4.

BOX 16.4 Protocol for evaluating hemodialysis arm access postoperatively

- Measure volume flow in the brachial or subclavian artery supplying the access
- Scan the circuit from subclavian artery through the fistula/graft to the draining veins to central veins
- Note any abnormality (thrombus, aneurysms, pseudoaneurysms, collections)
- Note any abnormal flows (unusual flow velocities or pulsatility, flow direction in veins)
- If there are multiple venous paths, draw them and state approximately the flow through each. Note where flow returns to the deep veins
- Measure vein diameter and depth, especially if there are needling problems. Note any sudden change in vein direction and the presence of thrombus/intimal flaps in the needling area
- Note any stenoses and measure them on B-mode and with peak systolic velocity and ratios of stenosis to pre/poststenosis velocities

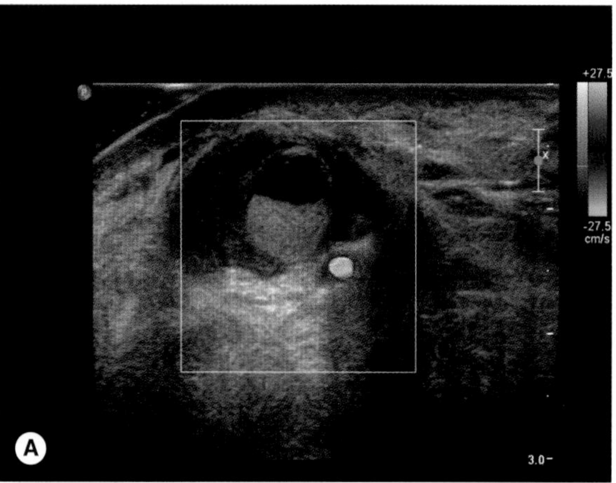

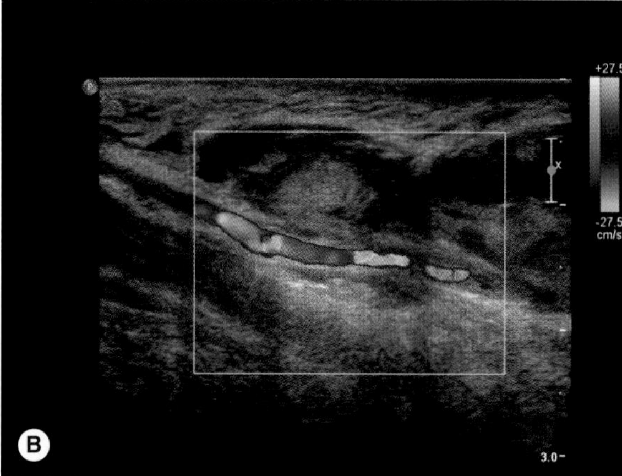

Figure 16.25 • Transverse (A) and longitudinal (B) image of a cephalic vein compressed by hematoma in the immediate postoperative period following fistula formation.

Steal

Steal may occur in hemodialysis with inadequate flow to distal tissue, resulting in pain in the hand and fingers and, if severe, tissue changes associated with ischemia. Ultrasound can be used to determine vascular anatomy, vessel patency, and qualitative evaluation of the circulation in the arm and hand. It has been shown that steal is associated with a high incidence of arterial stenosis in the arterial supply to the hand (Leon & Asir 2007). Ultrasound is effective in identifying this and as an aid to planning therapy through angioplasty or surgical revision.

Other findings

Collections and hematoma should be noted. These can lead to difficulties when needling fistulas and can cause extrinsic compression of the access circuit (Fig. 16.25). Very high volume flows are possible and can lead to cardiac problems. Ultrasound can be used to quantify the flow and monitor therapy (Fig. 16.26).

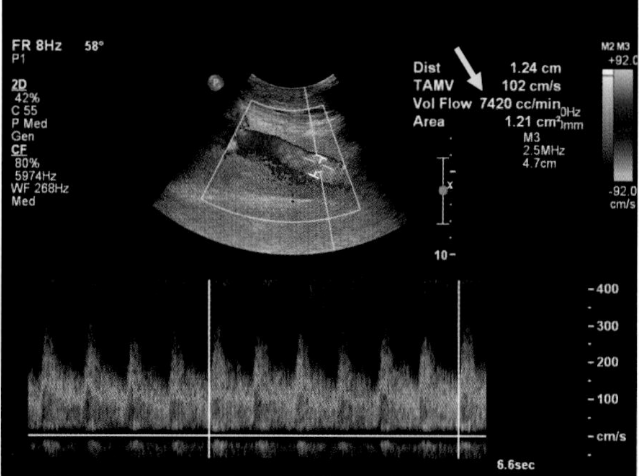

Figure 16.26 • Measured flow in this fistula exceeds 7 l/min, indicating the need for urgent revision to reduce flow.

REPORTING

The report should describe the flow and any significant changes to flow when compared with previous investigations. PSVs through stenoses should be described and ratios calculated. If diameters are clear on B-mode then these can also be used to describe the stenosis. The presence of thrombus, aneurysms/pseudoaneurysms, and collections should be noted and dimensions recorded. The diameter of the vein should be determined and, in cases where needling is difficult, its depth. If the fistula flow returns through more than one pathway then this should be described. It is important to report unusual flow pathways and flow in unsuspected directions.

We use diagrams of the access to aid dialysis staff where needling is difficult or as a guide for planning radiological intervention or surgery (Fig. 16.27).

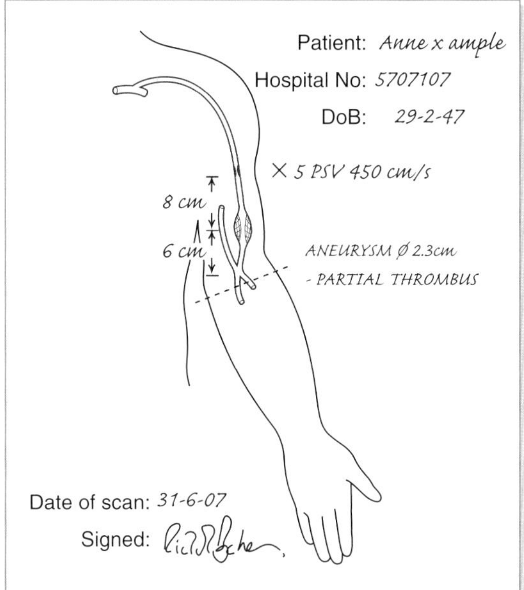

Figure 16.27 • A diagram of the fistula circuit aids understanding of the ultrasound examination and is helpful when planning intervention. PSV, peak systolic velocity.

References

Leon C, Asir A 2007 Arteriovenous access and hand pain: the distal hypoperfusion ischemic syndrome. Clinical Journal of the American Society of Nephrology 2: 175–183

Lockhart M E, Robbin M L, Allon M 2004 Preoperative sonographic radial artery evaluation and correlation with subsequent radiocephalic fistula outcome. Journal of Ultrasound Medicine 23: 161–168

Malovrh M 2002 Native arteriovenous fistula: preoperative evaluation. American Journal of Kidney Disease 39: 1218–1225

National Kidney Foundation 2006 NKF-K/DOQI clinical practice guidelines for vascular access: update 2006. American Journal of Kidney Disease 48 (suppl. 1): S177–S277

Older R A, Gizieski T A, Wilcowski M J et al. 1998 Hemodialysis access stenosis: early detection with color Doppler US. Radiology 207: 161–164

Tordoir J H M, Rooyens P, Dammers R et al. 2003 Prospective evaluation of failure modes in autogenous radiocephalic wrist access for hemodialysis. Nephrology Dialysis Transplantation 18: 378–383

Tordoir J, Canaud B, Haage P et al. 2007 EBPG on vascular access. Nephrology Dialysis Transplantation 22 (Suppl. 2): ii88–ii117

Appendix A
Decibel scale

The decibel scale allows the large range of values of ultrasound intensities, or signal voltages, to be expressed by a smaller range of numbers, as shown in Table A.1. The decibel scale expresses the ratios of intensities, or voltages, using a logarithmic scale. The decibel scale is used to describe ultrasound attenuation and amplifier gain.

INTENSITY RATIO (I/I_0)	DECIBEL (dB)	AMPLITUDE RATIO (V/V_0)
1 000 000	60	1000
10 000	40	100
100	20	10
10	10	3
2	3	1.4
0.5	–3	0.7
0.1	–10	0.3
0.01	–20	0.1
0.000 1	–40	0.01
0.000 001	–60	0.001

Intensity I (relative to I_0) in dB $= 10 \log_{10} (I/I_0)$.
Gain in dB $= 20 \log_{10}(V/V_0)$.

Table A.1 Decibel scale applied to intensity and voltage (or echo amplitude)

Appendix B
Sensitivity and specificity

When a new test is developed, a threshold at which the results are considered to indicate the presence or absence of the disease has to be selected. To do this the results of the test are compared to another method of detecting the disease, often known as the 'gold standard.' Unfortunately, there is usually an overlap between the results obtained in the presence of the disease and the results obtained in the absence of disease. This means that some patients will be falsely diagnosed as having the disease whereas others will be falsely diagnosed as not having the disease. Selecting the best threshold for the test depends partly on the prevalence of the disease within the group tested and also on the consequence of a false classification (i.e., missing the disease or incorrectly diagnosing disease in a normal patient). The performance of a diagnostic test can be measured by its sensitivity and specificity, which are defined as follows:

$$\text{Sensitivity} = \frac{\text{Number of patients with the disease correctly diagnosed}}{\text{Number of patients with the disease}}$$

$$\text{Specificity} = \frac{\text{Number of patients without the disease correctly diagnosed}}{\text{Number of patients without the disease}}$$

The value of the sensitivity and specificity will vary as the threshold of the test is altered. For example, if the threshold is changed to improve sensitivity, the specificity will fall. Altering the threshold and calculating the specificity and sensitivity can permit the selection of the optimal threshold and allow the value of the diagnostic test to be assessed. Other closely related qualities of a test often quoted in the literature are the positive predictive value, the negative predictive value, and accuracy. The positive predictive value is the probability that a subject who has a positive test (i.e., disease is detected) will be correctly classified. The negative predictive value is the probability that a subject who has a negative test (i.e., no disease is detected) is correctly classified.

Further reading

Bland M 1995 An introduction to medical statistics. Oxford University Press, Oxford

Index

Note: page numbers in *italics* refer to figures, tables or boxes.

A

B

C

D

E

G

H

I

J

K

L

M

N

O

P

S

V